Renal Disease

Editor

CHRISTAL POLLOCK

VETERINARY CLINICS OF NORTH AMERICA: EXOTIC ANIMAL PRACTICE

www.vetexotic.theclinics.com

Consulting Editor
JÖRG MAYER

January 2020 • Volume 23 • Number 1

ELSEVIER

1600 John F. Kennedy Boulevard • Suite 1800 • Philadelphia, Pennsylvania, 19103-2899
http://www.vetexotic.theclinics.com

VETERINARY CLINICS OF NORTH AMERICA: EXOTIC ANIMAL PRACTICE Volume 23, Number 1
January 2020 ISSN 1094-9194, ISBN-13: 978-0-323-71275-0

Editor: Colleen Dietzler
Developmental Editor: Laura Kavanaugh

Veterinary Clinics of North America: Exotic Animal Practice (ISSN 1094-9194) is published in January, May, and September by Elsevier, Inc., 360 Park Avenue South, New York, NY 10010-1710. Subscription prices are $287.00 per year for US individuals, $545.00 per year for US institutions, $100.00 per year for US students and residents, $338.00 per year for Canadian individuals, $657.00 per year for Canadian institutions, $352.00 per year for international individuals, $657.00 per year for international institutions, $100.00 per year Canadian students/residents, and $165.00 per year for international students/residents. To receive student/resident rate, orders must be accompanied by name of affiliated institution, date of term, and the *signature* of program/residency coordinator on institution letterhead. Orders will be billed at individual rate until proof of status is received. Foreign air speed delivery is included in all *Clinics* subscription prices. All prices are subject to change without notice. **POSTMASTER:** Send address changes to *Veterinary Clinics of North America: Exotic Animal Practice*, Elsevier Health Sciences Division, Subscription Customer Service, 3251 Riverport Lane, Maryland Heights, MO 63043. **Customer Service: Telephone: 1-800-654-2452** (U.S. and Canada); **1-314-447-8871** (outside U.S. and Canada). **Fax: 1-314-447-8029. E-mail: journalscustomerservice-usa@ elsevier.com (for print support); journalsonlinesupport-usa@elsevier.com (for online support).**

Reprints. For copies of 100 or more of articles in this publication, please contact the Commercial Reprints Department, Elsevier Inc., 360 Park Avenue South, New York, New York 10010-1710. Tel.: 212-633-3874; Fax: 212-633-3820; E-mail: reprints@elsevier.com.

Veterinary Clinics of North America: Exotic Animal Practice is covered in *MEDLINE/PubMed (Index Medicus)*.

Printed in the United States of America.

Contributors

CONSULTING EDITOR

JÖRG MAYER, Dr med vet, MSc
Diplomate, American Board of Veterinary Practitioners (Exotic Companion Mammals);
Diplomate, European College of Zoological Medicine (Small Mammals); Diplomate,
American College of Zoological Medicine; Associate Professor of Zoological Medicine,
Department of Small Animal Medicine and Surgery, University of Georgia College of
Veterinary Medicine, Athens, Georgia, USA

EDITOR

CHRISTAL POLLOCK, DVM
Diplomate, American Board of Veterinary Practitioners (Avian Practice); Veterinary
Consultant, Lafeber Company, Cornell, Illinois, USA

AUTHORS

JOÃO BRANDÃO, LMV, MS
Diplomate, European College of Zoological Medicine (Avian); Department of Veterinary
Clinical Sciences, Center for Veterinary Health Sciences, Oklahoma State University,
Stillwater, Oklahoma, USA

LEIGH A. CLAYTON, DVM
Diplomate, American Board of Veterinary Practitioners (Avian); Diplomate, American
Board of Veterinary Practitioners (Reptile and Amphibian); Animal Care, New England
Aquarium, Boston, Massachusetts, USA

OPHÉLIE COJEAN, Dr méd vét, IPSAV (Zoological Medicine)
Referral Practitioner, Zoological Medicine Service, Clinique vétérinaire Benjamin Franklin,
Brech, France

NICOLA DI GIROLAMO, DMV, MSc, PhD
Diplomate, European College of Zoological Medicine (Herpetology); Oklahoma State
University, Center for Veterinary Health Sciences, Stillwater, Oklahoma, USA

STEPHEN J. DIVERS, BVetMed, FRCVS
Diploma in Zoological Medicine; Diplomate, European College of Zoological Medicine
(Zoo Health Management, Herpetology); Diplomate, American College of Zoological
Medicine; Department of Small Animal Medicine and Surgery, College of Veterinary
Medicine, University of Georgia, Athens, Georgia, USA

M. SCOTT ECHOLS, DVM
Diplomate, American Board of Veterinary Practitioners (Avian); Parrish Creek Veterinary
Practice, Centerville, Utah, USA; Medical Center for Birds, Oakley,
California, USA

RUTH MACKENZIE HALLMAN, DVM
Diplomate, American College of Veterinary Radiology; Department of Veterinary Clinical Sciences, Center for Veterinary Health Sciences, Oklahoma State University, Stillwater, Oklahoma, USA

PETER H. HOLZ, BVSc, DVSc, MACVSc
Diplomate, American College of Zoological Medicine; Faculty of Veterinary and Agricultural Sciences, University of Melbourne, Werribee, Victoria, Australia

JAMES G. JOHNSON III, DVM, MS, CertAqV
Diplomate, American College of Zoological Medicine; Staff Veterinarian, Department of Animal Health, Saint Louis Zoo, St Louis, Missouri, USA; Adjunct Assistant Professor, Department of Veterinary Preventative Medicine, College of Veterinary Medicine, The Ohio State University, Columbus, Ohio, USA

CORNELIA KONICEK, Dr med Vet
Resident ECZM, Clinic for Birds and Reptiles, University of Vienna, Vienna, Austria

MARIA-ELISABETH KRAUTWALD-JUNGHANNS, Dr med vet, Dr med vet habil, ML
Diplomate, European College of Zoological Medicine (Avian); Professor, Clinic for Birds and Reptiles, University of Leipzig, Leipzig, Germany

SYLVAIN LARRAT, Dr méd vét, MSc, DES
Diplomate, American College of Zoological Medicine; Referral Practitioner, Zoological Medicine Service, Clinique vétérinaire Benjamin Franklin, Brech, France

ANGELA M. LENNOX, DVM
Diplomate, American College of Veterinary Pathologists (Avian Practice, Exotic Companion Mammal Practice); Diplomate, European College of Zoological Medicine (Small Mammal); Avian and Exotic Animal Clinic of Indianapolis, Indianapolis, Indiana, USA

LISA M. MANGUS, DVM, PhD
Diplomate, American College of Veterinary Pathologists; Department of Molecular and Comparative Pathobiology, Johns Hopkins University, Baltimore, Maryland, USA

SUSAN E. OROSZ, PhD, DVM
Diplomate, American Board of Veterinary Practitioners (Avian); Diplomate, European College of Zoological Medicine (Avian); Bird and Exotic Pet Wellness Center, Toledo, Ohio, USA

CHRISTINE PARKER-GRAHAM, DVM, MA
US Fish and Wildlife Service, Lacey, Washington, USA

DAVID N. PHALEN, DVM, PhD
Associate Professor, Sydney School of Veterinary Sciences, University of Sydney, Sydney, New South Wales, Australia

DRURY R. REAVILL, DVM
Diplomate, American Board of Veterinary Practitioners (Avian Practice, Reptile and Amphibian Practice); Diplomate, American College of Veterinary Pathologists; Zoo/Exotic Pathology Service, Carmichael, California, USA

LAUREN SCHMIDT, DVM
Oklahoma State University, Center for Veterinary Health Sciences, Stillwater, Oklahoma, USA

ILSE SCHWENDENWEIN, DVM
Diplomate, European College of Veterinary Clinical Pathology; Head, Division of Clinical Pathology, Department of Pathobiology, University of Veterinary Medicine, Vienna, Austria

ALEXANDRA SCOPE, DVM
Assistant Professor, Department for Companion Animals and Horses, University of Veterinary Medicine, Vienna, Austria

PAOLO SELLERI, DMV, PhD
Diplomate, European College of Zoological Medicine (Herpetology and Small Mammals); Clinica per Animali Esotici, Roma, Italy

CLAIRE VERGNEAU-GROSSET, Dr méd vét, CES, IPSAV (Zoological Medicine)
Diplomate, American College of Zoological Medicine; Assistant Professor in Zoological Medicine, Department of Clinical Sciences, Zoological Medicine Service, Faculté de médecine vétérinaire, Université de Montréal, Saint-Hyacinthe, Quebec, Canada

MEGAN K. WATSON, DVM, MS
Diplomate, American College of Zoological Medicine; Associate Veterinarian, Department of Animal Health, Zoo New England, Boston, Massachusetts, USA

E. SCOTT WEBER III, VMD, MSc, Cert Aquatic Vet WAVMA
Diplomate, American College of Veterinary Preventive Medicine; Aquatic Animal Medicine Consultant, Veterinary Information Network, Conestoga, Pennsylvania, USA

STACEY LEONATTI WILKINSON, DVM
Diplomate, American Board of Veterinary Practitioners (Reptile and Amphibian); Avian and Exotic Animal Hospital of Georgia, Pooler, Georgia, USA

Contents

The Urinary and Osmoregulatory Systems of Birds   1

Susan E. Orosz and M. Scott Echols

> The avian kidney contains both cortical or reptilian and medullary or mammalian nephrons. The kidney filters up to 11 times the total body water daily. Approximately 95% of this volume is reabsorbed by tubular reabsorption, which likely results from a change in the rate of filtration and/or the rate of reabsorption. These changes can result because of the antidiuretic hormone arginine vasotocin. The urinary concentrating ability generally varies inversely with body mass; however, birds can concentrate their urine, often at 2 to 3 times the osmolality of plasma. Further concentration of urine may occur by retroperistalsis.

Diseases of the Avian Urinary System   21

David N. Phalen

> Diseases of the renal system can be caused by infectious and noninfectious processes. Creating a relevant differential diagnosis for kidney disease in the live or dead bird requires a structured approach where the list of differentials is narrowed based on the signalment of the bird; its history, including its diet and management; physical findings; and other diagnostic findings. This article aims to provide the reader not only a list of the diseases that occur in birds but also the guidelines on when a disease should be considered in a differential.

Laboratory Evaluation of Renal Function in Birds   47

Alexandra Scope and Ilse Schwendenwein

> Renal disease often remains undetected in living patients. Urinalysis might contribute to the diagnosis of some kinds of renal and metabolic diseases. Blood uric acid concentrations reflect the excretory functional capacity of the renal proximal tubules. In contrast, blood urea concentrations are significantly affected by the bird's hydration status and have been proposed as a useful variable to detect prerenal causes for renal impairment in birds. Measurement of exogenous creatinine excretion shows promising preliminary results to become a useful test for the assessment of renal excretion in birds.

Diagnostic Imaging of the Avian Urinary Tract   59

Maria-Elisabeth Krautwald-Junghanns and Cornelia Konicek

> Due to the special anatomy and physiology of the avian urinary system, the value of diagnostic imaging techniques differs from the use in mammals. The diagnostic imaging methods regularly used in practice to evaluate

the avian kidneys are often limited to traditional radiography and ultraso-nography, whereas other imaging modalities (urography, scintigraphy, computed tomography, MRI) are rarely used. Furthermore endoscopy may be performed and taking a renal biopsy may be considered. The article describes common indications for imaging techniques used to diag-nose urinary tract disease as well as its anatomic and pathologic demonstration.

evaluation of urinary tract disease. The use of radiographs, ultrasonography, computed tomography, MRI, and endoscopy is discussed and compared for the evaluation of urinary tract disease in reptiles.

Stacey Leonatti Wilkinson and Stephen J. Divers

Renal disease is one of the most common medical conditions encountered in captive reptiles. In most cases, signs of disease are nonspecific and often not present until the condition is advanced. Many factors contribute to the development of renal disease, and the etiology often is multifactorial. Diagnosis of renal disease by traditional methods used in small animals is not as straightforward as in reptiles; often many tests may be needed to reach a firm diagnosis. Prevention is preferred to treatment. Understanding the pathophysiology, potential causes, diagnostic tests available, and treatment options is essential for the reptile veterinarian to manage this condition.

Drury R. Reavill and Angela M. Lennox

Diseases of the urinary tract are reviewed, covering infectious (bacterial, viral, parasitic), degenerative, congenital, metabolic, nutritional, neoplastic, obstructive, and toxic causes. Some clinical presentations and diagnostic procedures are described for ferrets, rabbits, guinea pigs, hamsters, mice, rats, chinchillas, hedgehogs, and sugar gliders, as well as therapies.

Ruth Mackenzie Hallman and João Brandão

Radiographs can be used to easily visualize common types of urinary calculi in all parts of the urinary tract. Positive-contrast excretory urography and cystourethrography are sensitive to diseases within the ureters and urethra, most commonly obstruction. Ultrasound is widely available and noninvasive and can be used to evaluate renal architecture, ureteral dilation, urinary bladder wall disease, and urolithiasis. Computed tomography is increasing in availability and provides a large amount of cross-sectional information quickly and noninvasively. Multiple imaging modalities can be used to estimate or quantify glomerular filtration rate.

Christine Parker-Graham, Leigh A. Clayton, and Lisa M. Mangus

Amphibians are a remarkably diverse group of vertebrates with lifestyles ranging from fully aquatic to entirely terrestrial. Although some aspects of renal anatomy and physiology are similar among all amphibians, species differences in nitrogenous waste production and broad normal variation in plasma osmolality and composition make definitive antemortem diagnosis of renal disease challenging. Treatment is often empirical and aimed at addressing possible underlying infection, reducing abnormal fluid accumulation, and optimizing husbandry practices to support metabolic and fluid homeostasis. This article reviews amphibian renal anatomy and physiology, provides recommendations for diagnostic and therapeutic options, and discusses etiologies of renal disease.

E. Scott Weber III

The number of fish as pets far exceeds the populations of any other companion animal. As our knowledge of aquatic animal species and aquatic animal medicine continues to expand, veterinary expertise is becoming more critical to the client, researcher, fisheries biologist, aquarist, farmer, and fish hobbyist. Similar to other vertebrates, fish are susceptible to infectious and noninfectious renal disease. This article compares vertebrate renal anatomy and physiology and highlights some renal disease examples.

VETERINARY CLINICS OF NORTH AMERICA: EXOTIC ANIMAL PRACTICE

SERIES OF RELATED INTEREST

Veterinary Clinics of North America: Small Animal Practice
Available at: https://www.vetsmall.theclinics.com/

THE CLINICS ARE NOW AVAILABLE ONLINE!
Access your subscription at:
www.theclinics.com

Preface

Renal Disease in Special Species

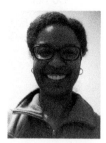

Christal Pollock, DVM, DABVP (Avian Practice)
Editor

Renal disease is a relatively common condition in clinical practice. Given the variety of exotic animal species encountered in exotic animal medicine, the breadth and depth of knowledge that is required to meet the challenge of managing this disease can be intimidating. This issue is intended to serve as a clinical aid for the veterinary practitioner.

Building on the principle of 1 medicine, a clear understanding of renal disease in domestic animals serves as a strong foundation for our understanding of this condition in exotic animal patients. We can often directly extrapolate the basics of anatomy and physiology, diseases, and even management of renal disease to exotic animal patients, particularly exotic companion mammals. Therefore, this issue contains only 2 articles on renal disease in exotic companion mammals. One article is an extensive review on renal diseases in small mammals. The other article is a more focused look at diagnostic imaging in small mammals.

An understanding of renal disease in birds and reptiles carries special challenges due to the unique nature of these taxonomic groups. Therefore, the avian and reptile content in this issue begins with clinically relevant reviews on renal anatomy and physiology. Additional content featured in this issue includes summaries of common renal diseases in both birds and reptiles, reviews of diagnostic imaging techniques in birds and reptiles, as well as laboratory evaluation of renal disease in birds. I am particularly excited by content that summarizes the best practices in clinical management of renal disease in bird and reptile patients, from medical treatment and supportive care to nutritional management and surgery. This issue also addresses the basics of renal

Vet Clin Exot Anim 23 (2020) xiii–xiv
https://doi.org/10.1016/j.cvex.2019.10.001
1094-9194/20/© 2019 Published by Elsevier Inc.

vetexotic.theclinics.com

disease in amphibians and fish, with comprehensive clinical reviews by experts in the field.

Christal Pollock, DVM, DABVP (Avian Practice)
Lafeber Company
Cornell, IL 61319, USA

E-mail address:
cpollock@lafeber.com

The Urinary and Osmoregulatory Systems of Birds

Susan E. Orosz, PhD, DVM, DABVP (Avian), DECZM (Avian)[a],*,
M. Scott Echols, DVM, DABVP (Avian)[b,c]

KEYWORDS

- Osmoregulation • Avian • Kidney • Nephrons • Glomerular filtration
- Urine concentration • Uric acid • Salt gland

KEY POINTS

- The kidneys of birds are fixed under the area of the synsacrum and are composed of divisions not lobes.
- Birds osmoregulate using their kidneys; intestinal tract; and, in some birds, salt glands.
- Avian nephrons are of 2 main types: the cortical, loopless, or reptilian nephrons and the medullary or looped nephrons. Knowing this anatomy, along with that of the renal portal system, is important in understanding the pharmacodynamics of drugs in birds.
- The kidney filters up to 11 times the total body water per day. Although the nephrons do not concentrate urine to the extent of mammals, they use the large intestine and/or the colon for resorption of ureteral urine. In addition, urates are modified by special colonic bacteria and some products produced are recycled through the renal portal system.
- There are some birds, particularly marine species, that are able to remove excess sodium through a countercurrent system in the salt glands. Angiotensin II has been shown to inhibit secretion of sodium chloride, whereas atrial natriuretic peptide enhances secretion.

INTRODUCTION

All animals require adequate water in their extracellular fluid compartment to regulate cellular functions, whether they live in the desert or in aquatic environments, which include fresh, brackish, or even marine water. Each environment presents challenges that require a variety of strategies to maintain the appropriate internal milieu for life.

Disclosure: Dr S.E. Orosz has nothing to disclose. Dr M.S. Echols is the creator of BriteVu and owner of Scarlet Imaging, mentioned in **Figs. 6** and **9**.
[a] Bird and Exotic Pet Wellness Center, 5166 Monroe Street, Suite 306, Toledo, OH 43623, USA;
[b] Parrish Creek Veterinary Practice, 86 North 70 West Street, Centerville, UT 84014, USA;
[c] Medical Center for Birds, 3805 Main Street, Oakley, CA 94561, USA
* Corresponding author.
E-mail address: drsusanorosz@aol.com

When discussing the urinary system and its unique aspects in birds, the important consideration is the question of how birds osmoregulate.

Within vertebrates, there are several organs used to maintain internal homeostasis. However, mammals have only 1 organ system that provides this osmoregulatory homeostasis: the kidney. In contrast, reptiles use their kidneys, bladder, and intestine for regulatory function. Although mammals can lose water and electrolytes through the skin, respiratory tract, and gastrointestinal (GI) tract, these organs do not provide any osmoregulatory function. Birds are between mammals and nonmammalian vertebrates with respect to osmoregulation. Many avian species have salt glands that perform an important osmoregulatory function, particularly in a marine environment. Like reptiles, birds also use the lower portion of the GI tract as an important component for osmoregulation. In addition, birds have a unique kidney that plays an important role in osmoregulation.[1] These organs are discussed here from an anatomic and physiologic perspective for clinicians.

EXTERNAL ANATOMY OF THE KIDNEY

The renal system consists of the kidneys, ureters, and the urodeal portion of the cloaca (**Fig. 1**). The kidneys of birds, which are fixed in ventral depressions of the synsacrum called the renal fossae, are symmetric and retroperitoneal. The kidneys extend from the proximal end of the synsacrum just distal to the caudal extent of the lungs to the cranial end of the synsacrum.[2] There can be diverticula of the abdominal air sacs that extend between the kidneys and the pelvis.

Renal Divisions

Unlike mammalian kidneys, the kidneys of birds are not divided into lobes grossly but into divisions. Birds tend to have 3 divisions: cranial, middle, and caudal. The external

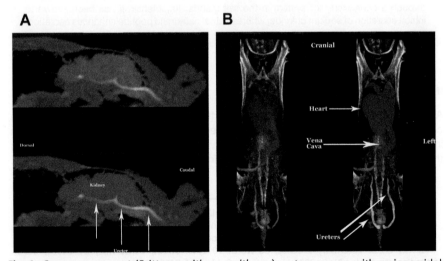

Fig. 1. Congo gray parrot (*Psittacus erithacus erithacus*) ureters as seen with an iopamidol 370 contrast computed tomography (CT) study. (*A*) Sagittal and (*B*) coronal views are used to identify the ureters, which course along the ventral middle aspect of each kidney. The ureters terminate caudally into the urodeum. Notice the air space dorsal to the kidney and ventral to the thin overlying synsacral bone on the sagittal view (*A*). (*Courtesy of* M. Scott Echols, DVM, DABVP-Avian, Centerville, UT.)

iliac artery cranially and the ischiatic (or ischiadic) artery caudally run through the kidney to form the 3 divisions[2] (**Figs. 2** and **3**). The portion of kidney cranial to the external iliac artery is the cranial division, the portion between the 2 arteries is the middle division, and that portion caudal to the ischiatic artery is the caudal division. In chickens and many parrot species, these divisions are distinct. The middle division in passerines blends with the cranial and more often the caudal division. In puffins, penguins, and herons, the caudal divisions are fused on the midline.[2]

The spinal nerves from the lumbar and sacral plexuses move through the renal parenchyma to provide motor and sensory innervation to muscles of the lower body wall and the leg. This anatomy is important clinically, because swelling or dorsally directed pressure on the kidneys causes reduction in nerve function, which results in altered muscle function in the leg. Clinically, the bird appears to not bear weight on the leg and, /although a fracture is suggested, none is detected on palpation. Often there is loss of muscle, and sometimes bone mass, most commonly over the lateral femur,

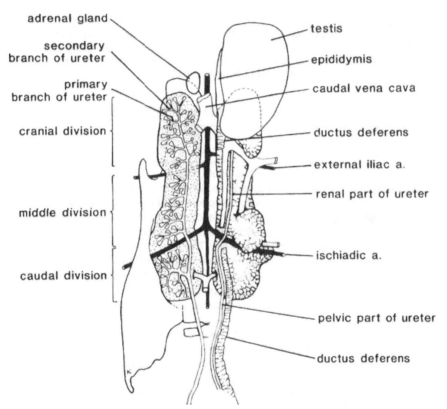

Fig. 2. Ventral view of the kidneys of the domestic cock. The right kidney is drawn as though transparent to show the primary branches of the ureter and some of its secondary branches. At the end of each secondary branch of the ureter the diagram shows a conical expansion. Each such conical expansion represents the encapsulated cone-shaped assembly of medullary collecting tubules, which forms the medullary part of a lobe. The proximal part of the left ductus deferens has been removed. a., artery. (*From* King AS, McLelland J. Urinary system. In: Birds: their structure and function, 2nd edition. London: Bailliere Tindall; 1984. p. 176; with permission.)

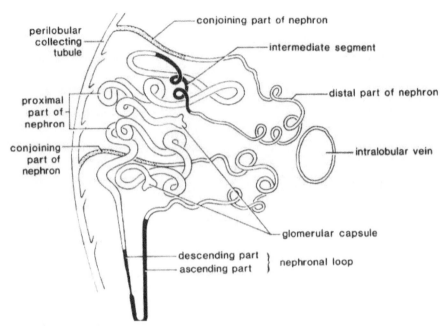

Fig. 5. The disposition of the various parts of a cortical (reptilian) type of nephron (*above*), and a medullary (mammalian) type of nephron (*below*). (*From* King AS, McLelland J. Urinary system. In: Birds: their structure and function, 2nd edition. London: Bailliere Tindall; 1984. p. 180; with permission.)

species living in an arid environment tend to have smaller kidneys, a larger medullary volume, and/or a smaller cortical volume.[5,6]

Both types of nephron have a renal corpuscle at their proximal ends. The corpuscle consists of a glomerular capsule that is indented by a tuft of capillaries, the glomerulus. The renal corpuscles lie about midway between the interlobular and intralobular veins. All nephrons have a proximal and distal portion, but only the mammalian type have the loop of Henle.[2]

In cortical nephrons, the proximal tubule is found in the outer portion of the lobule and it forms approximately half the length of the nephron. The middle segment of this nephron is poorly defined but is short and convoluted. The distal tubule of the reptilian nephron has compact convolutions near the intralobular veins.[2]

The medullary nephrons have, as their intermediate segment, the loop of Henle, which is anatomically similar to the short mammalian nephron type with the proximal

Table 1
The 2 basic types of nephrons found in birds

Nephron Type	Reptilian	Mammalian
Region of the kidney located	Cortical	Medullary
Loop of Henle present	No	Yes
Produces	Uric acid	Urine
Capable of concentrating urine to some degree	No	Yes
Makes up most of the nephrons in birds	Yes	No

descending loop enlarging before the bend.[2] Many species do not have a well-defined arrangement of their loops of Henle and collecting tubules because the components intermingle. However, passerines usually have their descending limbs just medial to an outer ring of perilobular collecting tubules. An inner ring is formed by the ascending limbs of the loops of Henle.[2]

The outer ring of collecting tubules of each lobule consists of perilobular collecting tubules, whereas those that are part of the medullary region are termed medullary collecting tubules. Commonly, these medullary tubules combine to form a single larger collecting duct. When several collecting ducts combine, they form a secondary branch of the ureter.[2]

Birds, like mammals, have a juxtaglomerular apparatus, which includes a macula densa, which is an epithelial thickening at the beginning of the distal convoluted tubule. This macula densa makes anatomic contact with the afferent arteriole through their secretory juxtaglomerular cells, which secrete renin. The third component of the juxtaglomerular apparatus is the extraglomerular mesangium, a collection of modified connective tissue found between the macula and the specialized cells of the afferent arterioles.[2]

ARTERIAL SUPPLY TO THE KIDNEYS

The cranial, middle, and caudal divisions of the kidney are supplied by their respective arteries that arise from the abdominal aorta. The caudal division has a branch off the aorta that bifurcates on the surface of the kidney, resulting in 2 arteries that enter the parenchyma of this larger division.[1] These arteries then branch within the substance of the kidneys to eventually form the intralobular arteries. The intralobular arteries are found in the lobule approximately half-way between the interlobular and intralobular veins.[2]

The intralobular arteries form the short afferent glomerular arteries that immediately coalesce to form the glomerulus. Each of these capillary tufts is simpler and much smaller than in mammals, because they consist of only 2 to 3 capillaries that have limited interconnections compared with mammalian capillary tufts. The afferent arteriole forms a single capillary loop that widens to form an efferent arteriole. When observing the arrangement of the glomeruli, capillary tufts transition from very simple in the outer cortex to increasing complexity in the medullary region, but are still less complex than mammalian glomeruli.[1]

Mammalian red blood cells are more deformable than avian red blood cells and can fold and bend while moving through the smaller space of their glomerular capillaries. Nucleated avian red blood cells are fusiform, larger (about 8×15 μm), and are more rigid than those of mammalian red blood cells (7–8 μm). Because avian capillaries are larger, to accommodate the size of the avian nucleated red blood cells, the capillary tufts of avian glomeruli are also larger than in mammals. This tuft of capillaries folds into the visceral layer of the Bowman capsule. The Bowman capsule is the sac that represents the beginning of the nephron. Associated with this visceral layer are cells called podocytes that have slits that act as pores for the movement of solutes from the blood into the Bowman space of the nephron. In the chicken, these fenestrations or pores are about 40% to 80% larger than those in mammals,[1] which allows more solutes to enter the nephrons. In addition, there is less of a polyanionic charge on the filtration barrier in the chicken, and this also contributes to greater flow, thereby allowing larger particles to pass. For this reason, the ureteral urine of birds normally contains about 100 times more protein (5 mg/mL) than that of mammalian ureteral urine.[7]

The arterial supply continues as efferent glomerular arterioles. These arterioles divide to form the peritubular capillary plexus, which surrounds the epithelium of the convoluted tubules in the cortical region. In the medullary region, the efferent glomerular arterioles form arteriolar recta that lie alongside the loops of Henle before forming the venulae recta that drains the area.[1,2]

VENOUS SUPPLY TO THE KIDNEYS

Blood from the area around the loops of Henle is drained by the venulae recta into the intralobular veins. The intralobular veins drain blood into the efferent renal veins or branches. Blood then flows into renal veins of the appropriate division (**Fig. 6**). In the cranial division of the kidney, there can be several cranial renal veins that drain into the common iliac vein after the renal portal valve or into the abdominal vena cava directly (**Figs. 7** and **8**). The caudal renal vein (**Fig. 9**) drains the middle and caudal divisions of the kidneys. The caudal renal vein, like the cranial renal vein, empties into the common iliac vein after the renal portal valve.

Renal Portal System

The renal portal system is involved in the secretion of urates into the blood so that uric acid can be excreted by the kidneys in birds. The renal portal system supplies venous blood to the peritubular capillary plexuses that surround the proximal convoluted tubules at the periphery of the lobule. These tubules are responsible for the secretion of urates. Urates are also filtered by the glomerulus but its rate is insufficient. It has been suggested that the renal portal system provides about two-thirds of the blood supply to the kidneys that bypasses the glomeruli.[2] This suggestion has important ramifications for the removal of urates along with other components, including drugs.

The renal portal system forms a venous ring with both kidneys. It consists of the right and left cranial and caudal renal portal veins. At the cranial end, the right and left cranial renal portal veins are connected via the internal vertebral venous sinus, which drains the vertebral column. The caudal end of the ring is completed by its anastomoses with the caudal mesenteric vein. There are numerous small venous branches that originate from this ring to penetrate the parenchyma of the kidney. Each afferent renal branch has a muscular sphincter at its base to control the volume of blood that enters the kidney. These afferent renal venous branches connect with the interlobular veins,

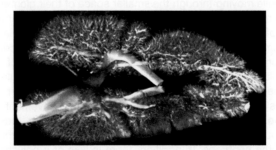

Fig. 6. Juvenile cassowary perfused with BriteVu contrast agent, kidneys removed, and then CT scanned. This maximum intensity view shows the renal vasculature and general layout of the cassowary kidneys. Cranial is to the left and the left kidney is at the top. The overlying veins were transected during organ removal. (*Courtesy of* M. Scott Echols, DVM, DABVP-Avian, Centerville, UT and Scarlet Imaging, Murray, UT and Scarlet Imaging, Murray, UT.)

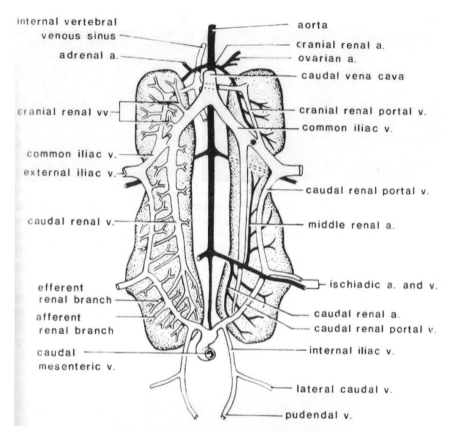

Fig. 7. Ventral view of the kidneys of the domestic fowl showing the blood supply. The kidneys are drawn as though transparent, in order to reveal the vessels. The left side of the diagram shows the renal portal veins and the efferent veins; the right side shows the arteries. The asterisk marks the site of the renal portal valve in the left kidney. In the right kidney the conical valve is shown diagrammatically. (*From* King AS, McLelland J. Urinary system. In: Birds: their structure and function, 2nd edition. London: Bailliere Tindall; 1984. p. 181; with permission.)

which in turn connect to the peritubular capillary plexus at the periphery of each lobule.[2]

In addition to the valves in the afferent renal venous branches, there are renal portal valves that control blood flow as well. These valves are found within the lumen of the common iliac veins between the renal and portal veins. Blood can enter the portal venous ring from the external iliac veins, the internal iliac veins, the caudal mesenteric vein, and the ischiatic veins. Each valve is innervated by adrenergic and acetylcholine receptors. If the valves are open, then blood flows directly into the caudal vena cava and not the kidney. Valve closure is inhibited by norepinephrine and epinephrine so that with flight there is available venous return to the heart. When the valve is closed, blood flows into the parenchyma of the kidney. Acetylcholine stimulates its closure.[2]

From a clinical perspective, understanding these connections with the renal portal system helps explain the spread of neoplasia and infectious agents to other parts of

A   **B**

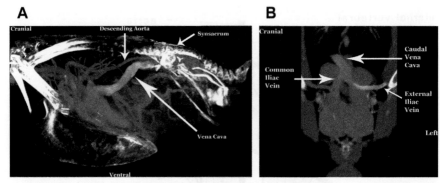

Fig. 8. Congo gray parrot (*P erithacus erithacus*) coelom as seen with an iopamidol 370 contrast CT study. (*A*) Sagittal and (*B*) coronal views of the local renal vasculature are noted. The left and right external iliac veins draining the leg divide the cranial and middle renal divisions on the ventral surfaces of the kidneys. The 2 external iliac veins course cranially to become common iliac veins, eventually combining to form the caudal extent of the vena cava. (*Courtesy of* M. Scott Echols, DVM, DABVP-Avian, Centerville, UT.)

the body. Blood from the renal portal system can flow through the portal valve into the vena cava, into the caudal mesenteric vein to the liver, and/or into the internal vertebral venous plexus within the vertebral canal. This shunt can result in the bypass of the kidney completely but often is only partially activated so that blood may go in a variety of directions.

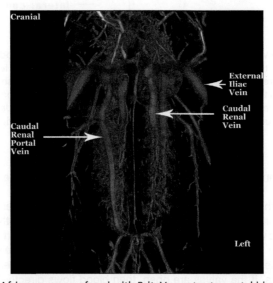

Fig. 9. Domestic African goose perfused with BriteVu contrast agent, kidneys removed, and then CT scanned. The external iliac veins draining the leg are joined by the caudal renal portal veins (lateral) and caudal renal veins (medial) to form the common iliac vein (not shown here) on the ventral surfaces of the kidneys. False color was used to highlight the venous vasculature as distinct from the overlying renal tissue. The common iliac veins and caudal vena cava were transected when the kidneys were removed. (*Courtesy of* M. Scott Echols, DVM, DABVP-Avian, Centerville, UT and Scarlet Imaging, Murray, UT.)

FUNCTIONAL ANATOMY OF THE RENAL CORPUSCLE

Glomerular filtration occurs in the renal corpuscle. The renal corpuscle consists of a blind-ended sac of the renal tubule with a tuft of capillaries invaginating its surface (**Fig. 10**). The sac consists of a visceral layer and a parietal layer. The parietal layer is an external layer of the sac that consists of a single layer of squamous epithelial cells. It is not part of the filtration barrier. The visceral layer of the renal tubule is composed of podocytes with fenestrated arms that surround the tufts of capillaries. The basal lamina of these podocytes is continuous with the basal lamina of the capillary endothelium. Fluid and solutes move through the endothelium, through the fenestrae, and into the Bowman space.

The macula densa is located in the distal convoluted tubule. These specialized epithelial cells detect sodium concentrations in the fluid of the tubule as it leaves the renal corpuscle.[2] When, for example, sodium levels decrease, this causes relaxation of the afferent arteriole, which, in turn, increases glomerular blood flow, thereby increasing glomerular hydrostatic pressure and hence the filtration rate of that renal tubule.[1] The second function of the macula densa is to signal the release of renin from specialized myocytes in the afferent arterioles called JG cells. Renin increases blood pressure via the renin-angiotensin-aldosterone system.[1] Macula densa cells are histologically distinct from the remaining cells of the distal convoluted tubule. These cells are taller with more prominent nuclei and appear darker and therefore appear denser, hence the name macula densa.

The renal corpuscle (see **Fig. 10**) consists of the blind-ended sac of the renal tubule, invaginated by a tuft of capillaries. The vascular pole, where the blood vessels enter and exit the corpuscle, consists of an afferent and efferent arteriole. The

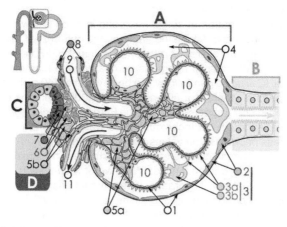

A – Renal corpuscle
B – Proximal tubule
C – Distal convoluted tubule
D – Juxtaglomerular apparatus
1. Basement membrane (Basal lamina)
2. Bowman's capsule – parietal layer
3. Bowman's capsule – visceral layer
3a. Pedicels (Foot processes from podocytes)
3b. Podocyte

4. Bowman's space (urinary space)
5a. Mesangium – Intraglomerular cell
5b. Mesangium – Extraglomerular cell
6. Granular cells (Juxtaglomerular cells)
7. Macula densa
8. Myocytes (smooth muscle)
9. Afferent arteriole
10. Glomerulus Capillaries
11. Efferent arteriole

Fig. 10. A renal corpuscle. (*Courtesy of* Michael Komorniczak Medical Illustrations - Creative Commons 3.0 Attribution-ShareAlike (CC BY_SA 3.0) via Wikimedia Commons; with permission.)

juxtaglomerular apparatus or JG apparatus is also located at the vascular pole. The JG apparatus consists of altered smooth muscle cells in the afferent arteriole and specialized epithelial cells in the distal convoluted tubule, called the macula densa. The macula densa sits between the afferent and efferent arterioles and detects changes in sodium concentration in the fluid of the tubule as it leaves the renal corpuscle. Macula densa cells also signal the release of renin in the specialized myocytes in the afferent arterioles: the JG cells. These JG cells in the afferent arteriole secrete renin, which increases blood pressure via the renin-angiotensin-aldosterone system. Baroreceptors in the afferent arterioles can also cause the JG cells to release renin.[1]

The urinary pole sits opposite the vascular pole and it is where the proximal tubule originates as the blind-ended sac. The sac consists of a parietal layer, which consists of a single layer of squamous epithelial cells, and a visceral layer. The visceral layer of the renal tubule is composed of fenestrated arms that surround the capillary tufts. The basal lamina of these podocytes is continuous with the basal lamina of the capillary endothelium. Fluid and solutes move through the endothelium through the fenestrae into the Bowman space.

GLOMERULAR FILTRATION

The movement of fluid and solutes across the filtration barrier is a function of hydrostatic pressure produced by the heart. Hydrostatic pressure favors movement across the barrier, but the colloid osmotic pressure of the plasma proteins tends to keep fluid in the capillary space. The charges on the fenestra and the size of the openings oppose the movement of large, negatively charged proteins, such as albumen. As described previously, the size of the fenestra and the complexity of the glomerular tufts are much reduced in class Aves.[1]

The rate of glomerular filtration of single nephrons in birds is low compared with mammals of similar body mass. Allometric analysis has determined that total kidney glomerular filtration rates (GFRs) are not different. This single GFR seems to be offset by birds having a larger number of nephrons compared with mammals of a similar mass. In desert quail (Callipepla gambelii) with a body mass of 140 g, there are approximately 48,000 nephrons, whereas a 300-g rat has 32,000 nephrons.[8] Single GFRs have been quantified in only 2 species of birds, the European starling (Sturnus vulgaris) and the desert quail. Although the techniques used were different, the data suggest that, with the loopless nephrons, the values are similar (Table 2).

Whole-kidney GFRs of birds are more variable than those of mammals and seems to be most dependent on hydration status. With water deprivation, the GFR can decrease up to 65% of that at full hydration. It seems that changes in GFR are regulated by the antidiuretic hormone of birds, arginine vasotocin (AVT).[1] AVT functions to conserve water by altering the tone of the renal vasculature and the tubular epithelium.[9,11] Some birds, such as hummingbirds, are able to alter their GFRs diurnally based on the consumption of food. When they consume large quantities of sugars

| Table 2 | | |
| Single-nephron glomerular filtration rate for small loopless nephrons | | |
Species	Desert Quail[9] (C gambelii)	Starling[10] (S vulgaris)
Single-nephron GFR (nL/min)	6.4 (average 14.6)	0.25–0.5
Technique	Ferrocyanide	In vivo micropuncture

in water, they are able to extract and use the energy of the sugars while excreting water.[12]

AVT is a peptide hormone released by the neurohypophysis. The most common reason for AVT release is an increase in extracellular fluid osmolality. As plasma osmolality increases by 1 mmol/kg, there is a subsequent increase of 0.25 to 2.0 pg/mL in AVT level.[13] A decrease in extracellular fluid volume using a hemorrhage model results in the release of AVT.[14] Dehydration also results in an increase in circulating levels of AVT, which in turn decreases GFR[15] and results in a reduction of urine flow not only because of reduced filtration but indirectly by enhanced tubular reabsorption. Reptilian or cortical nephrons are most sensitive to AVT, which is important because these nephrons lack a loop of Henle and therefore the ability to concentrate urine.

If, instead of water deprivation, there is water overload and/or an increased extracellular fluid expansion, there is an increased GFR to compensate. However, the mechanism is not known.[16]

There have been limited studies investigating renal blood flow in birds; however, there seems to be autoregulation of renal blood flow over a wide range of systemic blood pressures. In domestic fowl, systemic blood pressures as low as 50 mm Hg can allow continued maintenance of GFR.[1,2]

ANATOMIC DIAGNOSES OF SEVERAL DISEASE STATES

Based on an understanding of the physiology of the kidney and its blood supply, diagnosis of a variety of disease states can be determined with the use of computed tomography. Tumor masses adjacent to the kidney can be more easily distinguished from the kidney itself (**Fig. 11**). Cysts within renal parenchyma can also be visualized (**Fig. 12**). Ureteroliths and renal mineralization leading to secondary parenchymal atrophy can also be observed (**Fig. 13**).

NITROGEN EXCRETION AND URIC ACID IN AVIAN URINE

The major end product of nitrogen catabolism in birds is uric acid. Uric acid accounts for about 70% to 80% of the nitrogen excreted in ureteral urine, along with minor amounts of creatinine, amino acids, and urea.[17] Uric acid is considered to be a highly

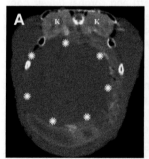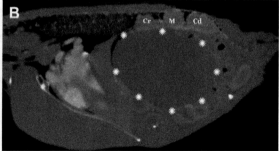

Fig. 11. Male eclectus (*E roratus*) with a nondifferentiated testicular tumor as seen with an iopamidol 370 contrast CT study on (*A*) transverse and (*B*) sagittal views. The testicular mass is outlined with white asterisks (*), whereas the kidney tissue is identified as K (on transverse view) and further defined as cranial (Cr), middle (M), and caudal (Cd) renal divisions on sagittal view. The renal tissue is displaced dorsally, completely filling the normally air-filled dorsal diverticulum of the abdominal air sac immediately ventral to the synsacrum. (*Courtesy of* M. Scott Echols, DVM, DABVP-Avian, Centerville, UT).

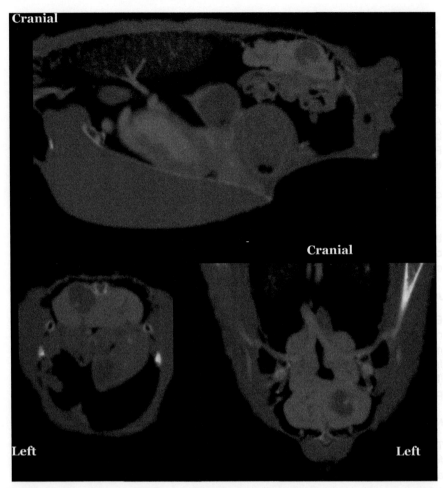

Fig. 12. Timneh gray parrot (*Psittacus erithacus timneh*) renal cyst as seen with an iopamidol 370 contrast CT study in sagittal (*top*), transverse (*lower left*) and coronal (*lower right*) planes. The cyst is in the left caudal renal division and is seen as a radiolucent (relative to the more normal and radiodense surrounding renal tissue) spherical lesion. A blood vessel carrying contrast agent can be seen coursing through the cyst in all 3 planes. (*Courtesy of* M. Scott Echols, DVM, DABVP-Avian, Centerville, UT.)

efficient excretory product because it has low solubility and removes 4 nitrogen atoms per molecule. However, the metabolic cost to synthesize uric acid is much higher than that of ammonia and urea.

Although uric acid has low aqueous solubility, it does remain soluble in the blood at pH 7.4.[1] Urate is a small molecule of 186 molecular weight that freely passes the fenestrae of the glomerulus. However, there are about 5 times more urates excreted by the renal tubules than are filtered. Micropuncture studies showed marked secretion of urate by the loopless nephrons.[18]

At normal urate levels, albumen plays an important role in taking urates out of solution and preventing crystal formation. Small, spherical structures begin to form in the proximal tubule and, by the time they reach the ureter, they range in size from 1 to 14 μm. Most spheres consist of 65% urates. Once taken out of solution, urate does

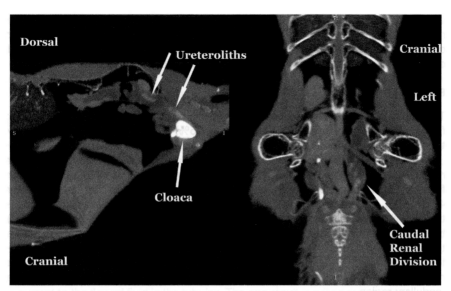

Fig. 13. Gyrfalcon (*Falco rusticolus*) with ureteroliths, renal mineralization, and renal atrophy as seen with an iohexol 240 contrast CT study. The sagittal (*left*) and coronal (*right*) images show the atrophied left kidney. There are multifocal mineralizations in the left caudal renal division and ureteroliths in the left ureter. The cloaca is filled with contrast. (*Courtesy of* C. Hebel, DVM, Dubai and P. Wencel, DVM, Lublin, Poland.)

not contribute to the osmolality of urine. Therefore, the mammalian urine/plasma osmolar ratios cannot be compared with avian systems because nitrogen metabolism is not contributed equally from an osmolality perspective.[1]

As the concentration of urates secreted into the lumen increases past its solubility limit, there is the potential for crystal formation in the proximal tubule.[1] This potential has important implications for clinicians because normal patient hydration provides a GFR sufficient to reduce the risk of possible sludge formation or obstruction. Maintaining adequate levels of dietary vitamin A also helps to keep the reptilian portion of the avian kidneys healthy by reducing the incidence of squamous metaplasia, which would also cause plugging.

INTAKE OF WATER AND SOLUTES

Drinking is important for many birds; however, there are species that meet their water needs from food items (carnivores and frugivores) or from metabolic water (xerophilic).[19] It has been estimated that a 100-g bird drinks about 5% of its body weight daily. As body mass decreases to 10 to 20 g, the drinking rate increases to 50%.[20,21] Birds with salt glands typically need an increased volume of water compared with those lacking these glands. Those species that require water are thought to have a minimum water requirement of one-third to one-half of the ad libitum drinking rate.[21]

The physiologic stimuli to initiate drinking are primarily cellular dehydration, extracellular dehydration, and angiotensin II. Cellular dehydration is determined in the periventricular nucleus of the hypothalamus and may respond to concentrations of Na+ in the cerebrospinal fluid.[22,23] Extracellular dehydration has been shown by models using hemorrhage or injection of nonabsorbed osmotically active substances to

5. Casotti G, Richardson KC. A stereological analysis of kidney structure of honey-eater birds (*Meliphagidae*) inhabiting either arid or wet environments. J Anat 1992;180:281–8.
6. Goldstein DL, Skadhauge E. Regulation of body fluid composition. In: Whittow GC, editor. Sturkie's avian physiology. San Diego (CA): Academic Press; 2000. p. 265–97.
7. Janes DN, Braun EJ. Urinary protein excretion in red jungle fowl (*Gallus gallus*). Comp Biochem Physiol A Physiol 1997;118:1273–5.
8. Yokota SD, Benyajati S, Dantzler WH. Comparative aspects of glomerular filtration in vertebrates. Ren Physiol 1985;8:193–221.
9. Braun EJ, Dantzler WH. Function of mammalian-type and reptilian-type nephrons in kidney of desert quail. Am J Physiol 1972;222(3):617–29.
10. Laverty G, Dantzler WH. Micropuncture of superficial nephrons in avian (*Sturnus vulgaris*) kidney. Am J Physiol 1982;243:F561.
11. Stallone JN, Braun EJ. Contributions of glomerular and tubular mechanisms to antidiuresis in conscious domestic fowl. Am J Physiol 1985;249:F842.
12. Del Rio CM, Schondube J, Mcwhorter TJ, et al. Intake responses in nectar feeding birds: digestive and metabolic causes, osmoregulatory consequences, and coevolutionary effects. Am Zool 2001;41:902–15.
13. Gray DA, Erasmus T. Plasma arginine vasotocin and angiotensin II in the water deprived kelp gull (*Larus dominicanus*), Cape gannet (*Sula capensis*) and jack-ass penguin (*Spheniscus demersus*). Comp Biochem Physiol A 1988;91:727–32.
14. Stallone JN, Braun EJ. Regulation of plasma arginine vasotocin in conscious water-deprived domestic fowl. Am J Physiol 1985;249:F842.
15. Braun EJ, Dantzler WH. Effects of ADH on single nephron glomerular filtration rates in the avian kidney. Am J Physiol 1974;226:1–12.
16. Roberts JR. Renal function and plasma arginine vasotocin during an acute salt load in feral chickens. J Comp Physiol B 1992;162:54–8.
17. Tsahar E, Del Rio CM, Izhaki I, et al. Can birds be ammonotelic? Nitrogen balance and excretion in two frugivores. J Exp Biol 2005;208:1025–34.
18. Dudas PL, Pelis RM, Braun EJ, et al. Transepithelial urate transport by avian renal proximal tubule epithelium in primary culture. J Exp Biol 2005;208:4305–15.
19. Bartholomew GA. The water economy of seed-eating birds that survive without drinking. Proceedings of the 15th Annual International Ornithological Congress. 1972. p. 237–54.
20. Bartholomew GA, Cade TJ. The water economy of land birds. Auk 1963;80: 504–39.
21. Skadhauge E. Osmoregulation in birds. New York: Springer Verlag; 1981.
22. Thornton SN. Osmoreceptor localization in the brain of the pigeon (*Columba livia*). Brain Res 1986;377:96–104.
23. Thornton SN. The influence of central infusions on drinking due to peripheral osmotic stimuli in the pigeon (*Columba livia*). Physiol Behav 1986;36:229–33.
24. Takei Y, Okawara Y, Kobayashi H. Control of drinking in birds. In: Hughes MR, Chadwick A, editors. Progress in avian osmoregulation. Leeds (UK): Leeds Philosophical and Literary Society; 1989. p. 1–12.
25. Campbell C, Braun EJ. Cecal degradation of uric acid in Gambel quail. Am J Physiol 1986;251:R51–62.
26. Barnes EM, Impey CS. The isolation and properties of the predominant anaerobic bacteria in the caeca of chickens and turkeys. Br Poult Sci 1970;11:467–81.
27. Karasawa Y, Maeda M. Effect of colostomy on the utilisation of dietary nitrogen in the fowl fed on a low protein diet. Br Poult Sci 1992;33:815–20.

28. Vranish JR, Braun EJ. Isolation of a putative osmoreceptor from the avian GI tract. FASEB J 2011;25:1047.3.
29. Brummermann M, Braun EJ. Effect of water deprivation on colonic motility of white leghorn roosters. Am J Physiol 1995;268:R690–8.
30. Shuttleworth TJ. Intracellular signals controlling ionic and acid-base regulation in avian nasal gland cells. Adv Comp Environ Physiol 1995;22:185–206.
31. Gray D, Downing C, Sayed N. Endogenous plasma atrial natriuretic peptide and the control of salt gland function in the Pekin duck. Am J Physiol 1997;273: R1080–5.

Diseases of the Avian Urinary System

David N. Phalen, DVM, PhD*

KEYWORDS

- Bird • Disease • Renal • Urinary

KEY POINTS

- The urinary system of the bird is difficult to assess because the kidneys cannot be palpated and are rarely visible by ultrasound.
- Disease diagnosis generally depends on a detailed history, biochemical and hematological findings, and increasingly on endoscopy and renal biopsy.
- As with all other species, diseases of the renal system can be degenerative, anomalous, nutritional, neoplastic, infectious, immune-mediated, caused by toxins, and as the result of trauma.
- Diagnosing renal disease requires knowledge of the processes that can affect the kidney and the ability to rule out diseases that would not be expected.

INTRODUCTION

There are many diseases of the renal system. They can be caused by infectious and noninfectious processes, and they can be of primary renal origin, the result of extension of disease occurring in adjacent organ systems, or part of a systemic disease. Creating a relevant differential diagnosis for kidney disease in the live or dead bird requires a structured approach where the list of differentials is narrowed based on the signalment of the bird; its history, including its diet and management; physical findings; and other diagnostic findings. The objective of this article is not only to provide a list of the diseases that occur in birds but also to provide the reader guidelines on when a disease should be considered in a differential.

DEGENERATIVE DISEASES OF THE URINARY SYSTEM
Context

- Based on the author's experience, there is usually an underlying cause for end-stage kidney disease in birds. End-stage kidney disease associated with age, as is seen in dogs and cats, is rare.

Disclosure Statement: The author has nothing to disclose.
Sydney School of Veterinary Sciences, University of Sydney, Sydney, New South Wales, Australia
* 425 Werombi Road, Camden, New South Wales 2570, Australia.
E-mail address: David.phalen@sydney.edu.au

End-stage kidney disease occurs in all animals. It is characterized by the gradual loss of normal functioning tissue that is replaced by fibrosis and is most commonly seen in older animals. The cause of kidney degeneration is generally not known but often there is some degree of accompanying inflammation. In mammals, degenerate kidneys are small. In birds and reptiles they are enlarged. Through the endoscope or at necropsy, in addition to being enlarged, end-stage kidneys in birds will have a surface that contains many diffuse hyperreflective foci or short linear streaks that represent urate tophi (**Fig. 1**) in the parenchyma and urate distended tubules (renal gout) (**Fig. 2**). Birds in renal failure will generally also have visceral gout with urate deposition on mesangial surfaces such as the pericardium, liver capsule, air sacs, joint capsules, and tendon sheaths (**Fig. 3**).

ANOMALOUS DISEASES OF THE URINARY SYSTEM
Context

- Anomalous diseases of the urinary system are rare but are most likely to occur in highly inbred birds and certain stains of chickens and other gallinaceous birds.[1]
- Aplastic and hypoplastic changes in the kidney are often compensated for by hyperplasia of the remaining kidney tissue and are incidental findings at necropsy.[2]

The 2 most common anomalous diseases of the kidney are renal hypoplasia and cystic kidneys (**Fig. 4**). Renal hypoplasia and aplasia are typically unilateral and segmental, most commonly affecting the cranial division. Renal cysts vary from microscopic to macroscopic and from individual cysts to numerous cysts that may replace large amounts of the kidney.[1,3] If the kidney is largely replaced by cysts then birds may die from renal failure. Cystic changes can also be acquired secondary to renal trauma and necrosis or other diseases of the kidney that result in scarring.[4] Two rare anomalous diseases of the kidney are ureteral cysts and hydronephrosis secondary to stenosis of the ureter (**Fig. 5**).[1,2]

EXTRAMEDULLARY MYELOPOIESIS

Extramedullary myelopoiesis is a common and normal finding in the kidney of nestlings and can be extensive (**Fig. 6**). It may also occur in mature birds with chronic inflammatory diseases.[2]

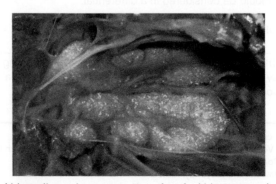

Fig. 1. End-stage kidney disease in a parrot. Note that the kidneys are enlarged and contain numerous bright reflective foci. The foci represent urate tophi and, in some instances, urate dilated tubules.

NUTRITIONAL DISEASES OF THE URINARY SYSTEM
Context

- Metastatic mineralization of the kidney, secondary to diets containing excess calcium, is a relatively common cause of renal failure in blue and gold macaws (*Ara ararauna*) and yellow-tailed black cockatoo chicks (*Calyptorhynchus funereus*) and adult and juvenile budgerigars, cockatiels (*Nymphicus hollandicus*), lovebirds (*Agapornis* spp.), and domestic pigeons (*Columba livia domestica*).

Calcium

It has been shown experimentally that diets containing more than 0.7% calcium will cause metastatic mineralization of the renal tubules and result in renal failure in budgerigar nestlings.[30] Other organs affected include the koilin of the ventriculus and the mucosa of the proventriculus. Similar lesions have been seen in hand-fed blue and gold macaws and yellow-tailed black cockatoos fed diets containing calcium concentrations in excess of 0.7%.[1] These lesions are also common in nestling and adult cockatiels and lovebirds fed all pelleted diet and the presumption is that at least some pelleted diets also contain excess calcium. Lesions similar to this occur sporadically in fledgling racing pigeons, but the exact diet fed to them is rarely known.[1]

Affected kidneys are grossly swollen and contain small widespread hyperreflective foci that represent mineral and urate tophi. Calcium deposits form in the tubules and cause necrosis of the tubular epithelium (**Fig. 8**). Calcium deposits may be abundant or relatively rare but should be considered to be significant even when they are infrequent. Glomeruli undergo degeneration and ultimately sclerosis. Typically, these kidneys contain extensive fibrosis and urate tophi (**Fig. 9**) are abundant. Similar lesions can be found in chickens and wild birds if they consume day-blooming jasmine (*Cestrum diurnum*).[31]

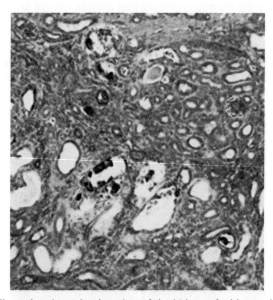

Fig. 8. Hematoxylin and eosin–stained section of the kidney of a blue and gold macaw (*Ara ararauna*) demonstrating renal calcification (purple concretions) with tubular endothelial cell necrosis and tubular dilation.

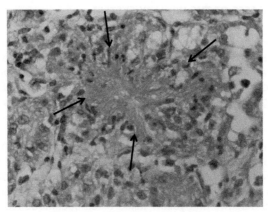

Fig. 9. Urate tophus in a hematoxylin and eosin–stained section of the kidney of a parrot (*arrows*).

Laying hen diets typically contain 1% calcium or more to replace the substantial calcium required to make egg shells. Metastatic mineralization of the kidney occurs in roosters that are fed laying diets and in hens that continue to eat laying diets after they cease laying. Urolithiasis, which is seen in chickens, is also likely to be caused by excess dietary calcium.[32] Uroliths partially or completely obstruct the ureters causing tubule dilation, loss of nephrons, and ultimately renal failure (**Fig. 10**).[33]

Vitamin D
Vitamin D_3 poisoning can also cause metastatic mineralization of the kidney and renal failure; however this is rare. The one confirmed instance of this occurred in lorikeets fed a diet with a formulation error. The vitamin D_3 concentration in the diet was in excess of 40 times the minimum amount that allowed normal bone development in budgerigars.[30]

Vitamin A
Vitamin A deficiency can cause squamous metaplasia of the mucosa of the ureters, which in turn leads to partial or complete obstruction of the ureters themselves or

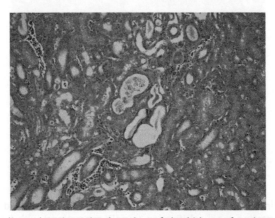

Fig. 10. Hematoxylin and eosin–stained section of the kidney of a pigeon (*Columba livia*) demonstrating dilated renal tubules containing protein and cellular casts.

branches of the ureters. Ureteral obstruction results in dilation of renal tubules, loss of glomeruli, and renal failure if not treated in time. It is the authors' impression that this only occurs in birds whose disease is advanced and therefore it is a very unusual histologic finding.

Iron

Iron storage disease is best known for causing iron accumulation in hepatocytes. In advanced cases, it also causes iron accumulation in renal tubules. Its functional impact is not known. Iron storage disease is common in captive ramphastids and sturnids; it rarely occurs in Psittacine birds.[1,7]

Moisture

Physiologic polyuria is common in birds that consume diets that contain a high amount of moisture. In rare instances, birds may drink water in an effort to cool themselves during periods of extreme heat and will subsequently be polyuric. The author has seen this behavior in ostrich chicks that drank so much water that they became edematous. A mild polyuria is common in birds that are stressed, particularly those that are taken to the veterinary hospital.

Birds compensate for dehydration by decreasing their glomerular filtration rate. Urates continue to be secreted by the proximal tubules, however, and the tubules become distended with urates and they can be seen grossly as white streaks in the kidney. With rehydration, this lesion will resolve. However, with advanced dehydration, tubules degenerate and urate tophi form resulting in renal failure. In poultry the formation of uroliths and nephritis has been associated with water deprivation during periods of elevated ambient temperature.[34]

INFECTIOUS DISEASE OF THE URINARY SYSTEM
Viral Diseases

Context

- Many viral diseases cause lesions in the kidneys. However, most of these viruses target other tissues causing significant disease in other organ systems or out rightly killing the bird. Therefore, evidence of renal disease is rarely helpful in making a diagnosis of a viral infection.
- The exception to this rule is pigeon paramyxovirus 1, which causes an interstitial nephritis. "Wet droppings" are often the first indicator of the presence of pigeon paramyxovirus in a loft.
- Avian polyomavirus,[35] the Gouldian finch polyomavirus,[36] the canary polyomavirus,[37] and some of the psittacine adenoviruses, particularly psittacine adenovirus-2,[38] infect cells in the kidney and can cause significant microscopic lesions.

Avian polyomavirus in hand-raised nestlings of large parrots causes an immune complex glomerulopathy, and the virus commonly infects mesangial cells (**Fig. 11**). These birds die acutely from liver necrosis and hemorrhage, so these lesions rarely have clinical relevance. In one instance, however, 2 nestling macaws with avian polyomavirus survived the acute form of disease and developed ascites that was secondary to renal failure characterized by glomerular sclerosis. Avian polyomavirus infects renal tubule cells in nestling budgerigars as well as many other tissues. Although kidney damage occurs in these birds, renal signs have not been reported. Chronic renal disease with glomerular sclerosis is seen in

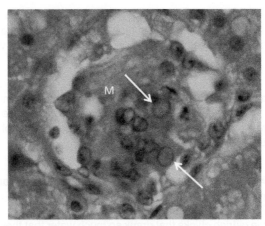

Fig. 11. Hematoxylin and eosin–stained section of the kidney of a nestling Alexandrine parrot (*Psittacula eupatria*) with avian polyomavirus. The section of a glomerulus shows mesangial cells that are exhibiting karyomegaly (*arrows*). The expanded mesangial matrix (M) is composed of virus-antibody complexes.

Gouldian finches that survive acute polyomavirus infection and theoretically they may show signs of kidney disease.[2]

By and large the adenoviruses that cause microscopic lesions in the kidneys (**Fig. 12**) seem to be reactivated when birds are concurrently infected with other infectious agents, for example, *Aspergillus* sp., and *Macrorhabdus ornithogaster*, and their presence is generally considered an incidental finding.[38] Lovebirds and budgerigars are 2 species where small numbers of infected renal tubular epithelial cells are commonly found in postmortem specimens. Increasing evidence suggests that subclinical infections with adenoviruses are widespread in captive and wild birds, meaning that their detection with modern molecular tools must be interpreted with caution (Phalen D, unpublished observations, 2018).

Pigeon paramyxovirus now has a global distribution. Although historically associated with neurologic signs, many variants now have a tropism for the pancreas and kidney. In the kidney, they cause a lymphocytic interstitial nephritis that is often associated with loss of tubules (**Fig. 13**). These birds will be polyuric.[1,39]

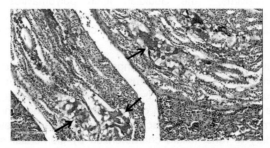

Fig. 12. Hematoxylin and eosin–stained section of the kidney from a Bourke's parrot (*Neopsephotus bourkii*) demonstrating Psittacid adenovirus 2 inclusions (*arrows*) in the collecting duct epithelial cells.

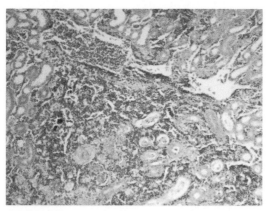

Fig. 13. Hematoxylin and eosin–stained section of the kidney from a pigeon with pigeon paramyxovirus (*Columbia livia*). Not the prominent lymphocytic interstitial nephritis.

West Nile Virus also causes an interstitial lymphoplasmacytic nephritis in many affected birds. However, in one study at least, signs of renal disease were not reported.[40] Avian bornavirus replicates in the avian kidney and is shed in the urine, but it is also not associated with renal signs.[41]

There are many viruses that infect poultry that can target the kidney.[42–46] These would result in significant flock morbidity and mortality and are best diagnosed by necropsy of a sick or recently dead bird by an experienced poultry pathologist or review of the comprehensive Diseases of Poultry 13th Edition.[46]

Bacterial Diseases

Context

- Systemic bacterial infections often cause kidney lesions.
- Ascending bacterial infections are rare and generally rapidly fatal.

Bacteria can enter the kidney either by ascending the ureters from the cloaca or by hematogenous spread.[47] A wide range of gram-positive and gram-negative bacteria are known to cause kidney disease, either as an ascending infection or as part of a systemic disease.[47,48] Staphylococci and Streptococci commonly cause disease in finches and canaries and less commonly in psittacine birds. Examples of other bacteria that can affect the kidney include members of Enterobacteriaceae, *Listeria* spp., *Erysipelothrix rhusiopathiae*, *Pasteurella* spp., *Mycobacteria* spp., and *Chlamydia psittaci*, but these bacteria are more likely to cause a systemic disease and generate signs associated with other organ systems.[7,49–52] Bacteria can be found in the kidney or interstitium when birds are bacteremic.[2,53] Disseminated intravascular coagulopathy can also result in thromboemboli formation in arteries and capillaries in the kidneys.[53] Inflammation of the kidney induced by bacterial infections may interfere with the ability of the kidney to concentrate urine.[54] Most bacterial infections of the kidney are diagnosed at necropsy; however, chronic bacterial diseases, for example, osteomyelitis, may result in chronic kidney lesions such as granulomas with possible -clinical significance (**Fig. 14**). Mycobacterial infections are characterized by granulomatous lesions of the liver, spleen, and lung but may also affect the kidney.[51,52,55]

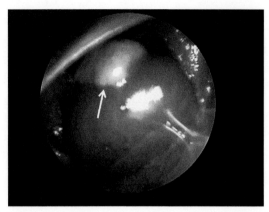

Fig. 14. Bacterial granuloma (*arrow*) on the surface of the kidney in a parrot as viewed through the endoscope. (*Courtesy of* L. Crosta, med vet, PhD, FNOVI, Camden, Australia.)

Fungal Diseases

Context

- The most common fungal lesion of the kidney is tissue invasion from an adjacent *Aspergillus* sp. air sac infection.

Aspergillosis is a common infection in many species of birds. Infection of the caudal thoracic and abdominal air sacs is common, but invasion through the air sac and into the kidney can occur when disease is severe (**Fig. 15**).[2] Affected birds show other systemic signs of disease and renal disease would be difficult to appreciate antemortem. *Aspergillus* sp. may also affect the kidney when they invade blood vessels and fragments of the mycelia cause thromboembolic disease that can affect the kidney.[56] Other fungi reported to affect avian kidneys as part of systemic disease include *Penicillium chrysogenum* and *Cryptococcus neoformans*.[1]

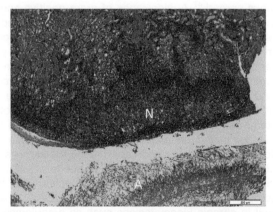

Fig. 15. Hematoxylin and eosin–stained section of the kidney from a Bourke's parrot (*Neopsephotus bourkii*). There is an extensive growth of an *Aspergillus* species on the surface of the kidney (A) as an extension of an infection from the adjacent air sac. The fungus is invading the kidney causing necrosis and a marked inflammatory response (N).

Parasitic Diseases

Context

- Most of the parasitic diseases of the kidney occur in wildlife. Many of these parasitic diseases are host adapted and cause minimal disease.
- Parasitic diseases of the kidney of captive birds are rare to uncommon, depending on the bird's husbandry, or cause little disease.

A summary of the most commonly reported parasitic diseases of the avian kidney is given in **Table 1**.[57-85] Parasites with direct life cycles can be maintained in cage and aviary birds, whereas parasites with intermediate hosts are more likely to affect wild birds or birds held in outdoor enclosures.

IMMUNE-MEDIATED DISEASE OF THE URINARY SYSTEM

Immune complex disease (glomerulonephrosis) of the avian kidney is an uncommon finding at necropsy. Often the affected bird will have a concurrent inflammatory or infectious disease. The lesions are typically mild to moderate and would not be expected to cause clinical signs. In other species with immune complex glomerulonephropathies, proteinuria is a common finding.[1,7] Protein loss can be seen in sections of kidneys with these lesions in birds and proteinuria may also occur in avian patients (**Fig. 16**).

TOXICOLGICAL DISEASES OF THE URINARY SYSTEM
Context

- Both endogenous and exogenous toxins can cause renal disease.
- Birds with liver disease, acute heavy metal exposure, crude oil ingestion, or diseases that cause rhabdomyolysis or hemolysis will have some degree of proximal tubular injury and require treatment that supports kidney function until regeneration occurs.
- Rodenticides containing vitamin D_3 or a vitamin D_3 analogue will cause metastatic mineralization of the kidney, and exposure to poisoned rodents is common in birds of prey.
- The renal lesions caused by many toxins, both acutely and after chronic exposure, are similar and therefore the cause of the lesion often cannot be differentiated histologically.

Pigmentary Nephropathies

Myoglobinuric nephrosis occurs after exertional rhabdomyolysis (capture myopathy) or severe crushing injuries in birds. Severe crushing injuries are most likely to occur in wild birds but also occur in poultry and pet and wild ducks and geese that have been attacked by dogs or foxes. Capture myopathy occurs in wild waterfowl that are rounded up for banding during molt or in long-legged birds after prolonged capture attempts or persistent struggling during restraint.[86] Muscle necrosis is a common phenomenon in ostriches that are unable to stand for any length of time.

Hemoglobinuric nephrosis occurs in birds with intoxications that cause hemolysis, including acute lead and zinc ingestion and[87] ingestion of crude oil,[88] and rarely in cage birds exhibiting an immune-mediated hemolytic anemia (**Fig. 17**).[89] Bile pigments may interfere with proximal tubular function, which is still hypothetical.[1]

Table 1
Most commonly reported parasitic diseases of the avian kidney

Parasite	Species	Prevalence	Pathogenicity	Lesions	Life Cycle
Coccidia (Eimeria and Isospora)[57–64]	Wild ducks and geese Shorebirds Raptors	Common Common Uncommon	Minimal in most cases	Developing organisms in renal tubular and ureteral epithelial cells	Direct
Cryptosporidia[65–73]	Psittacine birds Black-throated finches Pigeons Poultry	Rare[66] One report[67] Renal cryptosporidiosis is uncommon to rare	Variable but often severe	Microsporidia are predominately found in the collecting ducts and ureters where they can cause obstruction and renal failure	Direct
Encephalitozoon hellem[74–76]	Budgerigars, lovebirds Other parrots Wild birds	Infection is common, disease is rare Rare Rare	The number of organisms can vary from a few to many, but often there is little apparent effect on the host	E hellem infect the tubular epithelial cells and rarely the cells of Bowman's capsule and cause necrosis of the infected cell to varying degrees	Direct
Hematozoa,[1] Toxoplasmosis gondii,[77,78] atoxoplasmosis,[1] Sarcocystis species[1,79]	Many species	Uncommon	Part of a systemic disease. Urinary signs are unlikely	Mild multifocal lymphoplasmacytic interstitial nephritis. Organisms are typically rare and often not seen.	Indirect or insect vectors
Trematodes (several species)[80–85]	Many species Cage birds Wild birds intermediate host	Uncommon to rare must have exposure to the intermediate host Relatively common	In all susceptible species, the impact of infection can range from little to severe with extensive renal damage	Distention of ureters and collecting ducts compressing the adjacent normal kidney tissue. Severe inflammatory disease occurs in some instances. Obstruction of collecting ducts can cause disease of tubules and glomeruli of affected nephrons	Indirect

lovebirds treated with sodium benzoate for *M ornithogaster* (H. Baron, unpublished observation, 2016). Lesions seen in the great blue herons were generalized and include degeneration and necrosis of the epithelial cells of the proximal tubules. The most important lesion seen in the turkeys was extrarenal and was bilaterally symmetric areas of necrosis within the cerebral hemispheres. Renal lesions included "hyalinization of the glomerular capillary walls of the kidney and eosinophilic granular casts in the renal tubules."[115]

A summary of toxins affecting the kidney is shown in **Table 2**.

TRAUMATIC DISEASES OF THE URINARY SYSTEM
Context

- Trauma to the kidney is rare

The kidneys are found and firmly anchored within the renal fossae of the synsacrum and thus are protected from trauma in most circumstances. If a bird experiences sufficient trauma to damage the kidney, then it is likely that it will die or have other more life-threatening injuries.

REFERENCES

1. Schmidt R, Reavell D, Phalen DN, editors. Pathology of exotic birds. 2nd edition. Ames (IA): Iowa State University Press; 2015.
2. Siller WG. Renal pathology of the fowl- a review. Avian Pathol 1981;10:187–262.
3. Alstine V, Trampelor WG. Polycystic kidney in a pigeon. Avian Dis 1984;28: 758–64.
4. Sanchez C, Bush M, Montali R. Polycystic kidney disease associated with unilateral lameness in a Northern Pintail (*Anas acuta*). J Avian Med Surg 2004; 18:257–62.
5. Guo J-T, Aldrich CE, Mason WS, et al. Characterization of serum amyloid A protein mRNA expression and secondary amyloidosis in the domestic duck. Proc Natl Acad Sci U S A 1996;93:14548–53.
6. Meyerholz DK, Vanloubbeeck YF, Hostetter SJ, et al. Surveillance of amyloidosis and other diseases at necropsy in captive trumpeter swans (*Cygnus buccinator*). J Vet Diagn Invest 2005;17:295–8.
7. Phalen DN, Ambrus S, Graham DL. The avian urinary system: form, function, diseases. Proceedings Annual Conference Association Avian Veterinarians. Phoenix, AZ, September 10–15, 1990. p. 44–57.
8. Shientag LJ, Garlick DS, Galati E. Amyloidosis in a captive zebra finch (*Taeniopygia guttata*) research colony. Comp Med 2016;66:225–34.
9. Brayton C. Amyloidosis, hemochromatosis, and atherosclerosis in a roseate flamingo (*Phoenicopterus ruber*). Ann N Y Acad Sci 1992;653:184–90.
10. Hoffman AM, Leighton FA. Hemograms and microscopic lesions of herring gulls during captivity. J Am Vet Med Assoc 1985;187:1125–8.
11. Jansson DS, Broéjer C, Neimanis A, et al. Post mortem findings and their relation to AA amyloidosis in free-ranging Herring gulls (*Larus argentatus*). PLoS One 2018;13(3):e0193265.
12. Fox GA, Grasman KA, Campbell D. Health of herring gulls (*Larus argentatus*) in relation to breeding location in the early 1990s. II. Cellular and histopathological measures. J Toxicol Environ Health A 2007;70:1471–91.

13. Forbes NA, Cooper JE. Fatty liver and kidney syndrome of Merlins. In: Redig PT, Cooper JE, Remple D, et al, editors. Raptor biomedicine. Minneapolis (MN): University of Minnesota Press; 1993. p. 45–8.
14. Whitehead CC, Siller WG. Experimentally induced fatty liver and kidney syndrome in the young turkey. Res Vet Sci 1983;34:73–6.
15. Starkey SR, Wood C, de Matos R, et al. Central diabetes insipidus in an African Grey parrot. J Am Vet Med Assoc 2010;237:415–9.
16. Latimer KS, Ritchie BW, Campagnoli RP, et al. Metastatic renal carcinoma in an African grey parrot (Psittacus erithacus erithacus). J Vet Diagn Invest 1996;8: 261–4.
17. Mainez M, Cardona T, Such R, et al. Bilateral renal tubular neoplasm in a channel-billed toucan (Ramphastos vitellinus). J Avian Med Surg 2015;29: 46–50.
18. Neuman U, Kummerfeld N. Neoplasms in budgerigars (Melopsittacus undulatus): clinical, pathomorphological and serological findings with special consideration of kidney tumours. Avian Pathol 1983;12:353–62.
19. Okano T, Matsuura S, Kubo M, et al. Renal adenocarcinoma in a mountain hawk eagle (Spizaetus nipalensis) rescued for traffic accident. Jap J Zoo Wildl Med 2010;15:105–9.
20. Van Toor AJ, Zwart P, Kaal GTHF. Adenocarcinoma of the kidney in two budgerigars. Avian Pathol 1984;13:145–50.
21. Azmanis P, Stenkat J, Hübel J, et al. A complicated, metastatic, humeral air sac cystadenocarcinoma in a Timneh African grey parrot (Psittacus erithacus timneh). J Avian Med Surg 2011;27:38–43.
22. Dallwig RK, Whittington JK, Terio K, et al. Cutaneous mast cell tumor and mastocytosis in a black-masked Lovebird (Agapornis personata). J Avian Med Surg 2012;26:29–35.
23. Kajigaya H, Konagaya H, Ejima H, et al. Metastatic melanoma appearing to originate from the beak of a racing pigeon (Columba livia). Avian Dis 2010;54: 958–60.
24. Greenlee JJ, Nieve MA, Myers RK. Bronchial carcinoma in a red-shouldered hawk (Buteo lineatus). J Zoo Wildl Med 2011;42:153–5.
25. Williams SM, Williams RJ, Gogal RM. Acute lameness in a roller pigeon (Columba livia) with multicentric lymphosarcoma. Avian Dis 2017;61:267–70.
26. Furukawa S, Kenji Tsukamoto K, Maeda M. Multicentric histiocytosis related to avian leukosis virus subgroup J (ALV-J)- infection in meat-type local chickens. J Vet Med Sci 2014;76(1):89–92.
27. Kheirandish R, Azizi S, Salehi M, et al. Metastatic leiomyosarcoma originating in the thigh skeletal muscle of a Larry Breed Hen. J Avian Med Surg 2016;30: 141–5.
28. Osofsky A, Hawkins MG, Foreman O, et al. T-cell chronic lymphocytic leukemia in a double yellow-headed Amazon parrot (Amazona ochrocephala oratrix). J Avian Med Surg 2011;25:286–94.
29. Stenzel T, Gesek M, Paździor-Czapula K, et al. Cutaneous leiomyosarcoma with multiple visceral metastases in a domestic pigeon. Avian Dis 2017;61:274–8.
30. Phalen DN. The role of dietary calcium in the development of metastatic mineralization in parrots. Proceedings Association Avian Veterinarians Australasian Committee. Melbourne, Australia, November 25–27, 2009. p. 34-37.
31. Sarkar K, Narbaitz R, Pokrupa R, et al. The ultrastructure of nephrocalcinosis induced in chicks by Cestrum diurnum leaves. Vet Pathol 1981;18:62–70.

32. Blaxland JD, et al. An investigation of urolithiasis in two flocks of laying fowls. Avian Pathol 1980;9:5–19.

33. Mallinson ET, Rothenbacher H, Wideman RF, et al. Epizootiology, pathology, and microbiology of an outbreak of urolithiasis in chickens. Avian Dis 1983;28:25–43.

34. Julian R. Water deprivation as a cause of renal disease of chickens. Avian Pathol 1982;11:615–7.

35. Phalen DN, Wilson VG, Graham DL. Characterization of the avian polyomavirus-associated glomerulopathy of nestling parrots. Avian Dis 1996;40:140–9.

36. Circella E, Caroli A, Marino M, et al. Polyomavirus infection in Gouldian Finches (*Erythrura gouldiae*) and other pet birds of the family Estrildidae. J Comp Pathol 2017;156:436–9.

37. Halami MY, Dorrestein GM, Couteel P, et al. Whole-genome characterization of a novel polyomavirus detected in fatally diseased canary birds. J Gen Virol 2010; 91:3016–22.

38. Yang N, McLelland J, McLelland DJ, et al. Psittacid Adenovirus-2 infection in the critically endangered Orange-bellied Parrot (*Neophema chrysogastor*): a key threatening process or an example of a host-adapted virus? PLoS One 2019; 14(2):e0208674.

39. Barton JT, et al. Avian paramyxovirus type 1 infections in racing pigeons in California. I. Clinical signs, pathology, and serology. Avian Dis 1992;36:463–8.

40. Palmieri C, Franca M, Uzal FM, et al. Pathology and immunohistochemical findings of West Nile virus infection in Psittaciformes. Vet Pathol 2011;48(5):975–84.

41. Heatley JJ, Villalobos AR. Avian bornavirus in the urine of infected birds. Vet Med Res Rep 2012;3:19–23.

42. Cheng A-C, Wang MS, Chen XY, et al. Pathologic and pathological characteristics of new type gosling viral enteritis first observed in China. World J Gastroenterol 2001;7:678–84.

43. Guerin J-L, Gelfi J, Dubois L, et al. A novel polyomavirus (goose hemorrhagic polyomavirus) is the agent of hemorrhagic nephritis enteritis of geese. J Virol 2000;74:4523–9.

44. Ni Y, Kemp MC. A comparative study of avian reovirus pathogenicity: virus spread and replication and induction of lesions. Avian Dis 1995;39:554–66.

45. Wang HN, Wu QZ, Huang Y, et al. Isolation and identification of infectious bronchitis virus from chickens in Sichuan, China. Avian Dis 1997;41:279–82.

46. Swain DE, editor. Diseases of poultry. 13th edition. Hoboken (NJ): Wiley Blackwell; 2017.

47. Akkoc A, Kocabiyik L, Özgür M, et al. *Burkholderia cepacia* and *Aeromonas hydrophila* septicemia in an African grey parrot (*Psittacus erithacus erithacus*). Turk J Vet Anim Sci 2008;32:233–6.

48. Bounous DI, Schaeffer DO, Roy A. Coagulase-negative Staphylococcus sp. septicemia in a lovebird. J Am Vet Med Assoc 1989;195:1120–2.

49. Mutalib A, Keirs R, Austin F. Erysipelas in quail and suspected erysipeloid in processing plant employees. Avian Dis 1995;39:191–3.

50. Stoute ST, Cooper GL, Bickford AA, et al. *Yersinia pseudotuberculosis* in Eurasian Collared Doves (*Streptopelia decaocto*) and retrospective study of avian yersiniosis at the California Animal Health and Food Safety Laboratory System (1990–2015). Avian Dis 2016;60:82–6.

51. Saggese MD, Riggs G, Tizard I, et al. Gross and microscopic findings and investigation of the aetiopathogenesis of mycobacteriosis in a captive population of white-winged ducks (*Cairina scutulata*). Avian Pathol 2007;36:415–22.

52. Saggese MD, Tizard I, Phalen DN. Mycobacteriosis in naturally infected ring-neck doves (*Streptopelia risoria*): investigation of the association between feather colour and susceptibility to infection, disease and lesions type. Avian Pathol 2008;37:443–50.

53. Shibatana M, Suzuki T, Chujo M, et al. Disseminated intravascular coagulation in chickens inoculated with *Erysipelothrix rhusiopathiae*. J Comp Pathol 1997;117:147–56.

54. Gevaert D, Nelis J, Verhaeghe B. Plasma chemistry and urine analysis in Salmonella-induced polyuria in racing pigeons (*Columbia livia*). Avian Pathol 1991;20:379–86.

55. Mayahi M, Esmaeilzadeh S, Mosavari N, et al. Histopathological study of avian tuberculosis in naturally infected domestic pigeons with *Mycobacterium avium* subsp. *avium*. Iran J Vet Sci Technol 2013;5:45–56.

56. Tham VL, Purcell DA, Schultz DJ. Fungal nephritis in a grey-headed albatross. J Wildl Dis 1974;10:306–9.

57. Franson JC, Derksen DV. Renal coccidiosis in oldsquaws (*Clangula hyemalis*) from Alaska. J Wildl Dis 1981;17(2):237–9.

58. Gajadhar AA, Cawthorn RJ, Rainnie DJ. Experimental studies on the life cycle of a renal coccidium of lesser snow geese (*Anser c. caerulescens*). Can J Zool 1982;60:2085–92.

59. Gajadhar AA, Cawthorn RJ, Wobeser GA. Prevalence of renal coccidia in wild waterfowl in Saskatchewan. Can J Zool 1983;61:2631–3.

60. Gajadhar AA, Leighton FA. *Eimeria wobeseri* sp. n. and *Eimeria goelandi* sp. n. (Protozoa: Apicomplexa) in the kidneys of herring gulls (*Larus argentatus*). J Wildl Dis 1988;24:538–46.

61. Jankovsky JM, Brand M, Gerhold RW. Identification of a novel renal coccidian (Apicomplexa: Eimeriidae) from the great-horned owl (*Bubo virginianus*), USA. J Wildl Dis 2017;53:368–71.

62. Leighton FA, Gajadhar AA. *Eimeria fraterculae* sp. n. in the kidneys of Atlantic puffins (*Fratercula arctica*) from Newfoundland, Canada: species description and lesions. J Wildl Dis 1986;22:520–6.

63. Montgomery RD, Novilla MN, Shillinger RB. Renal coccidiosis caused by *Eimeria gavia* n. sp. in a common loon (*Gavia immer*). Avian Dis 1978;22:809–14.

64. Skirnisson K. Mortality associated with renal and intestinal coccidiosis in juvenile eiders in Iceland. Parassitologia 1997;39:325–30.

65. Abe N, Makino I. Multilocus genotypic analysis of Cryptosporidium isolates from cockatiels, Japan. Parasitol Res 2010;106:1491–7.

66. Blagburn BL, et al. Cryptosporidium sp. infection in the proventriculus of an Australian diamond firetail finch (Stagnopleura bella: Passeriformes, Estrilididae). Avian Dis 1990;34:1027–30.

67. Curtiss JB, Leone AM, Wellehan JFX, et al. Renal and cloacal cryptosporidiosis (Cyptosporidium genotype V in a Major Mitchell's Cockatoo (*Lophochroa leadbeateri*). J Zoo Wildl Med 2015;46:934–7.

68. Gardiner CH, Imes GD. *Cryptosporidium* sp. in the kidneys of a black-throated finch. J Am Vet Med Assoc 1984;185:1401–2.

69. Nakamura K, Abe F. Respiratory (especially pulmonary) and urinary infections of Cryptosporidium in layer chickens. Avian Pathol 1988;17:703–11.

70. Randall CJ. Renal and nasal cryptosporidiosis in a junglefowl (*Gallus sonneratii*). Vet Rec 1986;119:130–1.

71. Trampel DW, Pepper TM, Blagburn BL. Urinary tract cryptosporidiosis in commercial laying hens. Avian Dis 2000;44:479–84.

72. Werther K, de Sousa E, Alves JRF Jr, et al. *Cryptococcus gattii* and *Cryptococcus albidus* in captive domestic pigeon (*Columba livia*). Brazilian J Vet Pathol 2014;4:247–9.
73. Xiao L. Cryptosporidium spp. in pet birds: genetic diversity and potential public health significance. Exp Parasitol 2011;128:336–40.
74. Novilla MN, Kwapien RP. Microsporidian infection in the pied peach-faced lovebird (*Agapornis roseicollis*). Avian Dis 1978;22(1):198–204.
75. Pulparampil N, Graham D, Phalen D, et al. *Encephalitozoon hellem* in two eclectus parrots (*Eclectus roratus*): identification from archival tissues. J Eukaryot Microbiol 1998;45:651–5.
76. Snowden K, Daft B, Nordhausen BW. Morphological and molecular characterization of *Encephalitozoon hellem* in hummingbirds. Avian Pathol 2001;30: 251–5.
77. Biancifiori F, Rondini C, Grelloni V. Avian toxoplasmosis: experimental infection of chicken and pigeon. Comp Immunol Microbiol Infect Dis 1986;9(4):337–46.
78. Last RD, Shivaprasad HL. An outbreak of toxoplasmosis in an aviary collection of Nicobar pigeons (*Caloenas nicobaria*). J S Afr Vet Assoc 2008;79:149–52.
79. Smith JH, Neill PJG, Box ED. Pathogenesis of *Sarcocystis falcatula* (Apicomplexa: Sarcocystidae) in the budgerigar (*Melopsittacus undulatus*). III. Pathologic and quantitative parasitologic analysis of extrapulmonary disease. J Parasitol 1989;75:270–87.
80. Borah MK, Rahman T, Goswami S, et al. On the incidence and pathology of *Paratanaisia bragai* dos Santos, 1934 (Freitas, 1959) infection in domestic pigeon (*Columba livia*). J Vet Parasitol 2009;23:159–61.
81. Cheatum EL. *Dendritobilharzia anatinarum* n. sp., a blood fluke from the mallard. J Parasitol 1941;27:165–70.
82. Malik M, Goswami S, Upadhyaya TN, et al. Pathological and histochemical alterations of *Paratanaisia bragai* infection in domestic pigeon (*Columba livia*). Indian J Vet Pathol 2016;40:157–61.
83. Tavela AO, Carretta M Jr, Oliveira AR, et al. Parasitism by *Paratanaisia bragai* (Digenea, Eucotylidae) in common waxbill (*Estrilda astrild*). Arq Bras Med Vet Zootec 2014;66:1276–80.
84. Stunkard HW. Renicolid trematodes (Digenea) from the renal tubules of birds. Ann Parasitol 1971;46:109–18.
85. Xavier VB, Oliveira-Menezes A, Santos MAJ, et al. Histopathological changes in the kidneys of vertebrate hosts infected naturally and experimentally with *Paratanaisia bragai* (Trematoda, Digenea). Rev Bras Parasitol Vet 2015;24:241–6.
86. Smith KM, Murray S, Sanchez C. Successful treatment of suspected exertional myopathy in a rhea (*Rhea Americana*). J Zoo Wildl Med 2005;36:316–20.
87. Degernes LA. Toxicities in waterfowl. Sem Avian Exot Pet Med 1995;4(1):15–22.
88. Leighton FA. The toxicity of petroleum oils to birds. Env Res J 1993;1:92–103.
89. Bermudez AJ, Hopkins BA. Hemoglobinuric nephrosis in a rhea (*Rhea americana*). Avian Dis 1995;39:661–5.
90. Flammer K, Clark CH, Drewes LA, et al. Adverse effects of gentamicin in scarlet macaws and galahs. Am J Vet Res 1990;51:404–7.
91. Marshall KL, Craig LE, Jones MP, et al. Quantitative renal scintigraphy in domestic pigeons (*Columba livia domestica*) exposed to toxic doses of gentamicin. Am J Vet Res 2003;64:453–62.
92. Pereira ME, Werther K. Evaluation of renal effects of flunixin meglumine, ketoprofen and meloxicam in budgerigars (*Melopsittacus undulatus*). Vet Rec 2007; 160:844–6.

93. Sinclair KM, Chuch ME, Farver TB, et al. Effects of meloxicam on hematologic and plasma biochemical analysis variables and results of histologic examination of tissue specimens of Japanese quail (Coturnix japonica). Am J Vet Res 2012; 73:1720–7.

94. Montesinos A, Maria Ardiaca M, Carles Juan-Sallés C, et al. Effects of meloxicam on hematologic and plasma biochemical analyte values and results of histologic examination of kidney biopsy specimens of African grey parrots (Psittacus erithacus). J Avian Med Surg 2013;29:1–8.

95. Mulcahy DM, Tuomi P, Larsen RS. Differential mortality of male spectacled eiders (Somateria fischeri) and king eiders (Somateria spectabilis) Subsequent to anesthesia with propofol, bupivacaine, and ketoprofen. J Avian Med Surg 2003;17:117–23.

96. Oaks L, Gilbert M, Virani MZ, et al. Diclofenac residues as the cause of vulture population decline in Pakistan. Nature 2004;427:630–3.

97. Lumeij JT, Sprang EPM, Redig PT. Further studies on allopurinol-induced hyperuricemia and visceral gout in red-tailed hawks (Buteo jamaicensis). Avian Pathol 1998;27:390–3.

98. Bailey TA, Samour JH, Naldo J, et al. Lead toxicosis in captive houbara bustards (Chlamydotis undulata maqueenii). Vet Rec 1995;137:193–4.

99. Iichiro Fujii I, Waseda K, Onituka N, et al. Lead poisoning of gentoo penguins. J Japn Vet Med Assoc 2008;6:889–92.

100. Mateo R, Dolz JC, Aguilar Serrano JM, et al. An epizootic of lead poisoning in greater flamingos (Phoenicopterus ruber roseus) in Spain. J Wildl Dis 1997; 33:131–4.

101. Gulson B, Korsch M, Matisons M, et al. Windblown lead carbonate as the main source of lead in blood of children from a seaside community: an example of local birds as "canaries in the mine". Environ Health Perspect 2009;117:148–54.

102. Jackson A, Evers DC, Eagles-Smith CA, et al. Mercury risk to avian piscivores across western United States and Canada. Sci Total Environ 2016;568:685–96.

103. Chishti MA, Rotkiewicz T. Pathological changes produced in cockerels after mercuric chloride toxicity and then interaction with organophosphate insecticide. Arch Environ Contam Toxicol 1992;20:187–99.

104. Spalding MG, Bjork RD, Powell GV, et al. Mercury and cause of death in great white herons. J Wildl Manage 1994;58:735–9.

105. Sánchez-Virosta P, Espína S, García-Fernández AJ, et al. A review on exposure and effects of arsenic in passerine birds. Sci Total Environ 2015;512–513: 506–25.

106. Om A-S, Chung KW, Chung H-S. Effect of cadmium accumulation on renal tissue of broilers. Bull Environ Contam Toxicol 2002;68:297–301.

107. Afifi NA, Ramadan A. Kinetic disposition, systemic bioavailability and tissue distribution of apramycin in broiler chickens. Res Vet Sci 1997;62:249–52.

108. Pegram RA, Wyatt RD. Avian gout caused by oosporein, a mycotoxin produced by Chaetomium trilaterale. Poult Sci 1981;60:2429–40.

109. Manning RO, Wyatt RD. Toxicity of Aspergillus ochraceus contaminated wheat and different chemical forms of ochratoxin A in broiler chicks. Poult Sci 1984; 63:458–65.

110. Mohiuddin SM, Warasi SMA, Reddy MV. Haematological and biochemical changes in experimental ochratoxicosis in broiler chicken. Indian Vet J 1993; 70:613–7.

111. Mollenhauer HH, Corrier DE, Huff WE, et al. Ultrastructure of hepatic and renal lesions in chickens fed aflatoxin. Am J Vet Res 1989;50:771–7.

112. Sreemannarayana O, Frohlich AA, Marquardt RR. Acute toxicity of sterigmato-cystin to chicks. Mycopathologia 1987;97:51–9.
113. Dwivedi P, Burns RB. Pathology of ochratoxicosis A in young broiler chicks. Res Vet Sci 1984;36:92–103.
114. Bennett DC, Bowes VA, Hughes MR, et al. Suspected sodium toxicity in hand-reared great blue heron (*Ardea herodia*) chicks. Avian Dis 1992;36:743–8.
115. Wages DP, Ficken MD, Cook ME, et al. Salt toxicosis in commercial turkeys. Avian Dis 1995;39:158–61.

Laboratory Evaluation of Renal Function in Birds

Alexandra Scope, DVM[a],*, Ilse Schwendenwein, DVM, DECVCP[b]

KEYWORDS

- Avian nephrology • Diagnostics • Biochemistries • Urinalysis • Kidney • Uric acid
- Urea

KEY POINTS

- Lack of sensitive and specific biomarkers makes in vivo diagnosis of avian renal disorders difficult.
- Urinalysis is an underused tool in avian medicine, although it might contribute to the diagnosis of some kinds of renal and metabolic diseases in polyuric patients.
- The quest for sensitive and specific biomarkers continues. Uric acid levels increase when the functional capacity of the renal proximal tubules has been compromised, but only with extensive damage.
- Plasma uric acid concentrations are only mildly affected by a bird's hydration status, whereas blood urea concentration is a valuable indicator of hydration status. Urea has been proposed as a useful indicator for prerenal causes of renal impairment in birds.

INTRODUCTION

Although renal disease in avian patients is frequently encountered at necropsy, it often remains undetected under clinical conditions.[1] Assessment of renal function in birds is difficult because clinical signs are nonspecific and often subtle or absent until disease is quite advanced.[2] Lack of sensitive and specific biomarkers makes in vivo diagnosis of avian renal disorders difficult. Renal disease in avian patients may cause a variety of biochemical alterations but only a few of these changes can be considered specific for kidney diseases. In most cases, more than 1 laboratory test, complimented by clinical examination and diagnostic imaging, is necessary to confirm a renal disorder and establish a diagnosis.[3]

Birds have the unique ability to maintain renal blood flow, even with severe hemodynamic alterations or severe hemorrhage.[4] Glomerulopathies are well documented

Disclosure: The authors have nothing to disclose.
[a] Department for Companion Animals and Horses, University of Veterinary Medicine, Veterinärplatz 1, Vienna A-1210, Austria; [b] Division of Clinical Pathology, Department for Pathobiology, University of Veterinary Medicine, Veterinärplatz 1, Vienna A-1210, Austria
* Corresponding author.
E-mail address: alexandra.scope@vetmeduni.ac.at

in avian species,[5] but, because of the extensive renal blood supply, even severe chronic glomerulonephritis may persist without any clinical manifestation. Therefore, glomerulonephritis may be present in far more birds than are currently diagnosed in a clinical setting.[6]

Waste products from protein metabolism, such as uric acid (UA), are not eliminated by glomerular filtration but by active secretion into the proximal tubules. As a component of water conservation, birds have the ability to absorb significant amounts of excreted renal water in the colon and ceca.[7] This system also allows birds to compensate renal electrolyte loss.[8] This multitude of compensatory mechanisms unique to the avian kidney is a pivotal reason for the challenges in laboratory diagnosis of renal disease in birds.

URINALYSIS

In mammals, urinalysis is an established, indispensable tool for assessing renal function and identifying infection of the kidneys and lower urinary tract as well as metabolic diseases. Urinalysis is indicated in birds with increased plasma UA concentration or persistent polyuria.[9] In birds, urine consists of liquid and a more or less semisolid phase. Most of the UA is not in solution but is excreted as a colloid suspension. This suspension consists of small, spherical structures that range in diameter from 0.5 to 15 μm, and contain large amounts of protein.[10] Thus sampling of urine in birds requires modification to meet these peculiarities.[11] Data are scarce in the literature and, therefore, urinalysis is only rarely performed in avian medicine and its diagnostic potential remains to be investigated.

Sampling

Birds have no urinary bladder and the ureters empty into the cloaca where, in most species, urine and feces are eliminated together. Although cloacal cannulation techniques have been described,[12] free-catch urine samples are collected from clinical patients.

In practice, the ability to perform a urinalysis is in general dictated by the presence of polyuria.[6,11] Polyuria is a common clinical sign and the most important indication for urinalysis (**Fig. 1**). Stress is an important cause of polyuria, but there are many other possible causes, including renal disease. Birds with renal disease may be permanently polyuric because they are unable to concentrate urine.[11]

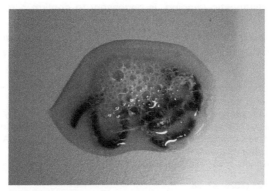

Fig. 1. Polyuria in an avian patient. Three components of the bird dropping can be seen: feces, creamy-white urates, and a large amount of urine.

Separation of urine from feces and UA in polyuric patients is easy: the liquid phase is aspirated from a nonabsorbent surface.[2,9] For birds with normal urine output, hematocrit capillary tubes or a tuberculin syringe may be used to collect a urine sample free of fecal matter.[9,11] A clean, urate-free sample increases the diagnostic quality of the results. Flocculent samples with fecal particles should be centrifuged for 15 to 30 seconds at 300 × g before analysis. The supernatant can be used for testing; however, microscopic evaluation of urinary sediment is impossible for contaminated samples.

Macroscopic Evaluation

Macroscopic evaluation is the first step in urinalysis. The amount, color, consistency, and clarity of the urine are assessed. Nonpolyuric birds produce only a small quantity of urine and a variable quantity of urates (**Fig. 2**). Avian urine is usually clear. A flocculent or cloudy sample usually indicates the presence of crystals, casts, or cells. The color of avian urine varies with specific gravity, as well as the presence of water-soluble vitamins and pigment-containing food or medications. Expected urate colors are pure white, off white, pale yellow, or light beige. With liver disease, urates may be greenish or yellowish to dark yellow (**Fig. 3**). Red or blue-tinged urates are frequently seen, caused by ingestion of berries or other staining foodstuffs (**Fig. 4**). Hemoglobinuria may be seen with lead toxicosis, which produces dark red, pink, or tan-brown urine (**Fig. 5**).[6,11]

Urine Specific Gravity

The renal capacity for water conservation is much less developed in birds than in mammals. Reference data on urine osmolality show great variability. Some investigators state that urine osmolality does not exceed plasma osmolarity because of the predominance of reptilian glomeruli, whereas others assume a maximal concentration ability between 2 or 2.5 times plasma osmolality.[7,10,13]

Urine specific gravity varies with hydration state and with certain disease conditions. Nonpolyuric birds excrete a semisolid UA waste product with a nonreadable specific gravity. In most polyuric birds, specific gravity ranges from 1.005 to 1.020 and is highly variable among different species.[9,14] Specific gravity has limited clinical relevance unless values are consistently low and do not increase with water deprivation[9]; however, more studies are needed to correlate osmolarity and specific gravity.[11]

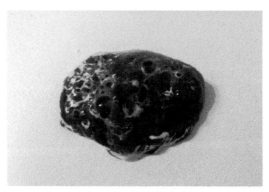

Fig. 2. A normal bird dropping showing a large amount of feces, creamy-white urates, and a small amount of urine.

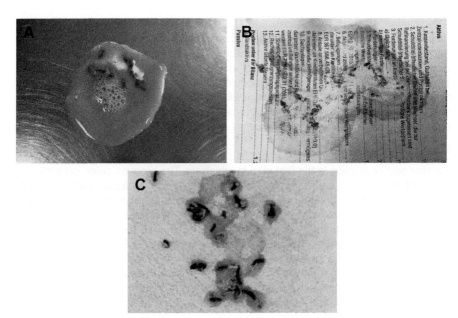

Fig. 3. Three examples of biliverdinuria in avian patients, showing (*A*) greenish, to (*B*) yellow, to (*C*) dark yellow urates.

Water deprivation testing has been used to evaluate the kidney's ability to concentrate urine to distinguish polyuria caused by psychogenic polydipsia from other causes of polyuria.[6] The bird is weighed and blood and urine are collected. Packed cell volume, total solids and osmolality of blood, and the specific gravity and osmolality of urine are evaluated. The bird is placed in a cage with no food or water for the duration of the test. Blood and urine variables should be evaluated every 3 to 24 hours over 12 to 48 hours, depending on the species and physical condition of the bird.[6] Strict observation of water loss (eg, by weight control) and behavioral changes is mandatory during water deprivation and the testing period must be terminated when clinical signs become obvious.

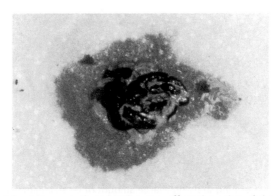

Fig. 4. Pigmented food items, such as berries, can affect the color of the urates.

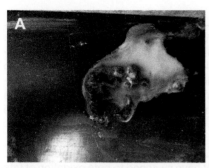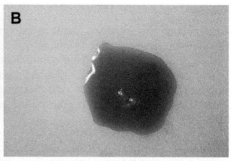

Fig. 5. Hemoglobinuria, which may be seen with lead poisoning, is associated with (*A*) dark red to blackish or (*B*) tan-brown urine in avian patients.

Chemical Analysis by Test Strips

Standard urine multitest reagent strips developed for humans may be used, but not all components are applicable to avian urine and therefore cautious interpretation is necessary.[9] Dipstick readings for nitrite, leukocytes, and specific gravity are unreliable and should be omitted. Test pads for pH, protein, glucose, ketones, blood, and urobilinogen can be used.[11] Because birds produce biliverdin instead of bilirubin, this analyte is not included in avian urinalysis.

Urine pH

Dictated by dietary constituents and cloacal contents, urine pH is highly variable in birds.[6,10,11] The pH of most companion birds ranges between 6.5 and 8.[9] Carnivores have consistently lower urine pH, whereas psittacine birds that consume plant material and grains often have higher pH values.[11] Urine pH is also influenced by egg laying, becoming acidic during calcium deposition and turning alkaline after the egg is laid or when calcium is not being deposited. Hypoxia may also decrease urine pH.[15] When using dipsticks, abnormal urine color can affect the results and create an abnormally high alkaline reading.[11]

Protein

In birds, most urinary protein is bound within the semisolid fraction of urine. Urate, a small molecule, is actively secreted by renal tubules. Crystal formation is prevented by the urate anion binding to serum albumin within the proximal tubules to form small, spherical colloid particles. A large amount of protein is found within this colloid matrix.[16] It is not known whether this protein is actively secreted within the tubules, like the Tamm-Horsfall protein in mammals, or passes through the glomerular barrier.

In wild birds, analysis of avian urate spheres may have potential value as a noninvasive sample collection method for biomonitoring environmental pollution and stress.[16]

In the liquid portion of avian urine, zero to trace levels of protein are expected.[11] A positive protein reading can be seen with fecal contamination,[11] hematuria, or hemoglobinuria, or possibly renal dysfunction. Persistent proteinuria is a clinicopathologic hallmark of chronic kidney disease in dogs and cats; however, numerous differences exist in this disease between birds and mammals.[6] For example, it is known that chicken leukocytes lack proteolytic enzymes that could potentially damage the glomerular basement membrane and allow protein leakage. Consequently, chickens, and possibly other birds, may not develop pathologic proteinuria with glomerulopathies.

Glucose

Most glucose readings are negative in avian patients. Trace readings should be considered suspicious. These values can suggest compromised tubular reabsorption (eg, tubular damage), fecal contamination, or increased glucose introduction (hyperglycemia). Urine dipstick glucose measurements are useful in screening polyuric birds for diabetes. Birds with diabetes mellitus routinely have blood glucose concentrations of more than 800 mg/dL and urine glucose concentrations more than 2000 mg/dL.[11]

Ketones

Normal avian urine is free of ketones. Birds that have switched to beta oxidation of fats caused by either starvation or normal metabolism during long-distance migratory flight may show urinary ketones. Ketonuria has also been reported in diabetic birds.[11,17]

Blood

Dipstick readings for blood or muscle pigment in avian urine samples should be negative. Nonhemolyzed trace readings, which appear as small dots on the test pad, indicate the presence of red blood cells in the sample, which is most likely caused by fecal or cloacal contamination. Hemolyzed trace readings, seen with a homogeneously stained test pad, suggest the presence of free hemoglobin or myoglobin and may indicate hemoglobin casts. Readings greater than trace are extremely rare and may suggest extreme kidney damage or failure.[11]

Urobilinogen

A positive reading for urobilinogen can indicate fecal contamination.[18] Increased readings may suggest severe liver disease or intravascular hemolysis.[11]

Urine Electrolytes and Enzymes

Urine electrolytes and other analytes, such as enzymes or specific proteins, can be measured, but there is limited information on their diagnostic meaning.[6] It has been suggested that measurement of urinary enzyme activity may be useful for detecting kidney damage because intracellular enzymes of damaged kidney cells are liberated into the urine.[13]

N-acetyl-β-D-glucosaminidase (NAG) is a renal tubular enzyme that has been identified in mammals and chickens. In humans, urinary NAG has been suggested as an early indicator of renal tubular damage and it may serve as a good noninvasive indicator of disease progression.[19] Urinary NAG has also been successfully evaluated in the chicken.[20] Although the investigators stated that NAG might be a potentially useful diagnostic marker of renal damage, this idea has not been further investigated.

Microscopic Examination of Urinary Sediment

Examination of urinary sediment is considered to be an essential diagnostic approach in renal disorders.[11] It is impossible to completely rid the urine of urates, and this major component usually obscures and destroys other elements of the sediment.[9] Vigorous centrifugation to clear urates damages casts. However, the use of stains greatly enhances the definition of cast components and other urine constituents.[11]

Normal bird urine is free of casts. Granular casts, hemoglobin casts, and others are reported in the literature but their clinical significance is controversial.[3,6,9,11] In our experience, the ability to detect leukocyte and erythrocyte casts is limited because of the difficulties mentioned earlier regarding preparing urinary sediments free of urates and other contaminants.

Small numbers of red blood cells may also be of concern; however, red cells can originate from the digestive tract, reproductive tract, or cloaca and not necessarily from the urinary tract. The presence of 2 or more red blood cells per high-power field may be significant, especially when the patient is showing signs of disease.

White blood cells are never a normal finding in avian urine, and their presence should always be considered a sign of infection or compromise.[11] Like erythrocytes, white blood cells and small numbers of bacteria can originate from the cloaca or gastrointestinal tract.[9,11,17]

PLASMA/SERUM ANALYTES

The application of inappropriate reference intervals may be one of the most important reasons for inefficiency or even failure of laboratory diagnostics.[21] For the interpretation of any laboratory test result, reported data should be compared with appropriate group-based reference limits, if available. For instance, the application of previously measured values from the same individual or from another healthy individual of the same species can be useful.[22] Laboratory-specific reference values are preferable to published reference limits established with different methods or without method specification. As a guideline, only reference intervals established by comparable analytical methods can be used safely.

Uric Acid

UA is produced and secreted predominately in the avian liver but also to a smaller extent in the kidney and pancreas.[23,24] Birds are uricotelic; 70% to 80% of total nitrogen is excreted in the form of UA.[25,26] As the major end product of nitrogen metabolism in birds, UA is the laboratory value most frequently used to screen birds for kidney disease.

One advantage of uricotelism is the ability to store this nitrogenous waste in the egg during development, where a water-soluble product such as urea would be toxic to the developing embryo.[8] Uricotelism also allows birds to minimize urinary water loss. Because UA is osmotically inactive, little water is required to excrete this nitrogenous waste.[8] The excretion of UA is 90% dependent on tubular secretion and largely independent of urine flow.[25] Blood UA concentrations are only mildly affected by hydration status but reflect the functional capacity of the renal proximal tubules.[6]

Although plasma UA can be useful as a screening tool for advanced renal disease, UA level does not increase significantly until there is extensive renal tubular damage.[6] It has been estimated that renal function must be less than 30% of its original capacity before hyperuricemia develops.[27] Increased UA level has been correlated with tubular nephrosis, dysfunctional proximal convoluted tubules, and interstitial nephritis.[5,28,29]

Published reference intervals differ considerably, ranging from approximately 2 to 14 mg/dL in granivorous birds. Variations caused by food intake and the possible inclusion of pathologic values are reasons for this wide reference interval. In the author's database, even with inclusion of diseased animals, 86% of granivorous birds have UA concentrations lower than 10 mg/dL, and 60% are less than 6 mg/dL. Thus, in our experience, repeated concentrations greater than 8 mg/dL are highly suggestive for major renal impairment in granivorous species.

It is a standard of care to repeat fasting UA concentrations on well-hydrated birds before a suggestion of renal disease is made.[6] In birds with suspect renal disease that have a single laboratory value of hyperuricemia, Echols[6] recommends

100 mL/kg of subcutaneous isotonic fluids every 12 to 24 hours for 2 days before rechecking the UA concentration. Birds with persistent hyperuricemia after fluid therapy and/or fasting are suspicious for some form of renal disease.[6]

In birds of prey, UA production is directly related to the amount of protein consumed and transient increases are noted following high-protein meals. Carnivorous and piscivorous birds show UA concentrations up to 29 mg/dL after feeding.[30] This significant postprandial increase in plasma UA concentration has been reported for up to 15 hours after feeding.[31] For this reason, 24-hour starving should be considered appropriate for all carnivorous and piscivorous avian species before blood UA testing.[32] Starving hyperuricemia indicates renal failure at least in peregrine falcons (*Falco peregrinus*).[13]

In parakeets, moderate protein concentrations of 13.2% to 25% in the feed had no effect on plasma UA concentrations.[33] Only extremely high protein levels (70%) led to a significant increase in serum UA in cockatiels (*Nymphicus hollandicus*). After feeding such high protein concentrations over 11 months, there was no evidence of visceral gout, articular gout, or renal disorder. The investigators concluded that high dietary protein concentrations are not associated with kidney dysfunction in this avian species.[34] In African grey parrots (*Psittacus erithacus*), plasma UA concentrations showed a positive correlation with a high dietary protein (30%) consumption.[35] In chickens, UA abnormalities may not be evident until very-high-protein diets (40%–60%) are fed.[5,36] It can be concluded that, in granivorous birds, only very-high-protein diets cause hyperuricemia and this increase is caused by reduced renal tubular secretion of UA and not by excessive production, as can occur in humans.[5,36]

Urea

Birds produce very little urea and it does not serve as an important end product of protein metabolism.[9] The avian urea cycle is primarily restricted to renal detoxification processes and not nitrogenous waste excretion.[8] Nevertheless, in birds of prey, a postprandial increase in urea has been reported, which persists for up to 15 hours after a meat or fish meal.[31] In cockatiels, serum urea concentrations also increased linearly with an increase in dietary protein.[34]

During normal hydration, 100% of urea is excreted by glomerular filtration, but 99% is reabsorbed in the tubules during dehydration.[13,32] Blood urea concentrations are thus more significantly affected by the bird's hydration status than plasma UA concentrations.[9,32] Blood urea nitrogen has little value in the detection of renal disease in most birds,[31,37] but it has been proposed as a sensitive indicator of hydration and a useful variable to detect prerenal causes for renal impairment in birds.[32]

Creatinine

Measurement of plasma creatinine concentration serves as a crude assessment of the glomerular filtration rate (GFR) in mammals. In birds, physiologic plasma creatinine concentrations are mostly less than the limit of detection (<0.06 mg/dL) of commonly used assays because birds excrete mainly creatine before its conversion to creatinine.[9,38,39] Creatinine is filtered, actively secreted, and may be reabsorbed in healthy birds.[40]

A connection between plasma creatinine and hydration has been shown in pigeons,[32] although the relationship between creatine and creatinine in birds with renal disease is poorly understood and the difference does not seem to be clinically useful.[27,41,42]

In mammals, the best approach for obtaining detailed information on renal function is the determination of the GFR, which is done by measuring the clearance of a filtration marker in the plasma.[43,44] The most frequently used substance for GFR determination is inulin; however, availability is limited. Research shows that creatinine is a useful, inexpensive, readily available, and easily analyzed compound to test renal excretion in birds.[45] Comparison of creatinine with exoiohexol and endoiohexol revealed comparable plasma concentration–time profiles.[46] To overcome size differences between various bird species, the exogenous excretion rate may be indexed using body surface area.[46,47] The clinical relevance of this method has not yet been investigated.

Protein

Although hypoproteinemia can be associated with renal failure, few studies have evaluated serum protein concentrations in birds with renal disease.[13] Current analytical methods for albumin measurement do not accurately report avian albumin concentrations. Serum or plasma protein electrophoresis is indicated for accurate quantification of plasma proteins and is recommended if hypoalbuminemia is suspected.[41,48,49] Birds may develop dysproteinemias with some kidney disorders but there is limited information about changes in plasma or serum protein patterns in the course of renal disease.[6]

Minerals and Electrolytes

The avian kidney is responsible for electrolyte regulation, but it cannot concentrate sodium or other electrolytes at levels much greater than normal.[12] It is reasonable to assume that electrolyte disorders can develop in birds with renal disease,[6] but the effect of renal diseases on plasma electrolytes has been poorly studied in birds. The proper interpretation of clinical biochemistry results also depends on correct sample handling.[50] For instance, hyperphosphatemia can be caused by microhemolysis. A significant decrease in plasma potassium concentrations can occur if blood is stored at room temperature.[50] Immediate separation of cells from plasma is recommended.

   Possible findings with renal failure may include hyponatremia, hyperkalemia, hypocalcemia, and hyperphosphatemia[3]; however, increases in inorganic phosphate concentrations are not commonly recognized in avian renal disease.[41,51] Unpublished data from budgerigar parakeets (*Melopsittacus undulatus*) showed a significant increase in phosphorous concentrations in birds with different health problems, but not specifically with renal disesases (Scope A, Schwendenwein I. Hyperphosphatemia in Budgerigars with Various Diseases. Unpublished data, 2005.).

Hematology

Some hematologic changes may be associated with avian renal disease.[6] A relative heterophilia is the primary finding reported, but monocytosis, lymphopenia, and normocytic-normochromic anemia have also been observed.[6,51,52] These changes are nonspecific, and heterophilia can also be seen in healthy birds under stress alone.[53,54]

SUMMARY

Renal disease is a frequent necropsy finding in avian patients at necropsy but often remains undetected in living patients. Urinalysis is likely an underused tool in avian medicine, although it might contribute to the diagnosis of some kinds of renal and metabolic diseases. UA concentration is the variable most frequently applied to screen for kidney diseases in birds. Blood UA concentration is only mildly affected by the bird's hydration status, but reflects the excretory functional capacity of the renal proximal tubules. In contrast, blood urea concentration is significantly affected by the bird's hydration status. Urea concentration has been proposed as a useful variable to detect prerenal causes for renal impairment in birds. Plasma creatinine concentrations in birds are less than the limit of detection for commonly used assay methods. Measurement of exogenous creatinine excretion shows promising preliminary results to become a useful, inexpensive, readily available, and easily performed test for the assessment of renal excretion in birds.

REFERENCES

1. Schmidt RE. Types of renal disease in avian species. Vet Clin North Am Exot Anim Pract 2006;9:97–106.
2. Pollock C. Diagnosis and treatment of avian renal disease. Vet Clin North Am Exot Anim Pract 2006;9:107–28.
3. Lierz M. Avian renal disease: pathogenesis, diagnosis, and therapy. Vet Clin North Am Exot Anim Pract 2003;6:29–55.
4. Bottje WG, Holmes KR, Neldon HL, et al. Relationships between renal hemodynamics and plasma levels of arginine vasotocin and mesotocin during hemorrhage in the domestic fowl (Gallus domesticus). Comp Biochem Physiol A Comp Physiol 1989;92:423–7.
5. Siller WG. Renal pathology of the fowl - a review. Avian Pathol 1981;10:187–262.
6. Echols MS. Evaluating and treating the kidneys. In: Harrison GJ, Lightfoot TL, editors. Clinical avian medicine. 1st edition. Palm Beach (FL): Spix Publishing; 2006. p. 451–92.
7. Braun EJ. Integration of renal and gastrointestinal function. J Exp Zoolog 1999; 283:495–9.
8. Wideman RF. Avian kidney anatomy and physiology. CRC Critical Reviews in Poultry Biology 1988;1:133–76.
9. Phalen D. Avian renal disorders. In: Fudge AM, editor. Laboratory medicine avian and exotic pets. Philadelphia: WB Saunders; 2000. p. 61–8.
10. Braun EJ. Comparative renal function in reptiles, birds, and mammals. Semin Avian Exot Pet Med 1998;7:62–71.
11. Lane RA. Avian urinalysis a practical guide to analysis and interpretation. In: Rosskopf WJ, Woerpel RW, editors. Diseases of cage and aviary birds. Baltimore (MD): Williams and Wilkins; 1996. p. 783–94.
12. Dorrestein GM. Physiology of the urogenital system. In: Altman RB, Clubb SL, Dorrestein GM, editors. Avian medicine and surgery. Philadelphia: WB Saunders; 1997. p. 622–5.
13. Lumeij JT. Pathophysiology, diagnosis and treatment of renal disorders in birds of prey. In: Lumeij JT, editor. Raptor biomedicine III. Lake Worth (FL): Zoological Education Network; 2000. p. 169–78.
14. Neumann U, Kummerfeld N. Neoplasms in budgerigars (melopsittacus undulatus): Clinical, pathomorphological and serological findings with special consideration of kidney tumours. Avian Pathol 1983;12:353–62.
15. Frazier DL, Jones MP, Orosz SE. Pharmacokinetic considerations of the renal system in birds: part I. Anatomic and physiologic principles of allometric scaling. J Avian Med Surg 1995;9:92–103.
16. Clapp JB. Urate spheres: a non-invasive method to biomonitor environmental pollution and stress in birds. [Thesis]. United Kingdom: Newcastle University; 2010.

17. Styles DK, Phalen DN. Clinical avian urology. Semin Avian Exot Pet Med 1998;7: 104–13.
18. Harr KE. Clinical chemistry of companion avian species: a review. Vet Clin Pathol 2002;31:140–51.
19. Costigan MG, Rustom R, Bone JM, et al. Origin and significance of urinary N-acetyl-β,D-glucosaminidase (NAG) in renal patients with proteinuria. Clinica Chim Acta 1996;255:133–44.
20. Forman MF, Beck MM, Kachman SD. N-Acetyl-β-D-glucosaminidase as a marker of renal damage in hens. Poult Sci 1996;75:1563–8.
21. Scope A, Schwendenwein I. Standardization of methods in enzymology and its consequences illustrated on budgerigars (Melopsittacus undulatus Shaw 1805). Tierarztl Prax Ausg K Kleintiere Heimtiere 2005;33:126–30.
22. Scope A, Schwendenwein I, Gabler C. Short-term variations of biochemical parameters in racing pigeons (Columba livia). J Avian Med Surg 2002;16:10–5.
23. Herzberg GR, Coady K, Maddigan B, et al. Uric acid synthesis by avian exocrine pancreas. Int J Biochem 1987;23:545–8.
24. Chin TY, Quebbemann AJ. Quantitation of renal uric acid synthesis in the chicken. Am J Physiol 1978;234:446–51.
25. Skadhauge E. Osmoregulation in birds. Berlin: Springer; 1981.
26. Braun EJ. Osmoregulatory systems of birds. In: Scanes CG, editor. Sturkie's avian physiology. 6th edition. London: Academic Press; 2015. p. 285–300.
27. Murray MJ, Taylor M. Avian renal disease: endoscopic applications. Semin Avian Exot Pet Med 1999;8:115–21.
28. Stoev SD, Daskalov H, Radic B, et al. Spontaneous mycotoxic nephropathy in Bulgarian chickens with unclarified mycotoxin aetiology. Vet Res 2002;33:83–93.
29. Abbassi H, Coudert F, Chérel Y, et al. Renal Cryptosporidiosis (Cryptosporidium baileyi) in specific-pathogen-free chickens experimentally coinfected with Marek's disease virus. Avian Dis 1999;43:738–44.
30. Chitty J, Lierz M, editors. BSAVA manual of raptors, pigeons and passerine birds. Gloucester, (United Kingdom): BSAVA; 2008.
31. Lumeij JT, Remple JD. Plasma urea, creatinine and uric acid concentrations in relation to feeding in peregrine falcons (Falco Peregrinus). Avian Pathol 1991; 20:79–83.
32. Lumeij JT. Plasma urea, creatinine and uric acid concentrations in response to dehydration in racing pigeons (Columba livia domestica). Avian Pathol 1987; 16:377–82.
33. Angel R, Ballam G. Dietary protein effect on parakeet plasma uric acid, reproduction, and growth. In: 1st Annual Conference of the Nutrition Advisory Group of the American Zoo and Aquarium Association. Toronto, Canada, May 1&2, 1995.
34. Koutsos EA, Smith J, Woods LW, et al. Adult cockatiels (Nymphicus hollandicus) metabolically adapt to high protein diets. J Nutr 2001;131:2014–20.
35. Harper EJ, Skinner ND. Clinical nutrition of small psittacines and passerines. Semin Avian Exot Pet Med 1998;7:116–27.
36. Austic RE, Cole RK. Impaired renal clearance of uric acid in chickens having hyperuricemia and articular gout. Am J Physiol 1972;223:525–30.
37. Speer BL. Diseases of the urogenital system. In: Altman RB, Clubb SL, Dorrestein GM, editors. Avian medicine and surgery. Philadelphia: WB Saunders; 1997. p. 625–44.
38. Bell DJ, Freeman BM. Physiology and biochemistry of the domestic fowl. New York: Academic Press; 1971.

39. Paton DN, Mackie W. The liver in relation to creatine metabolism in the bird. J Physiol 1912;45:115–8.
40. Sturkie PD. Kidneys, extrarenal salt excretion, and urine. In: Sturkie PD, editor. Avian physiology. 4th edition. New York: Springer New York; 1986. p. 359–82.
41. Fudge AM. Avian clinical pathology-hematology and chemistry. In: Altman RB, Clubb SL, Dorrestein GM, editors. Avian medicine and surgery. Philadelphia: WB Saunders; 1997. p. 142–57.
42. Orosz S, Dorrestein GM, Speer BL. Urogenital disorders. In: Altman RB, Clubb SL, Dorrestein GM, editors. Avian medicine and surgery. Philadelphia: WB Saunders; 1997. p. 614–44.
43. Stevens LA, Coresh J, Greene T, et al. Assessing kidney function - measured and estimated glomerular filtration rate. N Engl J Med 2006;354:2473–83.
44. Stevens LA, Levey AS. Measured GFR as a confirmatory test for estimated GFR. J Am Soc Nephrol 2009;20:2305–13.
45. Scope A, Schwendenwein I, Schauberger G. Plasma exogenous creatinine excretion for the assessment of renal function in avian medicine–pharmacokinetic modeling in racing pigeons (Columba livia). J Avian Med Surg 2013;27:173–9.
46. Caekebeke N, Montesinos A, Gasthuys E, et al. Comparative physiology of glomerular filtration in six different bird species. In: AAV, ed. Proceedings of the Third International Conference on Avian Herpetological and Exotic Mammal Medicine. Venice, Italy, March 25–29, 2017. p. 357.
47. Scope A. Exogenous creatinine clearance in birds – how to deal with different species? 3rd International Conference on Avian, Herpetological and Exotic Mammal Medicine (ICARE). Venice, Italy, March 25, 2017.
48. Lumeij JT. The diagnostic value of plasma proteins and non-protein nitrogen substances in birds. Vet Q 1987;9:262–8.
49. Lumeij JT, de Bruijne JJ. Evaluation of the refractometric method for the determination of total protein in avian plasma or serum. Avian Pathol 1985;14:441–4.
50. Lumeij JT. The influence of blood sample treatment on plasma potassium concentrations in avian blood. Avian Pathol 1985;14:257–60.
51. Chandra M, Singh B, Gupta PP, et al. Clinicopathological, hematological, and biochemical studies in some outbreaks of nephritis in poultry. Avian Dis 1985; 29:590–600.
52. Blaxland JD, Martindale L. An investigation of urolithiasis in two flocks of laying fowls. Avian Pathol 1980;9:5–19.
53. Scope A, Filip T, Gabler C, et al. The influence of stress from transport and handling on hematologic and clinical chemistry blood parameters of racing pigeons (Columba livia domestica). Avian Dis 2002;46:224–9.
54. McRee AE, Tully TN, Nevarez JG, et al. Effect of routine handling and transportation on blood leucocyte concentrations and plasma corticosterone in captive hispaniolian amazon parrots (Amazona ventralis). J Zoo Wildl Med 2018;49: 396–403.

Diagnostic Imaging of the Avian Urinary Tract

Maria-Elisabeth Krautwald-Junghanns, Dr med vet, Dr med vet habil, DECZM (avian), ML[a],*,
Cornelia Konicek, Dr med Vet[b]

KEYWORDS

- Imaging techniques • Biopsy • Kidneys • Ureters • Radiography • Ultrasonography
- Urography • Urinary tract

KEY POINTS

- Diagnostic imaging of the urinary tract often begins with conventional radiographs. In the normal avian patient, the kidneys are indistinct in the ventral dorsal view and the cranial end of the kidney is superimposed by the gonad in the lateral view. The kidneys are rarely demonstrated in full length on either view.
- Ultrasonography should be the first diagnostic method in cases of abdominal swelling. Organomegaly, air sac compression, and ascites all facilitate transducer coupling and improve image quality. Patient safety is at risk when a patient with profound abdominal swelling is placed in dorsal recumbency.
- Oral administration of a nonabsorbable contrast agent, like barium sulfate, can help to radiographically differentiate the kidneys from surrounding structures, particularly the gastrointestinal tract.
- The existence of the renal portal system allows rapid excretion of contrast in the normal avian patient. During a urographic examination, the kidneys and ureters are demonstrated 30 to 60 seconds after injection.

INTRODUCTION

Due to the special anatomy and physiology of the bird's urinary system, the value of diagnostic imaging techniques differs from their use in mammals. The paired avian kidneys are embedded retroperitoneally on either side of the vertebral column within a depression on the ventral surface of the synsacrum, which partially hinders noninvasive imaging. Each kidney has cranial, middle, and caudal divisions; however, this 3-part structure is often clearly seen only with computed tomography (CT), MRI (**Fig. 1**), or endoscopy. Neither a urinary bladder nor a urethra is present in birds. Excrement is

Disclosures: None.
[a] Clinic for Birds and Reptiles, University Leipzig, An den Tierkliniken 17, 04103 Leipzig, Germany; [b] Clinic for Birds and Reptiles, University of Veterinary Medicine Vienna, Veterinärplatz 1, A-1210 Vienna, Austria
* Corresponding author.
E-mail address: krautwald@vogelklinik.uni-leipzig.de

Vet Clin Exot Anim 23 (2020) 59–74
https://doi.org/10.1016/j.cvex.2019.08.003
1094-9194/20/© 2019 Elsevier Inc. All rights reserved.

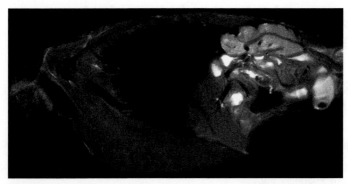

Fig. 1. MRI, longitudinal scan, T2 weighted in a gray parrot (*Psittacus erithacus*) illustrating the trilobed kidney and vessels.

discharged directly from the ureters into the cloaca via the urodeum, and this function of the urinary system can only be demonstrated using contrast techniques (**Fig. 2**) or, to some extent, direct endoscopy.

The diagnostic imaging methods regularly used in practice to evaluate the kidneys are often limited to traditional radiography and ultrasonography, whereas other imaging modalities are rarely used. Endoscopy is an invasive technique that requires an avian veterinarian familiar with this procedure. Taking a renal biopsy via endoscopy or celioscopy is often only performed as a last resort to diagnose renal neoplasia before euthanasia, as the risk of massive bleeding and functional disturbance have to be considered.

INDICATIONS

Anamnestic hints, such as a predisposition to renal neoplasia in older budgerigar parakeets or a history of polydipsia, a prolonged period without access to water, intoxication, or extensive dietary problems, can all serve as indications for diagnostic imaging of the urinary tract.

Severe clinical signs are also an important indication for diagnostic imaging of the urinary tract. These clinical findings can include polydipsia, polyuria, discoloration of the urates, vomiting, dehydration, an abnormal, hunched posture, chronic disturbances in feather growth, and/or skin alterations. Dyspnea, secondary to air sac compression, or paresis of the hind limb, caused by compression of the ischiatic nerve, may be observed in advanced cases of renal enlargement.[1] Abdominal swelling may also be detected during the clinical examination and this can indicate hyperplasia of the kidneys.

Abnormal laboratory results, such as uric acid levels that are consistently above reference range or show an increasing trend, can also be an indication for further diagnostic testing of the urinary system.[1] An imaging technique may also be indicated in some confirmed cases of systemic infectious disease involving the urinary tract, like polyomavirus, or in suspected cases of nephrocalcinosis (often associated with bacterial nephritis).

Conventional Radiography

In most cases, diagnostic imaging of the urinary tract begins with conventional radiographs, which may be followed by further steps, like contrast imaging and sonography

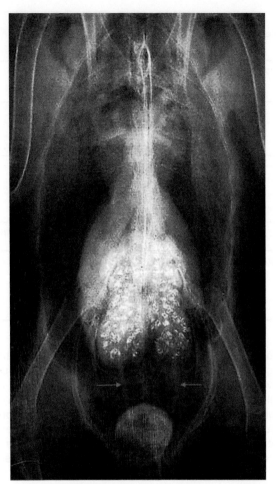

Fig. 2. Urography in a blue-fronted Amazon parrot (*Amazona aestiva*): ventro-dorsal view, 1-minute post installation of iopamidol, outlining kidneys, ureters (*arrows*) and cloaca, and spotted areas of increased radiodensity (hypercalcification) throughout the renal parenchyma.

(**Table 1**). An important exception to this rule of thumb occurs with abdominal swelling, most commonly caused by neoplasia, in which sonography is often performed as the first diagnostic step.

In cases with diffuse radiographic abdominal soft tissue swelling, oral administration of a nonabsorbable contrast agent like barium sulfate can be used to radiographically differentiate the kidneys from surrounding structures,[2,3] such as ovarian cysts or gonadal tumors (**Figs. 3** and **4**).

Urography

Anatomic and functional differences between the avian and mammalian excretory system limit the usefulness of urographic investigations in birds; however, renal contrast radiography is indicated in some instances to obtain information about functional disturbances of the urinary tract (see **Fig. 2**).[3] Suspected dysfunction of the urinary tract

Table 1
Imaging techniques and possible diagnostic findings

Method	Demonstration of...
Conventional radiography	Enlargement Increased radiodensity Crystalline deposits
Ultrasonography	Enlargement Tissue alterations Cysts Blood supply (via Doppler function)
Endoscopy	Enlargement Discolorations Uric acid accumulation Tissue alterations Ureter function impairment
Urography	Functional impairment, excretion (ureteroliths) Size, shape of kidneys
Computed tomography/MRI	Enlargement of defined renal areas Tissue assessment Functional impairment Contrast demonstration Blood supply

can be associated with massive polyuria/polydipsia or alterations in the size and form of the kidneys (eg, acute nephritis) in which survey radiographs or ultrasonographic investigations have not provided a clinical diagnosis. Urography is also suitable for assessing ureteral function, when diagnosing obstruction or after the surgical removal of uroliths.[4] As a side benefit, urography can also help to detect abnormalities in other parenchyma through the concentration of contrast material in these organs. Urographic investigation is contraindicated in dehydrated birds unless the patient has been sufficiently rehydrated before the contrast agent is administered.[3]

Sonography

In cases of abdominal swelling, which is often due to reasons unrelated to the renal system, ultrasonography should be considered as the first diagnostic test (see earlier

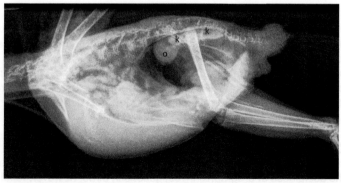

Fig. 3. Plain radiograph in a gray parrot (*Psittacus erithacus*): latero-lateral, follicle/active ovary (o = ovary, verified by sonography) superimposed to cranial pole of the kidneys (k).

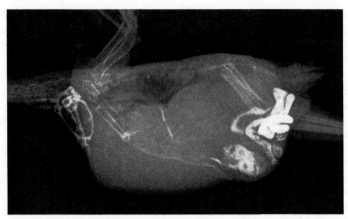

Fig. 4. Radiograph in a budgerigar parakeet (*Melopsittacus undulatus*): latero-lateral, increased radiodensity in the abdominal cavity, 1 hour post installation of 1 mL barium sulfate into the crop, outlining the displaced gastrointestinal tract from a mass in the renal region (final diagnosis: renal neoplasia). See also **Fig. 5**A and B.

in this article). Sonography can be used to assess renal vessels or parenchymal changes, which may allow the examiner to differentiate among neoplastic, cystic, or inflammatory changes (**Fig. 5**A, B).[5]

Computed Tomography and MRI

In the avian patient, CT is most commonly used to detect abnormalities of the skeletal system or respiratory tract[3]; however, CT can be used to diagnose renal disease or confirm a tentative diagnosis made by more conventional methods. The main advantage of CT is the ability to assess a 3-dimensional image without superimposing skeletal structure.[6] MRI can provide additional valuable information about renal parenchyma (see **Fig. 1**), but it carries serious limitations due to the loud noise during

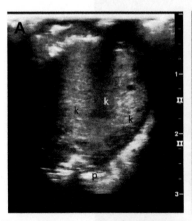
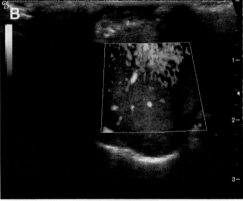

Fig. 5. (*A*) Sonography of a budgerigar (*Melopsittacus undulatus*): ventromedian approach, W-shaped pelvic structure (p) visible, renomegaly, renal parenchyma (k) inhomogeneous structure with partly anechoic areas (final diagnosis: renal neoplasia) (see **Fig. 4**). (*B*) Doppler sonography revealing typically spotted distribution of renal vessels.

examination and the long scanning time. Depending on bird size and the pathology present, the renal parenchyma, ureters, and large vessels can all be assessed in individual scanning planes with both techniques (see **Fig. 1**). Contrast enhancement with organic iodine compounds is also possible (see Urography section).[7]

Endoscopy or Laparotomy

More invasive diagnostic methods, like endoscopy or laparotomy, are indicated when a clinical diagnosis cannot be made by other diagnostic methods. Thus, endoscopic examination of the kidney is recommended in cases of persistent polyuria, anuria, or oliguria or where uric acid levels are permanently elevated.[8] Renal diseases that cause grossly visible alterations on the organ surface, such as swelling, discoloration, or uric acid accumulation can be visualized endoscopically (**Fig. 6**). An endoscopically performed biopsy with subsequent histologic examination of the bioptate is conceivable[9,10]; however, renal surgical biopsies are associated with the risk of massive bleeding (see **Table 1**).

CONVENTIONAL RADIOGRAPHY
Technique

A description on the performance and technical requirements for conventional radiography is available elsewhere, as this diagnostic standard technique is well established in birds.[2,3,11] When using digital radiology techniques, remember both results and interpretation depend on the technical system used as well as software processing of the data. One study has evaluated the potential uses and limitations of a digital imaging system in birds of medium and small size.[12] A major limitation with digital systems is low spatial resolution, particularly when compared with established conventional mammography systems.[12] Fortunately, newer digital systems can provide adequate resolutions, and this should be taken into account when acquiring new equipment.

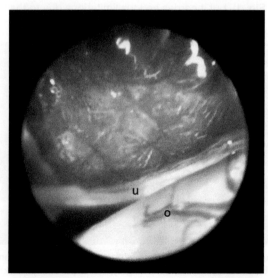

Fig. 6. Endoscopy in a racing pigeon (*Columba livia*), yellow-white deposits on the surface of the kidneys, consistent with dehydration (u, ureter; o, oviduct).

Anatomic Demonstration

The typical structural and functional divisions of the mammalian kidney are absent in the avian kidney. The avian kidneys are best visualized in the latero-lateral radiographic view along the vertebral column.[2,13] In ventro-dorsal radiographs, physiological-sized kidneys are often not visible or indistinct. In either view, the kidneys are rarely demonstrated in full length with conventional radiography. In lateral views, the cranial end of the kidney is superimposed by the gonad. The degree of superimposition depends on the bird's reproduction status as the genital tract can be markedly enlarged during the breeding season (see **Fig. 3**). The oral administration of a nonabsorbable contrast agent, like barium sulfate, can help to radiographically differentiate the kidneys from surrounding structures, especially the gastrointestinal (GI) tract (see **Fig. 4**).[2,3] The ureter and cloaca are not visible under normal, physiologic conditions.

Pathologic Alterations

Increased radiopacity

Increased opacity of the kidneys may be noted, especially on the lateral view (**Fig. 7**). This radiopacity may be caused by dehydration, vitamin A deficiency, or inflammatory processes, however this finding can be difficult to accurately assess due to summation of the pelvic girdle in this region. If available, use of a radiograph for comparison from another bird of the same species or the same radiographic procedure may be helpful for interpretation. The ureter and cloaca can appear radiopaque with certain disease conditions.

Changes in size

Renomegaly is a nonspecific finding that may be a consequence of an infectious process, vitamin A deficiency, cyst formation, or neoplasia. Massively enlarged kidneys are often associated with neoplasia. Renal neoplasia is identified radiologically in the lateral projection as an obviously enlarged shadow of the kidney or as a diffuse soft tissue swelling in the caudodorsal abdomen. Marked renomegaly can cause compression of the caudal air sacs and ventral displacement of the intestinal tract (see **Fig. 4**); however, extensive enlargement of the renal shadow can be difficult to distinguish from surrounding tissue. The highly enlarged gonads found in both sexes during the breeding season should not be falsely interpreted as renomegaly (see **Fig. 3**). A gastrointestinal contrast series after oral administration of barium sulfate (20 mL/kg) that reveals ventral displacement of the intestinal loops facilitates a diagnosis of renomegaly (see **Fig. 4**). In massive renomegaly, the radiographic shadows of the enlarged kidneys are also seen in the ventro-dorsal view (**Fig. 8**).[3,13]

Changes in contour

Although renomegaly is a common finding, alterations of the kidney's shape can rarely be seen on plain radiographs due to the manifold superimpositions of the skeletal system, gonads, and GI tract.

Hypercalcification

Radiopaque particles can be observed within the renal shadow in both standard radiographic projections (see **Fig. 2**). These radiopacities are a nonspecific sign of renal dysfunction, caused by hypercalcification, which often correlates with a rise in the patient's blood calcium values.[14]

Hypercalcification is distinct from visceral gout, or the crystallization of urates within the kidney. Prolonged dehydration can lead to visceral gout; however, gout is rarely

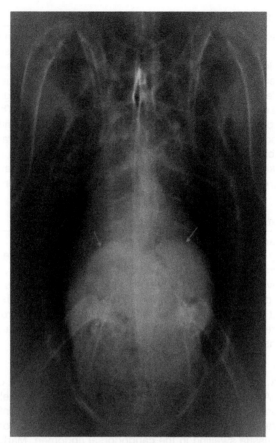

Fig. 7. Plain radiograph in an eclectus parrot (*Eclectus roratus*): increased radiodensity of the enlarged renal shadow (final diagnosis: advanced bacterial nephritis).

visible on radiologic images. Thus the diagnosis of visceral gout cannot be made radiographically.

UROGRAPHY
Technique

In case iodinated contrast is needed, select a nonionic contrast agent, such as iodixanol, iopamidol, or iotrolan (eg, Solutrast, Omnipaque). These agents have an iodine content between 300 and 400 mg iodine/mL. Higher concentrations produce stronger contrast, but the risk of adverse effects is also considered to be higher although this has not been seen in experimental studies nor described in the literature in diseased birds.[3,13] Hypertonicity is the main reason for iodinated contrast media induced side effects, therefore intravenous contrast procedures should not be performed on dehydrated animals or in birds with severe renal dysfunction.[3,13] Additional adverse reactions to ionic iodinated contrast media have been reported in the literature; however, they have not yet been described in birds.

The contrast agent must be warmed to body temperature for urography, then slowly administered intravenously (usually in the ulnar vein) to the sedated or anesthetized patient at a dosage of 2 mL/kg body weight.[3,15,16]

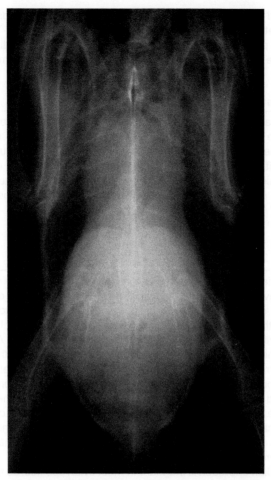

Fig. 8. Blue and gold macaw (*Ara ararauna*): Plain ventro-dorsal radiograph in a macaw illustrating severe renomegaly, enlarged heart silhouette (final diagnosis: herpesvirus infection).

The quality of the contrast image obtained depends on the concentrating capacity of the kidneys, the preparation used, and the iodine concentration of the medium. The high concentration, as compared with gastrography for instance, is necessary to achieve good contrast. As the renal venous system of the bird provides rapid elimination of the contrast agent, the procedure must be performed very rapidly. For instance, the patient should already be positioned on the plate when administering the contrast agent, so radiographs can be taken immediately afterward.[3]

Anatomic Presentation

Because the structure of the bird's urinary system lacks calices, a renal pelvis, or a bladder, strongly outlined kidneys, as seen in mammals, cannot be expected. The most significant radiographic feature is found in the renal portal system, as this allows rapid excretion of contrast during urographic investigations. The aorta, heart, and pulmonary arteries are demonstrated 10 seconds after injection. Kidneys and ureters are shown 30 to 60 seconds after injection. The ureters can be seen running parallel to the medial edge of the kidneys and ending in the cloaca (see **Fig. 2**). The cloaca and terminal gut are visualized 2 to 5 minutes after the injection.

Pathologic Alterations

Renal contrast radiography is indicated to obtain information about functional disturbances of the urinary tract. A reduction or complete absence of contrast flow through the kidney or ureter sometimes occurs when cysts, renal tumors, or ureteroliths are present.[4] Elimination of contrast medium is also retarded in cases of renal insufficiency, which can be due to a variety of causes, including trauma. Urographic recordings also make it possible to clarify changes in the shape or size of the kidneys.[5]

SONOGRAPHY
Technique

Whether the patient should be fasted before the ultrasonographic examination depends on the individual case. In general, an ingesta-filled GI tract can disturb the penetration of ultrasound waves, thereby reducing one's ability to image soft tissue organs, especially when the ventromedian coupling site is used. On the other hand, a relatively empty GI tract will allow the air sacs system to be more prominent. A major problem when imaging the kidneys sonographically is the air sac system that prevents the penetration of ultrasound waves into the deeper coelomic cavity. Therefore prolonged fasting can be counterproductive for kidney visualization. Furthermore, if the bird has been transported to the veterinarian without access to food, or if the bird has had a reduced appetite over a prolonged period, or is otherwise clinically diseased, fasting is neither necessary nor indicated. Sedation/Anesthesia is usually not necessary for ultrasonographic examination; however, the stress involved in handling the bird must be considered.[16]

The ventromedian approach is standard in most avian species, as this coupling site is easily accessible without plucking feathers, at least in psittacine birds. The transducer is placed immediately behind the sternum and directed dorsally, therefore penetrating the GI tract before reaching the kidneys. The parasternal coupling site can be particularly helpful for diagnosing renal alterations but is only possible in birds with enough space between the last rib and the pelvis, such as pigeons and some raptor species. The transducer is generally placed on the right or left side of the bird and the leg is drawn either forward or backward. The transducer is pressed lightly on the body wall to compress the air sacs lying below. Any plucking should be performed as judiciously as possible, particularly in aquatic birds, as excess feather loss can lead to hypothermia.

In larger birds, with a body weight of more than 2 kg, an intracloacal ultrasonographic examination can be achieved using appropriate probes.[17] The cloaca and intestines must be extensively lavaged with warm water before the procedure. Ultrasound gel is then applied directly into the cloaca. This technique was reported in 266 unanesthetized birds of 20 different species in 1995, but has not been described since that time. This coupling site allows the kidneys and gonads (but not the ureters) to be well visualized.[17]

When sonographically examining ratites, transcutaneous coupling sites are generally used in conjunction with a linear, 3.5 MHz transducer in unsedated birds.

Anatomic Demonstration

With the exception of intracloacal probes, ultrasonographic imaging of the kidneys and ureters is generally not possible in most healthy birds,[5] as the air sac system interrupts the sound waves and prevents penetration. In some species, however, especially those feeding on soft food or fruits, the relatively large GI tract might allow visualization of healthy kidneys.

Pathologic Alterations

In contrast, the situation is completely different in diseased avian patients. Any organ enlargement, displacement of the air sacs, or fluid accumulation facilitates transducer coupling and improves image quality. The risk of placing birds with swollen abdomens in dorsal recumbency for radiographic imaging is an additional reason to use sonography as the first diagnostic test in birds with a swollen abdomen or circulatory insufficiency.

Enlarged kidneys can be clearly identified sonographically, and the renal parenchyma can be easily assessed without difficulty in both large and small birds. In cross-section, in which the scanning plane is vertical to the spine, the kidneys are found in a W-shaped area of total reflection formed by the bones of the pelvis and spine. In this projection, the kidneys appear round to oval in cross-section and size measurements can be determined. The 2 kidneys can also be compared with each other. By turning the transducer approximately 90°, the kidneys can be examined down their longitudinal axis (ie, along the spine). Placing a light degree of pressure on the transducer can aid imaging of the urinary tract as this will compress the air sacs, thereby reducing interference of the sound waves by these structures. A portion of the blood from the pelvic limb flows through the kidneys in the renal portal vein circulation. By using Doppler function, both the abdominal aorta, lying between the 2 kidneys, and the larger renal vessels can be visualized.[3]

Sonographically, the enlarged, inflamed kidney is often hypoechoic and there is a reduced ability to image nearby structures.[5]

Neoplasia

Tumors can occasionally be observed as homogeneously hyperechoic structures or as nonhomogeneous parenchyma with focal necrosis (see **Fig. 5**A) (**Table 2**); however,

Table 2	
Sonographic diagnosis and common associated alterations of the urinary tract	
Sonographic Diagnosis	**Sonographic Image**
Cyst, (focal necrosis)	Focal roundish anechoic area, distal enhancement of ultrasound
Hemorrhage	Diffuse heterogenous echogenicity with altering sonographic appearance
(Hypercalcification)	Hyperechoic spots, only demonstrated in combination with renal swelling
Neoplasia	Space-occupying structure with clear heterogenous echoic/echopoor or partly anechoic content
Nephritis	Mostly homogeneous renal parenchyma, often W-shape of the pelvis visible

Parentheses indicate rare findings.

determination of the exact origin and nature of the neoplasm is often not possible.[3,5] Using Doppler function, conclusions can be formed about the type and malignancy of the neoplastic mass (see **Fig. 5B**).[3]

Cyst

Renal cysts normally appear as a diffuse enlargement of the renal shadow on traditional radiographic images. Sonographically, renal cysts have a typical appearance that can be easily differentiated from the renal parenchyma. Renal cysts appear as hyperechoic structures, with smooth walls and hypoechoic contents (see **Table 2**). Cysts are also associated with the phenomenon of distal sound reinforcement.

Cysts can also affect the ureter or genital system. If there is difficulty in differentiating a renal cyst from an ovarian cyst, ultrasound-guided aspiration of the cyst cavity and cytologic examination of the collected sample can be performed.

Hemorrhage

Severe renal bleeding after trauma can be identified during the sonographic examination, however most birds die before a diagnosis can be made. As the blood clots, an irregular parenchymal echogenicity is quickly organized (**Fig. 9**) (see **Table 2**).

Gout

Urate deposits and/or calcification occasionally cause hyperechoic reflections in the ultrasonographic image with the renal tissue appearing nonhomogeneous (see **Table 2**), but these structural abnormalities are not visible until the kidneys are enlarged. Therefore, renal gout must be diagnosed using other methods, such as endoscopy or blood chemistry.

To achieve a definitive diagnosis, a biopsy or fine needle tissue aspiration for histologic and/or microbiological diagnostic interpretation is necessary. In the case of the urinary tract, this is performed quite rarely. The method used (ultrasound-guided vs endoscopy vs exploratory laparotomy) depends on the clinical

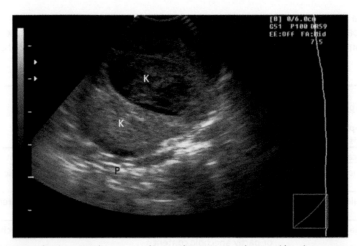

Fig. 9. Sonography in a Moluccan cockatoo (*Cacatua moluccensis*) using a ventromedian approach, renal parenchyma (k) showing large areas of varying echogenicity, sonographic picture altered in consequent examinations due to renal bleeding and blood clotting (p, pelvis).

situation as well as the examiner's skills. As surgical renal biopsies are associated with the risk of massive hemorrhage in avian patients, this procedure should be carefully considered. In contrast to ultrasound-guided liver biopsy, sonographically guided renal biopsy also carries a high risk for bleeding in birds. Therefore, when biopsies are obtained, it is usually during endoscopy (see **Table 2**).

ENDOSCOPY/BIOPSY
Technique

The traditional endoscopic approach is through the caudal thoracic air sac into the abdominal air sac, where the cranial and medial parts of the kidneys and associated structures can be visualized through the abdominal air sac. The technique is performed under general anesthesia, and has been described extensively elsewhere.[9,10,18] To investigate the caudal part of the kidneys, the endoscopic approach of choice is through a puncture site dorsal to the pubic bone and caudal to the ischium directly into the abdominal air sac.

Endoscopy-guided kidney biopsies are recommended when significant clinical findings are observed, such as uricacidemia,[13] or persistent polyuria and polydipsia without clinical explanation, or when gross abnormalities are detected during endoscopy.[19] The benefit of a potential diagnosis from an endoscopy-guided kidney biopsy must be carefully weighed against the risk to the patient as there is an increased chance of hemorrhage when biopsying an abnormal kidney. Biopsy samples should be collected through a working channel using cup-shaped flexible biopsy forceps, while keeping the location of larger vessels in mind.[13]

An alternative renal biopsy sampling technique (circa 1996) has been described by Suedmeyer and Bermudez.[20] A dorsal pelvic approach enables sample collection without expensive equipment; however, this technique is associated with an increased risk of tissue damage when compared with endoscopy-guided techniques. Another disadvantage is that the kidneys and other organs cannot be visualized.[20]

Anatomic Demonstration

Endoscopy allows the appearance of the kidney's surface to be assessed as well as renal size, shape, and color.[13] Most surrounding organs also can be evaluated and visceral gout may be detected.

Pathologic Alterations

One common pathologic finding is filled, swollen ureters due to dehydration or obstruction. The kidneys may appear brown-red-orange, with star-shaped collecting tubules filled with urates visible on the surface. Yellow-white deposits on the surface of the kidney often indicate renal gout or dehydration (see **Fig. 6**). Obesity can make the kidneys appear diffusely yellow. Abscesses or cysts may appear as large yellow spots.[19] To achieve a diagnosis, it is recommended to investigate both kidneys during endoscopy, as focal changes are not uncommon.[21]

SCINTIGRAPHY

Nuclear scintigraphy is a potentially useful diagnostic method for evaluating renal function. Older publications describe renal scintigraphy in several avian species[22,23]; however, this technique is currently used only for research purposes due to the challenge of sampling pure ureteral urine.[7]

COMPUTED TOMOGRAPHY AND MRI
Technique

CT and MRI techniques have been described extensively elsewhere.[6,7,24] In comparison with MRI, an important advantage to performing CT in the bird is the significantly shorter examination time of 1 or 2 minutes and the comparably less noisy examination procedure. Because of the small size of birds, thin slices can be used, preferably with a thickness of 0.6 to 1.0 mm. Positioning of the bird may be done transversal or parallel to the gantry (CT apparatus opening) to create transversal or longitudinal sections.[3,6,7,24,25]

Proper positioning is analogous to the positioning for ventro-dorsal radiography. The bird is placed in dorsal recumbency with slightly spread wings and the hind limbs extended as far caudal as possible. If possible, the examination should be done using general anesthesia[7]; however, a plexiglass positioning device in unsedated birds[3] or mild sedation using midazolam as described for conventional radiography can also be used.

MRI is only rarely used to diagnose diseases of the urinary tract in the avian patient. Given that most patients are already in an advanced stage of disease, the comparably long examination time, the extreme noise during the examination, and the problematic challenges of anesthetic monitoring during the procedure must all be weighed against the benefits of MRI. Newer devices allow shorter examination times and more detailed tissue demonstration, making this equipment more useful for this delicate examination.

In both CT and MRI, movement artifact greatly reduces the value of the examination. In birds in ventral recumbency, the back and pelvis move with the breathing cycle and prevent the linear demonstration of the organ after reformation of the slices. For the same reason, CT with the bird in a cage, as some hospitals report to perform as a first diagnostic step especially for assessment of the respiratory system, is not recommended.

Anatomic Demonstration

The main advantage of both CT and MRI is the ability to assess the kidneys and surrounding organs 3-dimensionally.[6] This prevents the superimposition of structures seen with conventional radiography, and allows possible enlargements to be assessed. Using CT, blood flow within the organ can also be demonstrated to some extent. MRI detects renal blood flow, perfusion, and changes in tissue signal intensity (see **Fig. 1**).

Pathologic Alterations

Enlargement of the kidneys may easily be detected with CT imaging, especially when contrast medium is used.[3,22] Calcifications can sometimes be seen but interpretation is difficult.

MRI is of special interest for the assessment of cysts, but also for detecting neoplastic alterations. The limitations of MRI mean there is still a lack of experience in demonstrating pathologic changes in the avian kidney.

SUMMARY

Although limited due to the anatomic peculiarities of birds, imaging diagnostic techniques can give some important information on the avian urinary tract. Whereas the conventional radiograph often provides only a rough impression, contrast radiography, as well as ultrasonography, is able to provide more precise information.

Nevertheless, in difficult, chronic cases, an endoscopy or renal biopsy is needed to confirm the diagnosis.

REFERENCES

1. Echols MS. Evaluating and treating the kidneys. In: Harrison G, Lightfoot T, editors. Clinical avian medicine, vol. II. Palm Beach (FL): Spix Publishing; 2006. p. 451–92.
2. Krautwald-Junghanns M-E, Tellhelm B. Advances in radiography of birds. Semin Avian Exot Pet Med 1994;3:115–25.
3. Krautwald-Junghanns M-E, Pees M, Reese S, et al. Diagnostic imaging of exotic pets. Hannover (Germany): Schlütersche Verlagsgesell; 2011. p. 26 (urinary tract), p. 32 (urography), p. 54–63 (computed tomography), p. 64–9 (MRI), p. 122–35 (urogenital tract).
4. Dennis P, Bennett R. Ureterotomy for removal of two ureteroliths in a parrot. J Am Vet Med Assoc 2000;217:865–8.
5. Hofbauer H, Krautwald-Junghanns M. Transcutaneous ultrasonography of the avian urogenital tract. Vet Radiol Ultrasound 1999;40:58–64.
6. Veladiano I, Banzato T, Bellini L, et al. Normal computed tomographic features and reference values for the coelomic cavity in pet parrots. BMC Vet Res 2016; 12:182.
7. Van Zealand Y, Schoemaker N, Hsu E. Advances in diagnostic imaging. In: Speer B, editor. Current therapy in avian medicine and surgery. St Louis (MO): Elsevier; 2016. p. 531–49.
8. Burgos-Rodriguez R. Avian renal system: clinical implications. Vet Clin North Am Exot Anim Pract 2010;13:393–411.
9. Taylor M. Endoscopic examination and biopsy techniques. In: Ritchie BW, Harrison GJ, Harrison LR, editors. Avian medicine. Principles and applications. Lake Worth (FL): Wingers Publishing; 1994. p. 327–54.
10. Taylor M. Endoscopic diagnosis. In: Olsen GH, Orosz S, editors. Manual of avian medicine. St Louis (MO): Mosby; 2000. p. 449–63.
11. Naldo J, Saggese M. Radiography. In: Samour J, editor. Avian medicine. 3rd edition. Edinburgh (United Kingdom): Elsevier Limited; 2016. p. 130–53.
12. Bochmann M, Ludewig E, Krautwald-Junghanns M-E, et al. Comparison of the image quality of a high-resolution screen-film system and a digital flat panel detector system in avian radiography. Vet Radiol Ultrasound 2011;52:256–61.
13. Lierz M. Avian renal diseases: pathogenesis, diagnosis, and therapy. Vet Clin North Am Exot Anim Pract 2003;6:29–55.
14. Morrow CJ, Browne AP, O'Donnell CJ, et al. Hypophosphatemic rickets and nephrocalcinosis in ostrich chicks brooded and reared on limestone sand. Vet Rec 1997;140:531–2.
15. Krautwald-Junghanns M-E, Schlömer J, Pees M. Iodine based contrast media in avian medicine. J Exot Pet Med 2008;17:189–97.
16. Krautwald-Junghanns M-E, Pees M. Ultrasonography. In: Samour J, editor. Avian medicine. 3rd edition. Edinburgh (United Kingdom): Elsevier Limited; 2016. p. 153–60.
17. Hildebrandt T, Pitra C, Göritz F, et al. Transintestinal ultrasonographic sexing. Proc 3rd Conference European Committee Assoc Avian Vet. Jerusalem, Israel, 1995. p. 37–41.
18. Samour J. Endoscopy. In: Samour J, editor. Avian medicine. 3rd edition. Edinburgh (United Kingdom): Elsevier Limited; 2016. p. 170–8.

19. Lierz M. Diagnostic value of endoscopy and biopsy. In: Harrison GJ, Lightfoot TL, editors. Clinical avian medicine, vol. II. Palm Beach (FL): Spix Publishing; 2006. p. 631–52.

20. Suedmeyer WK, Bermudez A. A new approach to renal biopsy in birds. J Avian Med Surg 1996;10:179–86.

21. Müller K, Göbel T, Müller S, et al. Use of endoscopy and renal biopsy for the diagnosis of kidney diseases in free-living birds of prey and owls. Vet Rec 2004;155: 326–9.

22. Marshall K, Craig L, Jones M, et al. Quantitative renal scintigraphy in domestic pigeons (*Columba livia f. domestica*) exposed to toxic doses of gentamicin. Am J Vet Res 2003;64:453–62.

23. Radin M, Hoepf T, Swayne D. Use of a single-injection solute-clearance method for determination of glomerular filtration rate and effective renal plasma flow in chickens. Lab Anim Sci 1993;43:594–6.

24. Schoemaker N, van Zealand Y. Advanced clinical imaging. In: Samour J, editor. Avian medicine. 3rd edition. Edinburgh (United Kingdom): Elsevier Limited; 2016. p. 161–70.

25. Gumpenberger M, Henninger W. The use of computed tomography in avian and reptile medicine. Sem Av Exot Pet Med 2001;10:174–80.

Clinical Management of Avian Renal Disease

Ophélie Cojean, Dr méd vét, IPSAV (Zoological Medicine)[a],
Sylvain Larrat, Dr méd vét, MSc, DES, Dipl ACZM[a],
Claire Vergneau-Grosset, Dr méd vét, CES, IPSAV (Zoological Medicine), Dipl ACZM[b],*

KEYWORDS

- Avian • Fluid therapy • Nutrition • Supportive care • Allopurinol • Antifungal drugs
- Chelation therapy • Chemotherapy

KEY POINTS

- Fluid therapy is one of the most important treatments in cases of kidney disorders in birds. The choice between oral, subcutaneous, intravenous, and intraosseous routes depends on the patient and its needs.

- Elevated dietary protein alone does not seem to be the underlying etiology of gout in all avian species because diets as high as 70% protein failed to induce gout in adult cockatiels.

- The efficacy of allopurinol remains controversial in avian medicine and its use has not been reported in many avian species.

- Surgical procedures, such as nephrectomy or renal transplantation, are not advisable in birds owing to the anatomic constraints of the avian kidney.

- No effective therapy is recognized in birds with renal neoplasia.

INTRODUCTION

As in mammals, avian renal disease may be classified as acute or chronic. Acute renal failure results from an abrupt decrease in renal function, often caused by an ischemic or toxic insult.[1] Chronic kidney disease is characterized by loss of functional renal tissue owing to a prolonged and usually progressive disease process.[2]

Causes of kidney disease may be classified as prerenal, renal, postrenal, or of mixed origin. A prerenal origin is characterized by hypoperfusion of the kidney. Conditions that commonly lead to the development of prerenal hyperuricemia include dehydration, hypovolemia, and congestive heart failure. Renal origin of kidney disease refers

Disclosure Statement: The authors have nothing to disclose.
[a] Zoological Medicine Service, Clinique vétérinaire Benjamin Franklin, 38 rue du Danemark, ZA Porte Océane II, Brech 56400, France; [b] Service de médecine zoologique, Département de sciences cliniques, Faculté de médecine vétérinaire, Université de Montréal, 3200 rue Sicotte, Saint-Hyacinthe, Quebec J2S 2M2, Canada
* Corresponding author.
E-mail address: claire.grosset@umontreal.ca

Vet Clin Exot Anim 23 (2020) 75–101
https://doi.org/10.1016/j.cvex.2019.08.004
1094-9194/20/© 2019 Elsevier Inc. All rights reserved.

to an intrarenal process, leading to a dramatic decrease in the glomerular filtration rate. In birds, a decrease in glomerular filtration rate can either be a sign of renal disease or an appropriate physiologic response to water restriction.[3] Causes of renal disease in the avian patient include infectious nephritis, hypovitaminosis A, heavy metal intoxication, and renal neoplasia. Postrenal hyperuricemia occurs when there is a disruption of the integrity of the urinary tract or an obstruction of urine outflow (eg, urolithiasis).[2]

The treatment of avian renal disease relies on supportive care such as fluid therapy and nutritional support. Analgesia and adaptations of the environment are indicated in cases of renal disease associated with painful joints or spinal nerve compression. Other treatments vary with the underlying etiology and may include systemic antibiotics, antifungal therapy, vitamin A supplementation, chelation therapy, and agents to lower uric acid levels such as allopurinol. Potentially nephrotoxic drugs should be used with extreme caution in patients with renal disease. Additionally, drugs that are excreted through the kidney may fail to reach therapeutic plasma levels in polyuric birds or reach toxic levels if drug excretion and elimination are impaired.[4]

GENERAL THERAPY FOR RENAL DISEASE
Fluid Therapy

As in mammals,[5] fluid therapy constitutes one of the most important treatments in cases of kidney disorders in birds. Uric acid is eliminated by active tubular secretion[6,7] and water is needed to flush the suspension through the renal tubules.[4] Without regular removal by diuresis, urates can accumulate within the kidneys.[8]

Fluid type is selected based on results of biochemical analyses, evaluation of blood electrolytes, glucose, and acid–base status. When these values are not known, a balanced isotonic crystalloid solution, such as lactated Ringer's solution may be used for rehydration and hemodynamic support.[9] Caution is recommended when using colloid fluids in patients with renal disease by extrapolation from mammals.

Route of administration

Depending on the clinical circumstance, fluids can be administered by oral, subcutaneous, intravenous (IV), and/or intraosseous (IO) routes. Fluids are often administered by mouth by gavage with liquid oral nutrition. This route is generally safe and adequate for avian patients that are not in shock or debilitated.[10] In birds with mild dehydration, fluids can also be provided subcutaneously. Subcutaneous fluids can be administered in the inguinal (**Fig. 1**), interscapular, or axillary regions. Volumes as great as 20 mL/kg may be administered in 1 location.[9] Subcutaneous fluids are easily delivered using a butterfly needle, which allows the animal to move without the needle being pulled out. Practitioners unfamiliar with avian anatomy should beware of the thin skin and the presence of abdominal air sacs close to the inguinal region. Thus, it is key to remain steady during the procedure and to firmly hold the leg in extension to avoid inadvertent coelomic puncture. Fluids given subcutaneously and by mouth are poorly absorbed if hypovolemic shock is present.

The vasculature in birds can be accessed via IV or intraosseous (IO) routes.[11] The choice between these routes depends on patient size, patient temperament, and the volume of fluids needed. IV catheters may be used for initial fluid therapy, but do not have the stability of an IO catheter. Permanent supervision of birds with IV catheters is also required to prevent fatal hemorrhage in case of accidental removal of the catheter.[11] IO catheters can be placed quickly, are stable and reliable, and are relatively easy to maintain, but placement is more painful. Fluids can also be provided

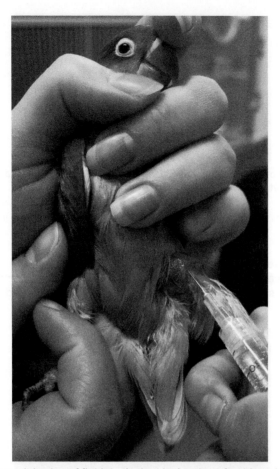

Fig. 1. Subcutaneous injection of fluids in the inguinal region of a Fisher's lovebird (*Agapornis fisheri*). An operator manually restrains the bird. The bird's leg is gently pulled forward, revealing a translucent cutaneous fold between the body and the leg, proximally and medially to the quadriceps muscle. (*Courtesy of* O. Cojean, méd vét, IPSAV, Saint-Hyacinthe, Canada).

in a larger bolus by the IO route than the IV route.[10] Unlike IV catheter placement, IO catheterization can also be performed even in very small birds.

IV catheters may be placed in ulnar (**Fig. 2**) and medial metatarsal veins (**Fig. 3**), or more rarely in the jugular vein.[11] IV catheterization often requires sedation or general anesthesia to avoid stressful physical restraint. Jugular and ulnar catheters must be sutured in place.[11] Medial metatarsal catheters can be secured using tape only.[11] All catheters should then be covered with a nonadhesive bandage. Wing catheters are protected with a figure-of-eight bandage (**Fig. 4**).[11]

IO catheter sites include the proximal tibiotarsus and the distal ulna (**Box 1**).[11] Pneumatized bones, such as the humerus and femur, should be avoided.[9] Rarely, in large birds such as pelicans, California condors (*Gymnogyps californianus*),[12] and turkey vultures (*Cathartes aura*),[13] the ulna is also pneumatized.

Some birds may benefit from an Elizabethan or cervical restraint collar; however, these devices can be extremely stressful to some birds and may adversely affect

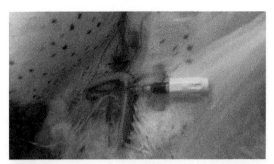

Fig. 2. Placement of a 26G catheter in the ulnar vein of a barn owl *(Tyto alba)*. (*Courtesy of* O. Cojean, méd vét, IPSAV, Saint-Hyacinthe, Canada.)

patient condition. The ability to tolerate a collar should be assessed in each patient[11] (see **Box 1**).

Fluid requirements

Daily maintenance fluid requirements have not been determined in birds; however, the recommendations of different authors range from 50 to 150 mL/kg/d, with the higher

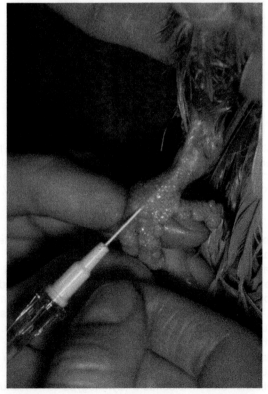

Fig. 3. Placement of a 24G catheter in the medial metatarsal vein of an Amazon parrot. The vein is manually occluded at the level of the proximal tibiotarsus. (*Courtesy of* I. Langlois, DVM, DABVP, Knoxville, TN.)

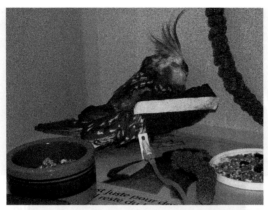

Fig. 4. A cockatiel (*Nymphicus hollandicus*) receiving fluid therapy via an IO catheter in the right ulna. The wing has been taped to the body. The patient is weak and thus does not need an Elizabeth collar. (*Courtesy of* C. Grosset, méd vét, CES, IPSAV, DACZM, Saint-Hyacinthe, Canada.)

end of the range expected in smaller species.[14,15] Maintenance plus one-half of the estimated fluid deficit is generally administered over the first 12 to 24 hours, with the remainder of the deficit replaced over the following 48 hours.[9] Fluids for maintenance and correction of dehydration are given as a constant infusion, using a pediatric

---

Box 1
IO catheter placement in the bird

Placement of an IO catheter in the distal ulna

- Palpate the styloid process of the distal ulna on the dorsal aspect of the wing.
- Pluck the feathers over the surrounding site and prepare aseptically.
- Ideally use a 20- to 25-gauge short spinal needle.
- Flex the distal wing tip and grasp the ulna between the fingers of one hand. With the other hand, the spinal needle is inserted just ventral to the condyle and directed proximally toward the elbow along the ulnar shaft (**Fig. 5**A, 5B).
- Apply gentle pressure as the bevel of the needle is rotated, allowing the needle to cut through the cortex of the bone and enter the medullary cavity.
- If the lumen of the needle becomes plugged, the needle may be removed and replaced.
- Check the patency of the catheter with a small amount of heparinized saline. Visualize flow in the ulnar vein as the fluid is injected (**Fig. 5**C).
- Two orthogonal radiographic views may also be obtained to confirm correct placement.
- Secure the catheter with butterfly taping and by suturing this tape to the skin, if necessary.
- Place a figure-of-eight wing bandage to minimize wing movement.

Placement of an IO catheter in the proximal tibiotarsus

- Flex the stifle, and palpate the cnemial crest at the proximal anterior surface of the tibiotarsus, just distal to the knee joint.
- Insert the needle at the cnemial crest at, or to either side of, the insertion of the patellar tendon, to avoid penetration of the stifle joint.
- Secure the catheter in place with tape.

Data from Refs.[9,10,12]

fatty acids (primarily linoleic acid) and limited in omega-3 fatty acids (**Table 1**). Of note, diets high in polyunsaturated fatty acids require additional antioxidants to prevent lipid peroxidation during storage.[14]

Incorporation of omega-3 into cockatiel red blood cells was greater after supplementation with fish oil[22,23]; however, the palatability of fish oil may be an issue when supplementing psittacine birds at home. Being carnivorous, some birds of prey are more likely to accept fish oil in their diet. In cases of concomitant gout, ensure the patient receives a plant-based source of EPA or docosahexanoic acid rather than a fish oil source, which may have higher purine levels[17] (see **Table 1**).

Management of Hyperuricemia

Severe dehydration and many forms of renal disease, including obstructed ureters, can result in decreased uric acid elimination thus causing hyperuricemia.[16] Fluid therapy (combined with medications for hyperuricemia if needed) is generally continued until uric acid decreases to either normal or mildly increased levels (10–20 mg/dL) and the bird demonstrates signs of improvement, such as eating or increased activity.[16]

The use of medications for hyperuricemia is extrapolated from human medicine, and the safety and efficacy of these treatments are often lacking in birds. These drugs have been poorly studied in psittacine birds and should only be used with close monitoring of uric acid levels.

Xanthine oxidase inhibitors

Xanthine oxidase inhibitors, such as allopurinol and febuxostat, decrease uric acid synthesis. The efficacy of allopurinol in avian medicine is controversial; information is available for only a limited number of species. In broilers, uricemia was reduced as well as xanthine oxidase and xanthine dehydrogenase activity in the kidney in birds treated with allopurinol (25 mg/kg by mouth).[24,25] Allopurinol was unable to completely inhibit xanthine oxidoreductase activity.[24]

Toxicity has been reported following administration of allopurinol in red-tailed hawks (*Buteo jamaicensis*). Vomiting developed at 50 mg/kg by mouth every 24 hours and was attributed to the accumulation of oxypurinol, a metabolite that worsens renal gout.[26] Allopurinol given at 25 mg/kg by mouth every 24 hours to red-tailed hawks was shown to be safe, but had no significant effect on plasma uric acid concentrations. Based on the lack of response at a dose of 25 mg/kg and the toxic effects at

Table 1
Omega-3 concentration and omega 3:omega 6 ratio of selected food items frequently offered as supplements to birds

Food Items	Omega 3 Concentration (g) Value per 100 g	Omega 3/Ω 6 Ratio Value per 100 g
Flax seeds	22.8	3.86
Chia seeds	17.6	3.03
Walnut	9.1	0.24
Soybean oil	6.8	0.13
Lafeber Senior Bird Nutri-Berries®	0.48	0.16
Edamame (green soybean)	0.3	0.16

Data from United States Department of Agriculture Agricultural Research Service Database (USDA). Available at: https://ndb.nal.usda.gov/ndb/.

50 mg/kg, allopurinol is not recommended in the red-tailed hawk.[27] It is unknown whether this finding should be extrapolated to psittacine birds.

Uricase
Uricase oxidizes uric acid to allantoin in humans. Little information is available in veterinary medicine. Poultry on a high-protein diet developed hyperuricemia, which was reversed with uricase injection.[28] In a more recent study, the uricolytic properties of uricase were studied in a granivorous bird (pigeon, *Columba livia domestica*) and a carnivorous avian species (red-tailed hawk). Plasma concentrations of allantoin and uric acid were determined in experimental groups before and after receiving 100, 200, and 600 UI/kg uricase intramuscularly once daily. All regimens caused a significant decrease in plasma uric acid concentrations within 2 days after the first administration, when compared with controls. Plasma allantoin concentrations were also significantly higher when compared with controls, suggesting a similar mechanism of action in these species.[29]

Xanthine dehydrogenase inhibitor
The xanthine dehydrogenase inhibitor, colchicine, is used for its antigout activity in humans.[16] Colchicine has also been used to treat amyloidosis and renal fibrosis in small animals.[16] In turkeys diagnosed with articular gout, colchicine administered at 0.18 mg/kg by mouth every 24 hours for 7 days failed to influence uric acid concentrations.[30] No controlled study on colchicine has been published in birds.

Uricosuric drugs
Uricosuric drugs, such as probenecid, promote uric acid excretion by the kidneys. Uricosuric drugs are contraindicated when tubular urate crystals are present, which is frequently seen in birds.[17] Probenecid has been shown to inhibit uric acid tubular secretion in chicken proximal tubule epithelium in vitro.[31] It has also been studied in vivo in chicken; depending on the dose given intravenously, the drug increased or decreased uric acid clearance.[7] Probenecid use has been reported anecdotally in psittacine birds and reptiles with gout,[32] but no efficacious dose is currently published.

Pain Management
Birds with renal disorders may suffer from pain caused by articular gout or nerve compression secondary to renal masses (**Fig. 6**). Affected birds are likely to spend more time on the cage floor and suffer from impaired locomotion. Husbandry adaptations and pain control are required to improve their quality of life.

Enclosure modifications
Water and food dishes can be placed as close to the bird as possible. Containers of different shapes and depths can stimulate consumption. Replace standard perches with perches of a larger diameter and ladders or ramps that allow the bird to use its beak. Once the bird is unable to perch normally, the claws may need to be trimmed and shaped more frequently than in a healthy bird. Patients with gout should not be restricted in their movements, and instead should be housed in as large a cage as possible. The minimum size considered adequate allows the bird enough space to spread its wings without hitting either the sides of the cage or other perches.[18]

Analgesia
Pain management is paramount in birds with articular gout or nerve compression by renal masses (**Table 2**). Long-term treatment with opioids may be considered. Intra-articular injections of corticosteroids are administered to humans with only 1 joint affected by gout,[17] but this treatment modality has not been investigated in birds.

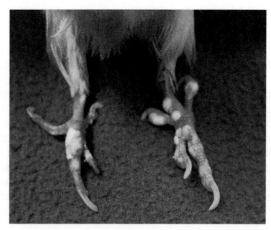

Fig. 6. Articular gout secondary to renal disease in a budgerigar parakeet (*Melopsittacus undulatus*). (*Courtesy of* C. Grosset, Dr méd vét, CES, IPSAV, DACZM, Saint-Hyacinthe, Canada.)

The effectiveness of intra-articular bupivacaine injections in the suppression of osteoarthritic pain has also been demonstrated in humans.[33] In an avian model of acute gouty arthritis, local anesthesia was effective in suppressing pain-associated behavior.[34] It was concluded that the optimum intra-articular dose of bupivacaine for the treatment of musculoskeletal pain in the domestic fowl was 3 mg bupivacaine in 0.3 mL saline.[34] Physical modalities such as thermotherapy and laser may also be used to diminish pain. Low-level laser therapy (660 nm, 9 J/cm^2) has been shown to decrease neuropathic pain.[35]

Alternatively, after discussion with owners of the safety versus quality of life balance, the use of nonsteroidal anti-inflammatory drugs may be considered as a palliative treatment. A study in Hispaniolan Amazon parrots (*Amazona ventralis*) indicated 1.3 mg/kg by mouth every 12 hours of meloxicam to be a therapeutic dosage for relief of arthritic pain.[39]

Both severe gout and renal tumors carry a poor prognosis; therefore, euthanasia must be considered when analgesia and husbandry modifications fail to ensure an appropriate quality of life for the patient.[17]

Miscellaneous Conditions Associated with Chronic Renal Disease

Hyperphosphatemia is poorly documented in birds in association with renal failure, but it has been reported in some instances.[40] If this condition develops, phosphate binders may be administered at doses extrapolated from small animals.

Table 2
Analgesic agents evaluated in Hispaniolan Amazon parrots (*Amazona ventralis*) by pharmacokinetic studies

Agent	Dosage	Route	Frequency	Comment
Tramadol hydrochloride[36]	30 mg/kg	PO	q6-12h	–
Butorphanol tartrate (long-acting poloxamer 407 gel formulation)[37]	12.5 mg/kg	SQ	q4-6h	–
Gabapentin[38]	15 mg/kg	PO	q8 h	Neuropathic pain, effects takes days to weeks

Abbreviations: PO, by mouth; SQ, subcutaneous; q, every.

Although rarely reported with renal disease in birds, gastric ulcers may be treated with omeprazole[41] (1–10 mg/kg by mouth every 12 hours) and sucralfate (25 mg/kg by mouth every 8 hours) staggered 2 hours apart from other oral treatments.

Chronic anemia owing to decreased erythropoietin secretion is challenging to manage because avian erythropoietin is structurally different from that of mammals.[42] The effect of epoetin alfa in birds has not been documented but it is likely to cause antibody production.

Colchicine may be administered long term to treat amyloidosis and limit renal fibrosis.[16] No controlled studies have been published in birds about this drug.

In mammals, peritoneal dialysis or hemodialysis is ideal for cases of renal disease not treatable with other medical options.[43] The use of dialysis has not been described in birds and coelomic dialysis is not possible in the avian patient owing to the presence of abdominal air sacs. Renal transplantation has also never been described in avian medicine and is unrealistic given the position of the kidneys immediately ventral to the synsacrum, adjacent to air sacs, and in close relation with pelvic nerves.

SPECIFIC THERAPY FOR RENAL DISEASE

In avian species, renal diseases are caused by various etiologies, including infectious nephritis (bacterial, viral, parasitic, fungal), renal neoplasms, toxic exposure, and nutritional disorders.[44] Specific treatment options vary depending on the cause.

Bacterial Nephritis

Many bacteria have been reported to cause nephritis in birds, including *Enterobacteriaceae, Pasteurella* spp., *Pseudomonas* spp., *Streptococcus* spp., *Staphylococcus* spp., *Listeria monocytogenes, Erysipelothrix rhusiopathiae*, and chlamydial organisms.[43,45] *Mycobacterium* spp. have also been rarely reported in the avian kidney.[43,46,47]

Antibiotics are indicated in suspected or confirmed cases of bacterial nephritis.[16] Drug choice should ideally be based on a susceptibility panel from blood or histopathologic samples.[16] Cloacal samples may also be used owing to the possibility of ascending infection but may not be reliable. In cats and dogs, bacterial nephritis is treated for at least 4 to 6 weeks.[5] This recommendation may be extrapolated to birds in the absence of controlled studies regarding duration of treatment in avian medicine.[16] Pending culture and sensitivity results, empirical broad-spectrum antibiotics that provide excellent therapeutic levels within renal tissue should be initiated such as β-lactams, trimethoprim-sulfamethoxazole, or fluoroquinolones.[44] Avoid potentially nephrotoxic antibiotics, such as aminoglycosides.[48,49]

Viral Nephritis

Among viral infections, polyomavirus often results in clinically relevant renal disease.[44] Polyomavirus is the most important cause of viral nephritis in the companion psittacine bird.[43] Many other viruses can cause renal lesions in psittaciformes including, but not limited to, paramyxoviruses,[43,44] bornavirus,[50,51] and West Nile virus.[52] In backyard chickens, infectious bronchitis virus is the most important cause of renal disease.[43] Treatment of viral nephritis usually relies on nonspecific supportive care.

Parasitic Nephritis

Renal coccidiosis is the most common cause of parasitic nephritis. Renal diseases caused by the coccidian *Eimeria* spp. have been reported in several species, including juvenile waterfowl,[53] domestic goose (*Anser anser domesticus*), and less commonly raptors.[43] Although rare, renal cryptosporidiosis has also been reported in birds.[44,54,55] Schizonts of *Leukocytozoon* spp., *Plasmodium* spp., and *Haemoproteus* spp. have been identified in avian renal tissue and associated with lymphoplasmacytic inflammation.[44,56] Renal trematodes and cestodes have also been reported in multiple species of bird housed outdoors, including order Columbiformes, Passeriformes, Anseriformes, Psittaciformes, and Galliformes.[44]

Parasitic diseases associated with the kidneys are typically diagnosed from a fecal parasite examination or renal biopsy.[44] Antiparasitic treatments vary greatly depending on the species and life cycle of the parasite, with ponazuril (20 mg/kg by mouth every 24 hours for 7 days) or toltrazuril (25 mg/kg by mouth once a week) being used for coccidia, and praziquantel (10 mg/kg subcutaneously 2 times 10 days apart) for trematodes and cestodes.[44,57–59] Although toltrazuril has been shown to successfully control coccidiosis in broilers with a single 2-day treatment course,[60] its use is not approved in food animal species in many countries. Practitioners should consult local regulations for approved anticoccidial agents. Monensin has been used for the treatment of renal coccidiosis, but is toxic in turkey and guinea fowl.[16] Reports on resistance of *Eimeria* isolates to anticoccidial drugs are increasing,[61–64] and rotation of anticoccidial drugs is recommended to minimize the risk of resistance. Natural products, such as cider vinegar, are also emerging as alternative strategies to control avian coccidiosis.[65–68]

Fungal Nephritis

Aspergillosis

Although predominantly a disease of the respiratory tract, systemic aspergillosis can occur.[69] Renal aspergillosis has been reported in several avian species, including chickens[66] and a black palm cockatoo (*Probosciger aterrimus*).[70] Fungal culture from a biopsy is recommended because treatment options can vary depending on the fungal organism involved.[44] Most systemic fungal infections require long-term therapy over a period of months.[71,72] Initial IV administration of antifungal drugs followed by oral therapy is recommended.[72]

Amphotericin B is a polyene macrolide that acts by binding to ergosterol, the principal sterol in the fungal cell membrane.[71] Amphotericin B has a broad antifungal spectrum, including *Aspergillus* spp. and *Cryptococcus* spp., although resistance has been reported.[73] IV administration quickly establishes fungicidal concentrations, making amphotericin B a frequent choice for initial therapy. The use of amphotericin B has been associated with nephrotoxicity in mammals[72]; however no evidence of nephrotoxicity has been documented in birds. This difference may be associated with the shorter elimination half-life in birds compared with mammals after IV administration of amphotericin B.[74]

In combination with early, systemic antifungal therapy, topical amphotericin B can be administered through a polypropylene tube during endoscopic or surgical procedures.[71] Topical therapy is recommended when renal lesions can be easily debrided to maximize drug concentrations in tissues; however, in many patients granulomas cannot be reached endoscopically.[71]

Itraconazole, fluconazole, and voriconazole are the most studied azoles in birds. The relative toxicity of an azole depends on the affinity to fungal cytochrome P450 enzyme, compared with its affinity to the avian cytochrome P450.[72] The most common adverse effects associated with azole administration in birds are anorexia, vomiting, and alterations in liver function.[71,72] Regular bile acid monitoring is recommended during treatment for early detection of hepatic adverse effects. Itraconazole is a first-generation triazole antifungal agent, commonly used in birds for treatment of aspergillosis.[75] Voriconazole is a third-generation triazole antifungal agent.[71,75] Voriconazole is increasingly used to treat invasive aspergillosis in birds, given the broad antifungal spectrum, which includes molds (fungicidal) and yeasts (fungistatic), and its rapid bioavailability.[72] Acquired resistance of *Aspergillus fumigatus* strains to both itraconazole and voriconazole has been reported.[73,76] Fluconazole is a water-soluble fungistatic agent that is rapidly absorbed with high bioavailability after oral administration.[69] A blue-fronted Amazon parrot with *Aspergillus* keratomycosis was successfully treated with oral and topical fluconazole.[77]

Terbinafine is an allylamine, fungicidal agent with activity against several fungal species, including *Aspergillus* spp.[75] and *Cryptococcus* spp.[78] Of note, the dose should be decreased in cases of impaired renal function.[57]

Studies have documented dose- and species-dependent variability, suggesting that different dosage regimens of antifungals may be required for different species of birds (**Table 3**).[71] Caution should be applied when extrapolating a dose to a different avian species.[75]

Cryptococcosis
Systemic cryptococcosis may also affect companion psittacine birds.[78,96] Partial response to treatment with fluconazole (15 mg/kg by mouth every 12 hours) and terbinafine (15–20 mg/kg by mouth every 12 hours) was described in an African gray parrot (*Psittacus erithacus*) with renal cryptococcosis.[96]

Microsporidiosis
Renal microsporidiosis has been reported in lovebirds (*Agapornis spp.*),[97] particularly in individuals positive for psittacine beak and feather disease,[98] as well as budgerigar parakeets (*Melopsittacus undulatus*), eclectus (*Eclectus roratus*),[99] red-bellied parrots (*Poicephalus rufiventris*),[98] and other avian species.[44] Treatment of renal microsporidiosis has not been reported in birds,[100] but an umbrella cockatoo (*Cacatua alba*) with keratoconjunctivitis associated with microsporidia was successfully treated with albendazole (25 mg/kg by mouth every 24 hours) for 90 days.[100] Clinicians should keep in mind potential toxicities associated with benzimidazoles in many birds.

Treatment of Intoxications Affecting Renal Function

Heavy metal intoxication
Lead and zinc toxicosis can cause renal nephrosis and acute tubular necrosis, respectively.[101,102] Treatment of heavy metal toxicosis must begin with removal of metal from the gastrointestinal tract to halt further absorption.[101] General supportive care is also important.[101] Diets higher in calcium decreased morbidity and mortality in experimentally lead-poisoned ducks.[103] Antioxidative therapies, such as supplemental vitamin C, may also be instituted, because lead induces free radicals.[101]

Various chelation agents have been used in avian species.[101] Careful monitoring of renal parameters is important for the duration of chelation therapy. Elevated uric acid levels can be observed with heavy metal poisoning and improvement of hyperuricemia with therapy has been reported.[102,104]

Calcium disodium salt of EDTA (CaEDTA) is the main chelator for lead and zinc poisoning in avian species.[101] CaEDTA must be administered parenterally because absorption from the gastrointestinal tract is poor.[101] In a study conducted with children, nephrotoxicity and inducement of acute renal failure were reported as an adverse effect of CaEDTA.[105] Although nephrotoxicity has not been reported in birds treated with CaEDTA, even at 40 mg/kg every 12 hours intramuscularly for 21 days,[106] fluid therapy is still recommended to minimize the risk of renal adverse effects.[102]

Table 3
Antifungal therapy in selected avian species

Antifungal Agent	Active Against	Pharmacokinetic Studies	Recommended Doses	Adverse Effects	Comments
Amphotericin B					
C	A	Domestic turkey, broad-winged hawk, red-tailed hawk, great-horned owl[74]	1–1,5 mg/kg IV q8–12 h	Renal toxicity considered lower than in mammals because elimination phase faster in birds[74]	
	Cr				
Itraconazole					
C	A	Humboldt penguin[82]	8.5 mg/kg PO q12 h	Anorexia, vomiting, and alterations in liver function are most common.[71,72]	Itraconazole is better absorbed in an acidic gastric pH[86]; thus, antacid medications should not be administered concomitantly.
ST			20 mg/kg PO q24 h		
		Blue-fronted Amazon parrot[83]	5 mg/kg PO q24 h		
		Racing pigeons[84]	6–26 mg/kg PO q12 h		
		Red-tailed hawk[85]	10 mg/kg PO q24 h		
		African gray parrot	If itraconazole is used owing to monetary constraints, doses of 2.5 mg/kg PO q12–24 h have been used safely with frequent monitoring of plasma bile acid levels	Voriconazole is usually preferred over itraconazole owing to toxicity reports in African gray parrots	

Drug / Spectrum	Species	Dosage		Comments
Voriconazole C (molds) ST (yeasts)	Red-tailed hawk[87,88]	10–12.5 mg/kg q8–12h	Anorexia, vomiting, and alterations in liver function are most common.[71,72]	Voriconazole induces its own metabolism via cytochrome P450 and doses should be increased over time.[95] Owing to toxicity reports in African gray parrots, voriconazole is usually preferred over itraconazole in this species.
	Timneh African gray parrot[89]	12–18 mg/kg PO q12 h		
	Hispaniolan Amazon parrot[90] Mallard duck[91] Chicken[92]	18 mg/kg PO q8 h 20 mg/kg PO q8–12h	Poor bioavailability in chickens[92]	
	African penguins[93] Falcon[94]			
Fluconazole ST	Cockatiel	5 mg/kg PO q24 h or 10 mg/kg PO q48 h or 100 mg/L in the drinking water	Fluconazole has the safest therapeutic index of the azoles.	Described doses resulted in plasma levels that exceeded human MIC for most strains of Candida albicans generally less effective against aspergillosis than itraconazole.[69]
Terbinafine C A[75] Cr[78]	Hispaniolan Amazon parrot[79] Red-tailed hawk[80] African penguin[81]	60 mg/kg q24 h 22 mg/kg q24 h 15 mg/kg q24 h	Regurgitation in red-tailed hawk[80]	Often combined with azoles[71] Dose should be decreased in cases on impaired renal function[57]

Abbreviations: A, Aspergillus spp; C, Fungicidal ST; Cr, Cryptococcus spp; Fungistatic MIC, minimum inhibitory concentration; PO, by mouth; q, every.
Data from Refs. [57,69,71,72,75,78–95]

Succimer (meso 2,3-dimercaptosuccinic acid or DMA) is an oral chelator, derived from British Anti-Lewisite capable of chelating lead from soft tissues, but not from bone.[107] Succimer is less efficient in cases of zinc intoxication.[101] Succimer has a narrow margin of safety, so accurate dosing is important. Doses as low as 15 mg/kg have been reported to be effective.[101] In an experimental trial with induced lead intoxication in cockatiels, a dose of 40 mg/kg by mouth every 12 hours was found to be safe, whereas a dose of 80 mg/kg by mouth every 12 hours was associated with a high mortality rate.[106]

Treatment of intoxication by drugs or plants

Potentially nephrotoxic drugs include aminoglycosides,[48,49] fenbendazole,[108] and nonsteroidal anti-inflammatory drugs, such as diclofenac[109] and flunixin meglumine.[110] Ingestion of rhubarb leaves and other oxalic-acid rich plants can also cause kidney failure.[102]

Treatment options for intoxications include crop lavage[111] or endoscopic removal of plant material when birds are presented within 1 to 6 hours of ingestion, depending on the avian species.[112–115] Fluid therapy and supportive care are also indicated. Some authors recommend the use of activated charcoal (1 g/kg or 1–3 mg/g body weight) as an adsorbent.[102] This treatment is not recommended for acids or corrosive alkaloid agents because it will be useless and may complicate retrieval from the crop. For more information regarding treatment of avian intoxications, the reader should refer to the excellent review by Lightfoot and Yeager.[116]

Treatment of Nutritional Diseases Affecting Renal Function

Hypovitaminosis A

Vitamin A deficiency is commonly reported in companion parrots fed seed-based diets.[20] Hypovitaminosis A can lead to squamous metaplasia of renal epithelium, ureteral mucosa, and collecting ducts leading to obstruction of the ureters and secondary hydronephrosis, hyperuricemia, and oliguric or anuric renal failure.[44] Vitamin A may be supplemented at 2000 to 5000 IU/kg intramuscularly, then repeated every 1 to 3 weeks depending on patient condition and response. Of note, fat-soluble vitamin A is considered safer than water-soluble vitamin A.[117] Vitamin A supplements are also available in powder form. Beta-carotenes and other provitamin A carotenoids can serve as a safer alternative to potentially toxic vitamin A in psittacine birds.[20] Seeds and nuts are generally low in carotenoids, whereas some orange-colored fruits and vegetables, such as carrots, melon, and butternut squash, can provide large quantities thereof.[14] A study in cockatiels demonstrated that vitamin A deficiency can be prevented with 4000 IU vitamin A/kg diet or 2.4 mg β-carotene/kg diet.[118] Levels of less than 10,000 IU vitamin A/kg do not significantly influence plasma levels in cockatiels.[118] Some avian species, such as recessive white canaries (Serinus canaria), are unable to convert β-carotene to vitamin A and require 3 times as much vitamin A as colored canaries.[119]

Hypervitaminosis D

Excess vitamin D_3 promotes metastatic mineralization of viscera, including the kidneys. Vitamin D_3 is considered toxic at 4 to 10 times the recommended dose. Any bird species can potentially be susceptible to hypervitaminosis D[16]; however the dietary requirements for vitamin D vary among avian species, with optimum levels at 200 IU/kg in poultry, 900 IU/kg in turkey, and 1200 IU/kg in Japanese quail.[14] In cases of hypervitaminosis D associated with hypercalcemia, fluid therapy and treatments stimulating calciuresis, such as bisphosphonates and corticosteroids, are recommended in dogs and cats.[120,121] Unfortunately, the use of corticosteroids is controversial in birds owing to the risk of associated immunosuppression and safe doses of bisphosphonate have not been described in birds. Because metastatic calcifications are irreversible, prognosis is guarded.

Iron overload

Iron storage disease results from the accumulation of iron in various tissues, including the kidneys.[122] High dietary iron has been implicated in the development of iron storage disease in susceptible species, such as hornbills, toucans, lories, and lorikeets, as well as mynahs and other Sturnidae.[122,123] It is generally recommended that the iron content of commercial diets be maintained at less than 100 mg/kg.[124] Iron-sensitive species require even lower amounts of iron, ranging from 19 to 25 mg/kg.[122] The high vitamin C content of many fruits also enhances dietary iron uptake. Frugivorous species should be offered fruits low in vitamin C to minimize uptake of iron from commercial diets.[122] Another common strategy is to soak commercial pellets in black tea (first discard the water after initial infusion to avoid caffeine administration, then add water again to the cup and let the pellets soak) to increase the amount of tannins in the food and thereby decrease iron absorption. Soaking should be done every other month to avoid causing other mineral deficiencies.

In case of renal hemochromatosis, treatments described in birds include therapeutic venipunctures to decrease hematocrit, oral deferiprone, or intramuscular deferoxamine injections (**Table 4**).

Treatments for Obstruction of Outflow

The underlying cause for urate concretions, such as a cloacolith or ureterolith, is rarely known.[128] In rare instances, changes to digestive microbial flora may affect the cloacal environment and contribute to the formation of cloacoliths. A cloacolith composed of 100% uric acid was reported in a blue-fronted Amazon parrot fed a mixture of table food, seeds, and pellets.[129] Cloacoliths can obstruct the ureteral opening and cause postrenal hyperuricemia. Cloacoliths can usually be disintegrated and removed with forceps via the cloaca with or without endoscopic assistance.

Ureteroliths have also been described in a double yellow-crowned Amazon parrot (*Amazona ochrocephala*), a chestnut-bellied seed finch (*Oryzoborus angolensis*), and in poultry.[130–132] Imbalances in dietary calcium and phosphorus content and coronavirus infection are reported causes of urolithiasis in poultry.[132,133] Treatment of ureteroliths requires a surgical approach[130]; lithotripsy may be an alternative treatment option.[134]

Treatment of Renal Neoplasia

Kidney neoplasms have been reported in several avian species[44]; however, budgerigar parakeets are overrepresented and renal neoplasms account for 17% to 20% of all neoplasms described in this species.[135] Renal carcinoma is the most common renal neoplasm reported. Other renal neoplasms reported include renal adenoma, nephroblastoma, cystadenoma, and lymphoma.[136]

Nephrectomy is the treatment of choice for unilateral renal tumors in dogs.[137] In birds, unless the renal neoplasm is contained and pedunculated, surgical removal is virtually impossible because of the kidney's dorsal location, its intricate relationship with adjacent vessels and nerves,[43] the limited access to the renal arteries, and the short distance between the renal artery and the aorta, which make ligation or hemostasis difficult if not impossible.[44] Regional invasion by renal neoplasms into the synsacrum bone and sacral nerve plexus is also reported,[138] precluding surgical excision.

Table 4
Treatments of hemochromatosis in selected avian species

Therapeutic agent	Species	Doses	Action	Adverse effects	Comments
Deferiprone	Chickens and pigeons	50 mg/kg PO q12 h	Significantly reduced iron concentration in liver and feces	Weight gain, decreased serum zinc levels, 30% mortality in chickens	Good gastrointestinal absorption at this dose
		70 mg/kg PO q24 h	Significantly reduced iron concentration in liver and feces	Weight gain, decreased serum zinc levels, 30% mortality in chickens	
	Hornbills (n = 3)	75 mg/kg PO q24 h for 90 d	Significantly decreased hepatic iron concentration		
Deferoxamine	Chestnut-fronted macaw (Ara severa) (n = 1)	50 mg/kg IM q12 h for 14 d	Reduced hepatic iron concentration		Associated with a low-iron diet

Abbreviation: PO, by mouth; q24 h, every 24 hours.
Data from Refs.[125–127]

No effective therapy for the management of renal tumors is recognized in birds.[136] Palliative treatment is often selected, including the use of analgesics (see Pain management) and corticosteroids.[43,44] Corticosteroids may predispose birds to opportunistic infections and should be used with caution.[135] Prophylactic antibiotic and antifungal therapy are recommended whenever immunosuppressive drugs are used in avian species.[139]

In mammals, chemotherapy has not been shown to be effective against renal tumors other than lymphosarcoma.[137] Chemotherapy has not been thoroughly evaluated for avian renal tumors. Carboplatin was used to treat renal adenocarcinoma in a budgerigar, resulting in a short-lived clinical improvement but the mass continued to grow.[140] In this case, carboplatin was used at 5 mg/kg IV every 4 weeks without side effects.[140] A few cases of lymphocytic leukemia affecting the kidneys and treated with chemotherapy have been described in psittacine birds.[141,142]

Radiation therapy for renal tumors has been rarely performed owing to questionable tolerance of adjacent tissues. In the case of a black swan (Cygnus atratus) presented with chronic T-cell lymphocytic leukemia affecting the kidneys, whole body radiation therapy with 2 Gy was performed over 31 days, in addition to chemotherapy with chlorambucil, followed by lomustine, L-asparaginase, and prednisone.[143] The swan survived more than 1 year after treatment initiation and was euthanized owing to hyperviscosity syndrome associated with the leukemia. The white blood cell count decreased after radiation therapy and no adverse effects to radiation were detected clinically or at necropsy in this swan. The dose received was much lower than tolerable radiation doses evaluated in ring-necked parakeets (Psittacula krameri).[144] Further studies are needed on the use of radiation therapy in birds for radiosensitive neoplasms.

SUMMARY

The clinical management of bird with renal disease may prove challenging. Treatment choice is highly impacted by the cause and chronicity of the disease. The specific physiology of avian kidneys, and the large variety of species encountered in clinic implies that only a small part of the knowledge about mammalian therapeutics can be extrapolated to birds. More studies on renal disease treatments and their specific applications are warranted.

REFERENCES

1. Grauer GF. Management of acute renal failure. In: Elliott J, Grauer GF, editors. Manual of canine and feline nephrology and urology. 2nd edition. Gloucester (England): BSAVA; 2007. p. 215–22.
2. Brown SA. Management of chronic kidney disease. In: Elliott J, Grauer GF, editors. Manual of canine and feline nephrology and urology. 2nd edition. Gloucester (England): BSAVA; 2007. p. 223–30.
3. Scope A, Schwendenwein I, Schauberger G. Plasma exogenous creatinine excretion for the assessment of renal function in avian medicine. Pharmacokinetic modeling in racing pigeons (Columba livia). J Avian Med Surg 2013;27: 173–9.
4. Lierz M. Avian renal disease: pathogenesis, diagnosis, and therapy. Vet Clin North Am Exot Anim Pract 2003;6:29–55.
5. Langston CE. Acute kidney injury. In: Ettinger SJ, Feldman EC, Côté E, editors. Textbook of veterinary internal medicine. 8th edition. Saint Louis (MO): Elsevier; 2017. p. 1919–34.

6. Koutsos EA, Smith J, Woods LW, et al. Adult cockatiels (*Nymphicus hollandicus*) metabolically adapt to high protein diets. J Nutr 2001;131:2014–20.

7. Nechay BR, Nechay L. Effects of probenecid, sodium salicylate, 2,4-dinitrophenol and pyrazinamide on renal secretion of uric acid in chickens. J Pharmacol Exp Ther 1959;126:291–5.

8. Speer B. Diseases of the urogenital system. In: Altman RB, Clubb SL, Dorrestein GM, et al, editors. Avian medicine and surgery. Philadelphia: WB Saunders; 1997. p. 628–9.

9. Powers LV. Common procedures in psittacines. Vet Clin North Am Exot Anim Pract 2006;9:287–302.

10. Jenkins JR. Critical care of pet birds. Vet Clin North Am Exot Anim Pract 2016; 19:501–12.

11. Lichtenberger M, Lennox A. Critical care. In: Speer BL, editor. Current therapy of avian medicine and surgery. 1st edition. Saint Louis (MO): Elsevier; 2016. p. 582–8.

12. Heard D. Anesthesia. In: Speer BL, editor. Current therapy of avian medicine and surgery. 1st edition. Saint Louis (MO): Elsevier; 2016. p. 601–15.

13. Kiang JH. Avian wing bones. UC San Diego Electronic Theses and Dissertations. 2013.

14. McDonald D. Nutritional considerations: nutrition and dietary supplementation. In: Harrison GJ, Lightfoot TL, editors. Clinical avian medicine, vol. 1, 2nd edition. Palm Beach (FL): Spix Publishing Inc; 2005. p. 86–107.

15. Mayer J, Donnelly TM. Renal disease. In: Mayer J, Donnelly TM, editors. Clinical veterinary advisor. Birds and exotic pets. Saint Louis (MO): Elsevier; 2013. p. 228–9.

16. Echols S. Evaluating and treating the kidneys. In: Harrison GJ, Lightfoot TL, editors. Clinical avian medicine, vol. 2, 2nd edition. Palm Beach (FL): Spix Publishing Inc; 2005. p. 451–92.

17. Duncan M. Gout in exotic animals. In: Miller RE, Fowler ME, editors. Fowler's zoo and wild animal medicine. 8th edition. Saint Louis (MO): Elsevier; 2015. p. 667–70.

18. Rupley AE, Simone-Freilicher E. Psittacine wellness management and environmental enrichment. Vet Clin North Am Exot Anim Pract 2015;18:197–211.

19. Bartges JW. Nutritional management of renal conditions. In: Ettinger SJ, Feldman EC, Côté E, editors. Textbook of veterinary internal medicine. 8th edition. Saint Louis (MO): Elsevier; 2017. p. 771–3.

20. Koutsos E, Gelis S, Echols MS. Advancements in nutrition and nutritional therapy. In: Speer BL, editor. Current therapy of avian medicine and surgery. 1st edition. Saint Louis (MO): Elsevier; 2016. p. 142–76.

21. Nettleton JA. Omega-3 fatty acids: comparison of plant and seafood sources in human nutrition. J Am Diet Assoc 1991;91:331–7.

22. Heinze CR, Hawkins MG, Gillies LA, et al. Effect of dietary omega-3 fatty acids on red blood cell lipid composition and plasma metabolites in the cockatiel, *Nymphicus hollandicus*. J Anim Sci 2012;90:3068–79.

23. USDA Food Composition Databases [Internet]. Available at: https://ndb.nal. usda.gov/ndb/. Accessed September 6, 2019.

24. Settle T, Carro MD, Falkenstein E, et al. The effects of allopurinol, uric acid, and inosine administration on xanthine oxidoreductase activity and uric acid concentrations in broilers. Poult Sci 2012;91:2895–903.

25. Carro MD, Falkenstein E, Radke WJ, et al. Effects of allopurinol on uric acid concentrations, xanthine oxidoreductase activity and oxidative stress in broiler chickens. Comp Biochem Physiol C Toxicol Pharmacol 2010;151:12–7.
26. Lumeij JT, Sprang EP, Redig PT. Further studies on allopurinol-induced hyperuricaemia and visceral gout in red-tailed hawks (*Buteo jamaicensis*). Avian Pathol 1998;27:390–3.
27. Poffers J, Lumeij JT, Timmermans-Sprang EPM, et al. Further studies on the use of allopurinol to reduce plasma uric acid concentrations in the red-tailed hawk (*Buteo jamaicensis*) hyperuricaemic model. Avian Pathol 2002;31:567–72.
28. Siller WG. Renal pathology of the fowl, a review. Avian Pathol 1981;10:187–262.
29. Poffers J, Lumeij JT, Redig PT. Investigations into the uricolytic properties of urate oxidase in a granivorous (*Columba livia domestica*) and in a carnivorous (*Buteo jamaicensis*) avian species. Avian Pathol 2002;31:573–9.
30. Snoeyenbos GH, Reynolds IM, Tzianabos T. Articular gout in turkeys: a case report. Avian Dis 1962;6:32–6.
31. Dudas PL, Pelis RM, Braun EJ, et al. Transepithelial urate transport by avian renal proximal tubule epithelium in primary culture. J Exp Biol 2005;208:4305–15.
32. Martinez-Silvestre A. Treatment with allopurinol and probenecid for visceral gout in a Greek tortoise, *Testudo graeca*. Bulletin of the Association of Reptilians and Amphibian Veterinarians 1997;7:4–5.
33. Creamer P, Hunt M, Dieppe P. Pain mechanisms in osteoarthritis of the knee: effect of intraarticular anesthetic. J Rheumatol 1996;23:1031–6.
34. Hocking PM, Gentle MJ, Bernard R, et al. Evaluation of a protocol for determining the effectiveness of pretreatment with local analgesics for reducing experimentally induced articular pain in domestic fowl. Res Vet Sci 1997;63:263–7.
35. Hawkins MG, Paul-Murphy J, Sanchez-Migallon Guzman D. Advances in anesthesia, analgesia, and surgery. In: Speer BL, editor. Current therapy of avian medicine and surgery. 1st edition. Saint Louis (MO): Elsevier; 2016. p. 616–30.
36. Souza MJ, Gerhardt L, Cox S. Pharmacokinetics of repeated oral administration of tramadol hydrochloride in Hispaniolan Amazon parrots (*Amazona ventralis*). Am J Vet Res 2013;74:957–62.
37. Laniesse D, Sanchez-Migallon Guzman D, Knych HK, et al. Pharmacokinetics of butorphanol tartrate in a long-acting poloxamer 407 gel formulation administered to Hispaniolan Amazon parrots (*Amazona ventralis*). Am J Vet Res 2017;78:688–94.
38. Baine K, Jones MP, Cox S, et al. Pharmacokinetics of compounded intravenous and oral gabapentin in Hispaniolan Amazon Parrots (*Amazona ventralis*). J Avian Med Surg 2015;29:165–74.
39. Cole GA, Paul-Murphy J, Krugner-Higby L, et al. Analgesic effects of intramuscular administration of meloxicam in Hispaniolan parrots (*Amazona ventralis*) with experimentally induced arthritis. Am J Vet Res 2009;70:1471–6.
40. Curtiss JB, Leone AM, Wellehan JFX, et al. Renal and cloacal cryptosporidiosis (*Cryptosporidium avian* genotype V) in a major Mitchell's cockatoo (*Lophochroa leadbeateri*). J Zoo Wildl Med 2015;46:934–7.
41. Hinrichsen JP, Neira M, Lopez C, et al. Omeprazole, a specific gastric secretion inhibitor on oxynticopeptic cells, reduces gizzard erosion in broiler chicks fed with toxic fish meals. Comp Biochem Physiol C Pharmacol Toxicol Endocrinol 1997;117:267–73.

42. Harrison GJ, Lightfoot TL, Flinchum GB. Emergency and critical care. In: Harrison GJ, Lightfoot TL, editors. Clinical avian medicine, vol. 1, 2nd edition. Palm Beach (FL): Spix Publishing Inc; 2005. p. 213–32.

43. Pollock C. Diagnosis and treatment of avian renal disease. Vet Clin North Am Exot Anim Pract 2006;9:107–28.

44. Johnson JG, Brandao J, Perry SM, et al. Urinary system. In: Mitchell MA, Tully TN, editors. Current therapy of exotic pet practice. 1st edition. Saint Louis (MO): Elsevier; 2016.

45. Mutalib A, Keirs R, Austin F. Erysipelas in quail and suspected erysipeloid in processing plant employees. Avian Dis 1995;39:191–3.

46. Sato Y, Aoyagi T, Matsuura S, et al. An occurrence of avian tuberculosis in hooded merganser (*Lophodytes cucullatus*). Avian Dis 1996;40:941–4.

47. Ackerman LJ, Benbrook SC, Walton BC. *Mycobacterium tuberculosis* infection in a parrot (*Amazona farinosa*). Am Rev Respir Dis 1974;109:388–90.

48. Junge RE, MacCoy DM. Amikacin therapy for *Pseudomonas cellulitis* in an Amazon parrot. J Am Vet Med Assoc 1985;187:417–8.

49. Flammer K, Clark CH, Drewes LA, et al. Adverse effects of gentamicin in scarlet macaws and galahs. Am J Vet Res 1990;51:404–7.

50. Leal de Araujo J, Rech RR, Heatley JJ, et al. From nerves to brain to gastrointestinal tract: a time-based study of parrot bornavirus 2 (PaBV-2) pathogenesis in cockatiels (*Nymphicus hollandicus*). PLoS One 2017;12:11.

51. Payne S, Shivaprasad HL, Mirhosseini N, et al. Unusual and severe lesions of proventricular dilatation disease in cockatiels (*Nymphicus hollandicus*) acting as healthy carriers of avian bornavirus (ABV) and subsequently infected with a virulent strain of ABV. Avian Pathol 2011;40:15–22.

52. Palmieri C, Franca M, Uzal F, et al. Pathology and immunohistochemical findings of west Nile virus infection in psittaciformes. Vet Pathol 2011;48:975–84.

53. Gajadhar AA, Cawthorn RJ, Wobeser GA, et al. Prevalence of renal coccidia in wild waterfowl in Saskatchewan. Can J Zool 1983;61:2631–3.

54. Randall CJ. Renal and nasal cryptosporidiosis in a junglefowl (*Gallus sonneratii*). Vet Rec 1986;119:130–1.

55. Gardiner CH, Imes GD. *Cryptosporidium* sp in the kidneys of a black-throated finch. J Am Vet Med Assoc 1984;185:1401–2.

56. Baker KC, Rettenmund CL, Sander SJ, et al. Clinical effect of hemoparasite infections in snowy owls (*Bubo Scandiacus*). J Zoo Wildl Med 2018;49:143–52.

57. Plumb DC. Plumb's veterinary drug handbook. 9th edition. Hoboken (NJ): Wiley-Blackwell; 2018.

58. Forbes NA, Fox MT. Field trial of a *Caryospora* species vaccine for controlling clinical coccidiosis in falcons. Vet Rec 2005;156:134–8.

59. Carpenter JW. Exotic animal formulary. 5th edition. Saint Louis (MO): Elsevier; 2018.

60. Mathis GF, Froyman R, Irion T, et al. Coccidiosis control with toltrazuril in conjunction with anticoccidial medicated or nonmedicated feed. Avian Dis 2003;47:463–9.

61. Sokól R, Galecki R. The resistance of *Eimeria* spp. to toltrazuril in black grouse (*Lyrurus tetrix*) kept in an aviary. Poult Sci 2018;97(12):4193–9.

62. Stephen B, Rommel M, Daugschies A, et al. Studies of resistance to anticoccidials in *Eimeria* field isolates and pure *Eimeria* strains. Vet Parasitol 1997;69:19–29.

63. Harfoush MA, Hegazy AM, Soliman AH, et al. Drug resistance evaluation of some commonly used anti-coccidial drugs in broiler chickens. J Egypt Soc Parasitol 2010;40:337–48.

64. Lan LH, Sun BB, Zuo BXZ, et al. Prevalence and drug resistance of avian *Eimeria* species in broiler chicken farms of Zhejiang province, China. Poult Sci 2017; 96:2104–9.

65. Ahad S, Tanveer S, Nawchoo IA, et al. Anticoccidial activity of *Artemisia vestita* (Anthemideae, Asteraceae), a traditional herb growing in the Western Himalayas, Kashmir, India. Microb Pathog 2017;104:289–95.

66. Hayajneh FMF, Jalal M, Zakaria H, et al. Anticoccidial effect of apple cider vinegar on broiler chicken: an organic treatment to measure anti-oxidant effect. Pol J Vet Sci 2018;21:361–9.

67. Malik TA, Kamili AN, Chishti MZ, et al. Synergistic approach for treatment of chicken coccidiosis using berberine, a plant natural product. Microb Pathog 2016;93:56–62.

68. Muthamilselvan T, Kuo TF, Wu YC, et al. Herbal remedies for coccidiosis control: a review of plants, compounds, and anticoccidial actions. Evid Based Complement Alternat Med 2016;2016:2657981.

69. Dahlhausen RD. Implications of mycoses in clinical disorders. In: Harrison GJ, Lightfoot TL, editors. Clinical avian medicine, vol. 2, 2nd edition. Palm Beach (FL): Spix Publishing Inc; 2005. p. 691–704.

70. Greenacre CB, Latimer KS, Ritchie BW. Leg paresis in a black palm cockatoo (*Probosciger aterrimus*) caused by aspergillosis. J Zoo Wildl Med 1992;23: 122–6.

71. Martel A, Wellehan JFX, Lierz M, et al. Infectious disease. In: Speer BL, editor. Current therapy of avian medicine and surgery. 1st edition. Saint Louis (MO): Elsevier; 2016. p. 22–106.

72. Antonissen G, Martel A. Antifungal therapy in birds: old drugs in a new jacket. Vet Clin North Am Exot Anim Pract 2018;21:355–77.

73. Ziołkowska G, Tokarzewski S, Nowakiewicz A. Drug resistance of *Aspergillus fumigatus* strains isolated from flocks of domestic geese in Poland. Poult Sci 2014; 93:1106–12.

74. Redig PT, Duke GE. Comparative pharmacokinetics of antifungal drugs in domestic turkeys, red-tailed hawks, broad-winged hawks, and great-horned owls. Avian Dis 1985;29:649–61.

75. Summa NM, Sanchez-Migallon Guzman D. Evidence-based advances in avian medicine. Vet Clin North Am Exot Anim Pract 2017;20:817–37.

76. Beernaert LA, Pasmans F, Van Waeyenberghe L, et al. Avian *Aspergillus fumigatus* strains resistant to both itraconazole and voriconazole. Antimicrob Agents Chemother 2009;53:2199–201.

77. Hoppes S, Gurfield N, Flammer K, et al. Mycotic keratitis in a blue-fronted Amazon Parrot (*Amazona aestiva*). J Avian Med Surg 2000;14:185–90.

78. Maccolini ÉO, Dufresne PJ, Aschenbroich SA, et al. A disseminated *Cryptococcus gattii* VGIIa Infection in a citron-crested cockatoo (*Cacatua sulphurea citrinocristata*) in Québec, Canada. J Avian Med Surg 2017;31:142–51.

79. Evans EE, Emery LC, Cox SK, et al. Pharmacokinetics of terbinafine after oral administration of a single dose to Hispaniolan Amazon parrots (*Amazona ventralis*). Am J Vet Res 2013;74:835–8.

80. Bechert U, Christensen JM, Poppenga R, et al. Pharmacokinetics of terbinafine after single oral dose administration in red-tailed hawks (*Buteo jamaicensis*). J Avian Med Surg 2010;24:122–30.

81. Bechert U, Christensen JM, Poppenga R, et al. Pharmacokinetics of orally administered terbinafine in African penguins (*Spheniscus demersus*) for potential treatment of aspergillosis. J Zoo Wildl Med 2010;41:263–74.

82. Bunting EM, Abou-Madi N, Cox S, et al. Evaluation of oral itraconazole administration in captive Humboldt penguins (*Spheniscus humboldti*). J Zoo Wildl Med 2009;40:508–18.

83. Orosz SE, Frazier DL, Schroeder EC, et al. Pharmacokinetic properties of itraconazole in blue-fronted Amazon parrots (*Amazona aestiva aestiva*). J Avian Med Surg 1996;10:168–73.

84. Lumeij JT, Gorgevska D, Woestenborghs R. Plasma and tissue concentrations of itraconazole in racing pigeons (*Columba livia domestica*). J Avian Med Surg 1995;9:32–5.

85. Jones MP, Orosz SE, Cox SK, et al. Pharmacokinetic disposition of itraconazole in red-tailed hawks (*Buteo jamaicensis*). J Avian Med Surg 2000;14:15–22.

86. Keller KA. Itraconazole. J Exot Pet Med 2011;20:156–60.

87. Parsley RA, Tell LA, Gehring R. Pharmacokinetics of a single dose of voriconazole administered orally with and without food to red-tailed hawks (*Buteo jamaicensus*). Am J Vet Res 2017;78:433–9.

88. Gentry J, Montgerard C, Crandall E, et al. Voriconazole disposition after single and multiple, oral doses in healthy, adult red-tailed hawks (*Buteo jamaicensis*). J Avian Med Surg 2014;28:201–8.

89. Flammer K, Nettifee Osborne JA, Webb DJ, et al. Pharmacokinetics of voriconazole after oral administration of single and multiple doses in African grey parrots (*Psittacus erithacus timneh*). Am J Vet Res 2008;69:114–21.

90. Sanchez-Migallon Guzman D, Flammer K, Papich MG, et al. Pharmacokinetics of voriconazole after oral administration of single and multiple doses in Hispaniolan Amazon parrots (*Amazona ventralis*). Am J Vet Res 2010;71:460–7.

91. Kline Y, Clemons KV, Woods L, et al. Pharmacokinetics of voriconazole in adult mallard ducks (*Anas platyrhynchos*). Med Mycol 2011;49:500–12.

92. Burhenne J, Haefeli WE, Hess M, et al. Pharmacokinetics, tissue concentrations, and safety of the antifungal agent voriconazole in chickens. J Avian Med Surg 2008;22:199–207.

93. Hyatt MW, Wiederhold NP, Hope WW, et al. Pharmacokinetics of orally administered voriconazole in African penguins (*Spheniscus demersus*) after single and multiple doses. J Zoo Wildl Med 2017;48:352–62.

94. Schmidt V, Demiraj F, Somma AD, et al. Plasma concentrations of voriconazole in falcons. Vet Rec 2007;161:265–8.

95. Sanchez-Migallon Guzman D. Advances in avian clinical therapeutics. J Exot Pet Med 2014;23:6–20.

96. Schunk RSK, Sitinas NE, Quesenberry KE, et al. Multicentric cryptococcosis in a Congo African grey parrot (*Psittacus erithacus erithacus*). J Avian Med Surg 2017;31:373–81.

97. Randall CJ, Lees S, Higgins RJ, et al. Microsporidian infection in lovebirds (*Agapornis* spp.). Avian Pathol 1986;15:223–31.

98. Barton CE, Phalen DN, Snowden KF. Prevalence of microsporidian spores shed by asymptomatic lovebirds: evidence for a potential emerging zoonosis. J Avian Med Surg 2003;17:197–202.

99. Pulparampil N, Graham D, Phalen D, et al. *Encephalitozoon hellem* in two eclectus parrots (*Eclectus roratus*): identification from archival tissues. J Eukaryot Microbiol 1998;45:651–5.

100. Phalen DN, Logan KS, Snowden KF. *Encephalitozoon hellem* infection as the cause of a unilateral chronic keratoconjunctivitis in an umbrella cockatoo (*Cacatua alba*). Vet Ophthalmol 2006;9:59–63.
101. Wismer T. Advancements in diagnosis and management of toxicologic problems. In: Speer BL, editor. Current therapy of avian medicine and surgery. 1st edition. Saint Louis (MO): Elsevier; 2016. p. 589–99.
102. Richardson JA. Implications of toxic substances in clinical disorders. In: Harrison GJ, Lightfoot TL, editors. Clinical avian medicine, vol. 2, 2nd edition. Palm Beach (FL): Spix Publishing Inc; 2005. p. 711–20.
103. Carlson BL, Nielsen SW. Influence of dietary calcium on lead poisoning in mallard ducks (*Anas platyrynchos*). Am J Vet Res 1985;46:276–82.
104. Pikula J, Hajkova P, Bandouchova H, et al. Lead toxicosis of captive vultures: case description and responses to chelation therapy. BMC Vet Res 2013;9:11.
105. Samour JH, Naldo J. Diagnosis and therapeutic management of lead toxicosis in falcons in Saudi Arabia. J Avian Med Surg 2002;16:16–20.
106. Denver MC, Tell LA, Galey FD, et al. Comparison of two heavy metal chelators for treatment of lead toxicosis in cockatiels. Am J Vet Res 2000;61:935–40.
107. Andersen O. Principles and recent developments in chelation treatment of metal intoxication. Chem Rev 1999;99:2683–710.
108. Gozalo AS, Schwiebert RS, Lawson GW. Mortality associated with fenbendazole administration in pigeons (*Columba livia*). J Am Assoc Lab Anim Sci 2006; 45:63–6.
109. Sharma AK, Saini M, Singh SD, et al. Diclofenac is toxic to the steppe eagle, *Aquila nipalensis*: widening the diversity of raptors threatened by NSAID misuse in South Asia. Bird Conserv Int 2014;24:282–6.
110. Cuthbert R, Parry-Jones J, Green RE, et al. NSAIDs and scavenging birds: potential impacts beyond Asia's critically endangered vultures. Biol Lett 2007; 3:90–3.
111. Coutant T, Vergneau-Grosset C, Langlois I. Overview of drug delivery methods in exotics, including their anatomic and physiologic considerations. Vet Clin North Am Exot Anim Pract 2018;21:215–59.
112. Kubiak M, Forbes NA. Fluoroscopic evaluation of gastrointestinal transit time in African Grey parrots. Vet Rec 2012;171:563.
113. Doss GA, Williams JM, Mans C. Determination of gastrointestinal transit times in barred owls (*Strix varia*) by contrast fluoroscopy. J Avian Med Surg 2017;31: 123–8.
114. Bloch RA, Cronin K, Hoover JP, et al. Evaluation of gastrointestinal tract transit times using barium-impregnated polyethylene spheres and barium sulfate suspension in a domestic pigeon (*Columba livia*) model. J Avian Med Surg 2010; 24:1–8.
115. Vink-Nooteboom M, Lumeij JT, Wolvekamp WTC. Radiography and image-intensified fluoroscopy of barium passage through the gastrointestinal tract in six healthy Amazon parrots (*Amazona aestiva*). Vet Radiol Ultrasound 2003; 44:43–8.
116. Lightfoot TL, Yeager JM. Pet bird toxicity and related environmental concerns. Vet Clin North Am Exot Anim Pract 2008;11:229–59.
117. Palmer D, Rubel A, Mettler F, et al. Experimentally induced skin changes in land tortoises by giving high doses of vitamin A parenterally. Zentralbl Veterinarmed A 1984;31:625.
118. Koutsos EA, Klasing KC. Vitamin A nutrition of growing cockatiel chicks (*Nymphicus hollandicus*). J Anim Physiol Anim Nutr 2005;89:379–87.

119. Wolf P, Bartels T, Sallmann HP, et al. Vitamin A metabolism in recessive white canaries. Anim Welf 2000;9:153–65.

120. Mellanby RJ, Mee AP, Berry JL, et al. Hypercalcaemia in two dogs caused by excessive dietary supplementation of vitamin D. J Small Anim Pract 2005;46: 334–8.

121. Wehner A, Katzenberger J, Groth A, et al. Vitamin D intoxication caused by ingestion of commercial cat food in three kittens. J Feline Med Surg 2013;15: 730–6.

122. Harrison GJ, McDonald D. Nutritional considerations: nutritional disorders. In: Harrison GJ, Lightfoot TL, editors. Clinical avian medicine, vol. 1, 2nd edition. Palm Beach (FL): Spix Publishing Inc; 2005. p. 108–40.

123. Lowenstine L, Stasiak IM. Update on iron overload in zoologic species. In: Miller RE, Fowler ME, editors. Fowler's zoo and wild animal medicine. 8th edition. Saint Louis (MO): Elsevier; 2015. p. 674–80.

124. Johnston GB. Iron storage disease (hemochromatosis) in softbilled birds. Journal of the American Federation of Aviculture 1999;26:25–8.

125. Whiteside DP, Barker IK, Mehren KG, et al. Clinical evaluation of the oral iron chelator deferiprone for the potential treatment of iron overload in bird species. J Zoo Wildl Med 2004;35:40–9.

126. Sandmeier P, Clauss M, Donati OF, et al. Use of deferiprone for the treatment of hepatic iron storage disease in three hornbills. J Am Vet Med Assoc 2012;240: 75–81.

127. Gancz AY, Wellehan JFX, Boutette J, et al. Diabetes mellitus concurrent with hepatic haemosiderosis in two macaws (Ara severa, Ara militaris). Avian Pathol 2007;36:331–6.

128. Taylor WM. Clinical significance of the avian cloaca; Interrelationships with the kidney and the hindgut. In: Speer BL, editor. Current therapy of avian medicine and surgery. 1st edition. Saint Louis (MO): Elsevier; 2016. p. 341–2.

129. Beaufrère H, Nevarez J, Tully TN. Cloacolith in a blue-fronted amazon parrot (Amazona aestiva). J Avian Med Surg 2010;24:142–5.

130. Dennis PM, Bennett RA. Ureterotomy for removal of two ureteroliths in a parrot. J Am Vet Med Assoc 2000;217:865–8.

131. Marietto-Gonçalves GA, Salgado BS. Post-mortem lesions of urolithiasis in a lesser seed finch (Sporophila angolensis). Acta Vet Bras 2012;6:52–5.

132. Wideman RF, Closser JA, Roush WB, et al. Urolithiasis in pullets and laying hens: role of dietary calcium and phosphorus. Poult Sci 1985;64:2300–7.

133. Brown TP, Glisson JR, Rosales G, et al. Studies of avian urolithiasis associated with an infectious bronchitis virus. Avian Dis 1987;31:629–36.

134. Machado C, Mihm F, Buckley DN. Disintegration of kidney stones by extracorporeal shockwave lithotripsy in a penguin. Proceeding of first international conference of zoological avian medicine. Oahu Hawaii, September 6–11, 1987. p. 343–9.

135. Simova-Curd S, Nitzl D, Mayer J, et al. Clinical approach to renal neoplasia in budgerigars (Melopsittacus undulatus). J Small Anim Pract 2006;47:504–11.

136. Robat CS, Ammersbach M, Mans C. Avian oncology: diseases, diagnostics, and therapeutics. Vet Clin North Am Exot Anim Pract 2017;20:57–86.

137. Brown S, Sandersen SL. Urinary system. In: Kahn CM, Line S, editors. The Merck veterinary manual. Non-infectious diseases of the urinary system in small animals. 9th edition. Summerset, (South Dakota): John Wiley and Sons; 2005. p. 1249–88.

138. Freeman KP, Hahn KA, Jones MP, et al. Right leg muscle atrophy and osteopenia caused by renal adenocarcinoma in a cockatiel (*Melopsittacus, undulatus*). Vet Radiol Ultrasound 1999;40:144–7.
139. Zehnder A, Graham J, Antonissen G. Update on cancer treatment in exotics. Vet Clin North Am Exot Anim Pract 2018;21:465–509.
140. Macwhirter P, Pyke D, Wayne J. Use of carboplatin in the treatment of a renal adenocarcinoma in a budgerigar. Exotic DVM 2002;4:11–2.
141. Hammond EE, Sanchez-Migallon Guzman D, Garner MM, et al. Long-term treatment of chronic lymphocytic leukemia in a green-winged macaw (*Ara chloroptera*). J Avian Med Surg 2010;24:330–8.
142. Osofsky A, Hawkins MG, Foreman O, et al. T-cell chronic lymphocytic leukemia in a double yellow-headed Amazon parrot (*Amazona ochrocephala oratrix*). J Avian Med Surg 2011;25:286–94.
143. Sinclair KM, Hawkins MG, Wright L, et al. Chronic T-cell lymphocytic leukemia in a black swan (*Cygnus atratus*): diagnosis, treatment, and pathology. J Avian Med Surg 2015;29:326–35.
144. Barron HW, Roberts RE, Latimer KS, et al. Tolerance doses of cutaneous and mucosal tissues in ring-necked parakeets (*Psittacula krameri*) for external beam megavoltage radiation. J Avian Med Surg 2009;23:6–9.

Anatomy and Physiology of the Reptile Renal System

Peter H. Holz, BVSc, DVSc, MACVSc, DACZM

KEYWORDS

- Reptile renal anatomy • Reptile renal physiology • Urinary bladder • Urea • Uric acid
- Reptile kidney • Cloaca • Renal portal system

KEY POINTS

- Reptile kidneys are relatively simple in structure compared with birds and mammals. They contain fewer nephrons and lack a Loop of Henle. Therefore, the kidneys cannot produce a hypertonic urine.
- Only chelonians, the tuatara, and some lizards have a urinary bladder.
- Additional fluids and electrolytes are excreted and absorbed through the cloaca and urinary bladder.
- Aquatic reptiles excrete predominantly urea, while terrestrial reptiles excrete predominantly uric acid to conserve water.
- All reptiles have a renal portal system, which can direct blood from the caudal extremities either through or around the kidneys. The renal portal system functions to prevent ischemic necrosis of the tubule cells during periods of water deprivation.

INTRODUCTION

The kidneys function to maintain a constant extracellular environment within the body. They excrete waste products, maintain normal concentrations of salt and water, regulate acid-base balance, and produce a variety of hormones and vitamins.[1] Reptiles are the first class of animals to lack an aquatic larval stage and to be capable of survival solely on dry land. An entirely terrestrial existence is possible only through the conservation of water and salt and the excretion of organic and inorganic metabolites. The kidney has evolved to perform these functions by filtering extracellular fluid, resorbing essential nutrients, and excreting waste products. Although some variations do occur, reptilian kidneys follow the basic vertebrate plan. The kidneys contain nephrons, which consist of glomeruli designed to filter the plasma, Bowman's capsules to collect the filtrate, and tubules to resorb most of the filtered water and nutrients while excreting waste metabolites.

Disclosure statement: The author has nothing to disclose.
Faculty of Veterinary and Agricultural Sciences, University of Melbourne, 250 Princes Highway, Werribee, Victoria 3777, Australia
E-mail address: prjlholz@gmail.com

GROSS ANATOMY

The reptilian urinary tract consists of paired kidneys, each connected to the cloaca by a ureter (**Fig. 1**).[2] A urinary bladder may be present. Unlike mammals, reptiles do not have separate openings for the discharge of urinary and digestive waste products. The end products of the digestive, urinary, and reproductive systems all enter a single chamber, the cloaca, and are discharged through a single opening, the vent.

The cloaca is divided into 3 regions.[3] The coprodeum is the most anterior section and receives the waste products of digestion from the rectum. The middle section, or urodeum, receives the ureters, urinary bladder, and genital ducts. In some species, the genital ducts and ureters penetrate the urodeum separately, but in others they fuse before entering the urodeum. Posterior to the urodeum is the proctodeum, which is the final stop before waste and reproductive products are discharged to the exterior through the vent.

Order Squamata: Suborder Sauria

In most lizards, the kidneys are located deep within the pelvic canal. Monitors are the exception to this rule of thumb, and their kidneys sit in the caudal coelom.[4] The kidneys are paired, symmetric, elongated, slightly lobulated, and flattened dorsoventrally. The caudal aspect of the kidneys is fused in many species and are fully separate in the water monitor (*Varanus salvator*) and chameleons.[2]

The literature regarding the presence of a urinary bladder in lizards is confusing and inconsistent. Well-developed urinary bladders, which connect to the ventral urodeum by a urethra, have been reported in slow worms (*Anguis* spp.); worm lizards (*Amphisbaena* spp.); wall lizards (Lacertidae); anoles (*Anolis* spp.); many Iguanidae, including the green iguana (*Iguana iguana*); geckos; chameleons; some skinks, including the shingleback skink (*Tiliqua rugosa*), blue-tongued skink (*Tiliqua scincoides*), and pygmy spiny-tailed skink (*Egernia depressa*); some agamids, including spiny-tailed lizards (*Uromastyx* spp.); and the Gila monster (*Heloderma suspectum*). A rudimentary bladder exists in the Teiidae, which include the ameivas, tegus, and whiptails. A bladder is not present in bearded dragons (*Pogona vitticeps*) or most monitors (*Varanus* spp.).[2,5–9] A urinary bladder was reported to exist in neonatal spiny lizards (*Sceloporus* spp.) but not in adults, having degenerated to a vestigial structure.[10]

The vent appears as a fold of skin on the ventral side of the tail, just caudal to the attachment of the tail base to the pelvic girdle. Depending on the species, the vent may be slitlike, with the opening running transversely across the tail base, or round, placed centrally just caudal to the pelvis. The vent is covered by multiple, single scales in iguanas, a single large scale on the anterior and posterior margin in skinks, or fleshy, soft skin in geckos. In males, 2 copulatory structures, the hemipenes, open on either

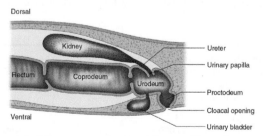

Fig. 1. Simplified model of the gross anatomy of the reptilian urinary tract and cloaca.

side of the vent. The hemipenes are tucked caudally into the tail and evert when engorged during mating.

Arterial blood is supplied to the kidneys by a variable number of renal arteries that branch off the aorta.[2] These renal arteries penetrate the medial aspect of the kidneys and branch into interlobular arteries. These interlobular arteries, in turn, branch to form afferent glomerular arterioles, which give rise to glomerular capillary loops. The capillaries rejoin to form efferent glomerular arterioles, which are also connected to the renal portal veins.[11]

Lizards, like all reptiles, have a renal portal system, which can potentially convey blood from the caudal regions of the body through the kidneys, before continuing to the heart (**Fig. 2**).[12–14] A single caudal vein drains the tail region and bifurcates to form 2 afferent renal portal veins. Two iliac veins drain the hind limbs and connect to the afferent renal portal veins via an anastomosis before continuing anteriorly as the pelvic veins. The afferent renal portal veins penetrate the kidneys and divide into a series of capillaries that perfuse only the renal tubule cells, not the glomeruli. Blood then leaves each kidney via the efferent renal portal veins. These efferent renal portal veins fuse to form the post caval vein, which becomes the vena cava and conveys blood back to the heart. The pelvic veins unite with the pubic vein and continue anteriorly as the abdominal vein, which conveys blood to the liver.

Suborder Serpentes

Snake kidneys are paired, flattened, and elongated organs containing 25 to 30 lobules,[15] except for dwarf boas (*Tropidophis* spp.) whose kidneys are not lobulated.[2] The right kidney lies cranial to the left.[4] The position of the kidneys has been calculated as a proportion of the distance between the snout and the cloaca (**Table 1**).[15,16] The kidneys occupy approximately 10% to 15% of the snake's body length. A ureter connects each kidney to the urodeum. Unlike the basic reptilian model the urodeum

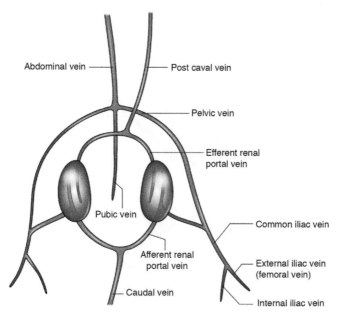

Fig. 2. Renal portal system of order Squamata, suborder Sauria.

Table 1
Kidney position as a proportion of the distance between the snout and the cloaca

Taxonomic Group	Distance Between the Snout and Cloaca
Boids	0.76–0.84
Colubrids	0.84–0.96
Elapids	0.80–0.92
Crotalids	0.84–0.96

lies dorsal to the coprodeum and is separated from it by a horizontal tissue septum. There is no urinary bladder.[4]

The vent is linear, with the slitlike opening running transversely across the tail base. Because there is no outwardly discernible pelvic girdle, except in boids, the vent is considered the beginning of the tail. There is a single scale covering the vent in boas and paired scales in pythons. A pair of hemipenes, similar to lizards, is present.

Arterial blood supply is the same as for the Sauria. The venous blood flow is also similar except for the absence of iliac veins (**Fig. 3**).[12] A large vein arises from each afferent renal portal vein caudal to its insertion in the kidney. These 2 veins unite to form the mesenteric vein, which carries blood to the liver. The abdominal vein is present but is only connected to the afferent renal portal veins in the African rock python (*Python sebae*). In other species, the abdominal vein has its origin in the fat bodies.

Order Rhynchocephalia

The kidneys of the tuatara (*Sphenodon punctatus*) are similar to lizards. They are paired, single lobed, crescentic in outline, and situated along the dorsal wall of the pelvic canal. The 2 kidneys meet posteriorly but do not fuse.[2] Blood supply is similar to lizards; however, there is no direct connection between the iliac veins and the abdominal vein. It has been postulated that a connection to the abdominal vein may exist within the body of the kidneys.[17] A bladder is present. The male does not have a copulatory organ.

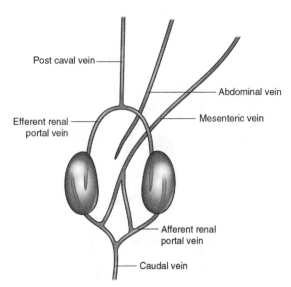

Fig. 3. Renal portal system of order Squamata, suborder Serpentes.

Order Testudines

Chelonian kidneys are paired and lie in the caudal coelom just ventral to the carapace. In marine turtles the kidneys are cranial to the pelvic girdle. The kidneys are flattened, lobulated, and symmetric.

Ureters leave the kidneys and enter the urinary bladder, as in mammals. The bladder is connected to the cloaca via the urethra.

The vent is circular and lies on the ventral aspect of the tail caudal to its attachment to the plastron. The skin is usually scaleless. The turtle has a single phallus situated cranial to the vent and ventral to the base of the tail. As a result, the vent in males is positioned more caudally than in females. In the female, the vent lies within the margins of the carapace. The vent in males is placed more distally on the tail such that it is beyond the outer margin of the carapace. This is a consistent finding across chelonians and is a reliable method for sex determination.

Arterial and venous blood supply is similar to lizards; however, there are 2 abdominal veins, which are linked by a transverse anastomosis.[12]

Order Crocodylia

Crocodilians have paired lobulated kidneys that lie against the dorsal body wall adjacent to the spinal column. The left kidney may be larger than the right kidney. Ureters enter the cloaca at the urodeum. There is no urinary bladder. Crocodilians have a single phallus, similar to that described for chelonians.

Arterial and venous supply is similar to the lizards[12]; however, there are 2 abdominal veins. Each abdominal vein connects to an iliac vein and, as for snakes, a mesenteric vein originates from the afferent renal portal veins.

MICROSCOPIC ANATOMY

Reptilian kidneys have no pelvis or pyramids, and are not divided into a medulla and cortex. The kidneys contain a few thousand nephrons, compared with 200,000 to 1,800,000 nephrons in humans, 4,000,000 nephrons in cattle, and 200,000 nephrons in cats.[1,2] Reptilian nephrons are 2 to 8 mm long, compared with approximately 18 mm for avian nephrons and 30 to 38 mm for human nephrons.[18] Each nephron is oriented at right angles to the long axis of the kidney and enters the collecting duct at right angles (**Fig. 4**).[19]

Structurally, reptilian glomeruli are poorly developed with a lower number of capillaries per gram body weight compared with birds.[18] The glomerulus is followed by the neck segment, proximal tubule, intermediate segment, and distal tubule. There is no loop of Henle. All of the segments, except the distal tubule, consist of ciliated, cuboidal cells. The cells of the distal tubule lack cilia.

The distal tubule is followed by the sex segment (**Fig. 5**). In all female reptiles and male chelonians, this consists of columnar mucous-secreting cells. In male snakes and lizards, the cells are flat and filled with mucus during the nonbreeding season. During the breeding season, these cells increase in height 2 to 4 times and are filled with large refractile granules that stain brightly eosinophilic with hematoxylin and eosin.[20] These granules contain acid phosphatase, phospholipids, glycoprotein, mucoprotein, and amino acids. The function of the secretions contained within the sex segment is unknown. A number of theories have been proposed. These secretions may act to produce a copulatory plug to prevent rivals from mating successfully. Alternatively, the secretions may block the tubules during copulation to keep semen and urine separate, or they may be a source of energy for the sperm.[18]

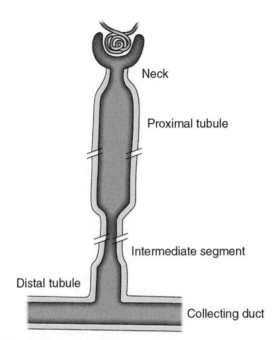

Fig. 4. Diagram of a reptilian nephron.

After the sex segment, the nephron ends with the collecting duct. These cells are similar to those contained within the sex segment except mucus is only present at the tip of the cell. The collecting ducts are oriented at right angles to the long axis of the kidney. They originate on the dorsolateral surface of each lobule, wrap around the lateral margin of the lobule, and pass ventrally into the ureter, which lies on the ventromedial surface of the kidney.

Blood supply to the nephron consists of an afferent arteriole forming the glomerular capillary tuft, which is surrounded by the Bowman's capsule. Blood exits in the efferent arteriole, which supplies blood to the tubule cells. Venous blood, via the renal portal system, mixes with the arteriolar blood at the start of the proximal tubule.

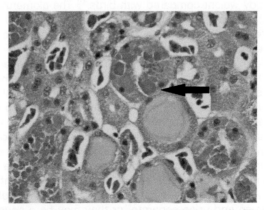

Fig. 5. Sex segment. Hematoxylin and eosin stain (× 400). Note cells filled with large refractive granules (*arrow*).

RENAL PHYSIOLOGY
Water Conservation

One of the major functions of the kidneys in terrestrial vertebrates is the conservation of water. Although reptiles can concentrate their urine, they do not have a loop of Henle, therefore they cannot produce hypertonic urine.[21] The only documented exception is the Lake Eyre dragon lizard (*Ctenophorus maculosus*), which can produce urine more concentrated than plasma; however, it accomplishes this not via the kidneys but by absorbing additional water through the coprodeum and rectum.[22]

In reptiles, regions distal to the kidney, such as the colon, cloaca, and urinary bladder, play a much greater role in water absorption than they do in mammals.[21] The coprodeum is a major site of water resorption with an extensive blood supply and a large number of folds, villi, and microvilli. The quantity of water resorbed by the coprodeum depends on the hydration state of the individual. For example, a well hydrated Rosenberg monitor (*Varanus rosenbergi*) absorbs approximately 8 mL of water per hour from its coprodeum, whereas a dehydrated monitor can absorb up to 21 mL of water per hour.[23]

Reptiles are also able to conserve water by decreasing the number of filtering glomeruli.[21] Reptile glomerular filtration rate (GFR) is normally lower than in other species, such as birds. Compare the GFR for blue-tongued lizards (15.9 mL/kg per hour) with that for starlings (*Sturnus vulgaris*) (169.8 mL/kg per hour).[21] Dehydration or salt loading further decreases the GFR by reducing the number of filtering glomeruli. This process is mediated through the action of arginine vasotocin, which is secreted by the pituitary gland and increases in the circulation with dehydration or salt loading. Conversely, prolactin increases the GFR by increasing the number of filtering glomeruli.[24] Arginine vasotocin constricts the afferent glomerular arterioles causing glomerular filtration to decrease with the potential for filtration to cease altogether. As blood ceases to flow through the nephron, the tubules collapse and transport across the tubular epithelium ceases.[25] In the freshwater turtle (*Pseudemys scripta*), total anuria occurs if plasma osmolality exceeds 20 mOsm. For the desert tortoise (*Gopherus agassizii*), this does not occur until osmolality exceeds 100 mOsm.[26]

The cessation of blood flow through the glomerulus leads to a lack of perfusion of the renal tubule cells, placing them at risk for ischemic necrosis. To minimize this risk, renal portal blood continues to perfuse the tubule cells. Blood from the caudal regions of the body can flow through the kidneys to sustain the tubule cells until glomerular blood flow resumes (**Fig. 6**); however, blood also can be diverted around the kidneys (**Fig. 7**). A valve responsible for regulating the direction of blood flow has been identified in poultry[27] and tentatively described in red-eared sliders (*Trachemys scripta elegans*)[28]; however, a valve has not been identified in iguanas or agamids.[11,13,14] In poultry, adrenaline causes the valve to open, diverting blood around the kidneys and acetylcholine causes it to close, shunting blood through the kidneys.[29] The method of control of renal portal blood flow in reptiles is not currently known.

Clinical implications of the renal portal system are not clear. Some investigators have suggested that drugs should not be injected into the caudal part of the reptilian body because the renal portal system conveys these drugs to the kidney,[30–32] potentially leading to premature excretion and/or nephrotoxicity. However, work on chelonians,[33,34] iguanas,[13] and pythons[35] has failed to substantiate this claim, with plasma drug concentrations being unaffected by injection site.

Nitrogenous Waste Excretion

As well as conserving water, the kidneys also excrete metabolic wastes, particularly the nitrogenous compounds that are the end product of protein metabolism. The

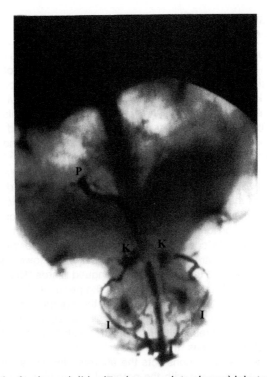

Fig. 6. Radiograph of red-eared slider (*Trachemys scripta elegans*) injected with radiopaque dye (diatrizoate meglumine 370 mg/mL, Hypaque-M, 76%, Sterling-Winthrop Inc., Markham, Ontario, Canada) in the dorsal coccygeal vein. Note dye perfused the kidneys. I, iliac vein; K, kidney; P, post caval vein.

simplest way of doing this is by complexing nitrogen with hydrogen to produce ammonia. This is the preferred method of nitrogenous waste excretion in fish[36]; however, ammonia is toxic to the central nervous system and requires large amounts of water for excretion.[19] Hence, the production of ammonia in reptiles is limited to aquatic species, such as marine turtles, alligators, and crocodiles.[37–39] Ammonia complexes with bicarbonate in crocodilians, resulting in the production of an alkaline urine.[37]

For mammals, the end product of protein metabolism is urea, a substance less soluble than ammonia but 40,000 times more soluble than uric acid.[19] Urea also must be excreted with water, which limits its production in reptiles to species such as freshwater turtles, which produce 45% to 95% of their waste nitrogen as urea.[38,39]

Most reptile species excrete nitrogenous wastes as uric acid, as this product is relatively insoluble and can be excreted with minimal amounts of water.[39] This includes crocodilians that can switch from ammonia to uric acid excretion in times of water deprivation.[37]

Uric acid is actively secreted into the proximal tubule. This process requires potassium, but is independent of sodium.[21] Uric acid secretion increases if blood pH increases, but does not decrease if pH decreases.[18] Once secreted into the tubule, uric acid forms a suspension by complexing with protein and either sodium in carnivorous lizards and snakes to produce an acidic urine or

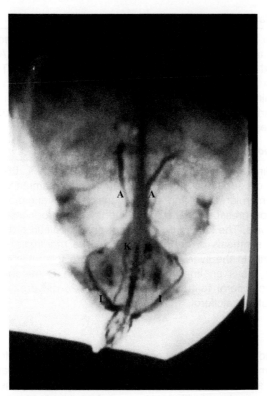

Fig. 7. Radiograph of red-eared slider (*Trachemys scripta elegans*) injected in the dorsal coccygeal vein with the same radiopaque dye as in **Fig. 6**. Note dye entered the abdominal veins and bypassed the kidneys. A, abdominal vein; I, iliac vein; K, kidney.

potassium in herbivorous lizards and terrestrial chelonians to produce an alkaline urine.[40]

This urate suspension contains spheres that are composed of approximately 65% uric acid and range in diameter from 2 to 10 μm.[41] The kidney secretes mucoid substances containing glycoprotein and mucopolysaccharides that aid in sphere formation and prevent clogging of collecting ducts with urates. Consequently, ureteral urine in reptiles contains large amounts of protein, compared with mammals that contain almost none.[19] This protein is not lost to the animal, as once ureteral urine enters the urodeum, it is moved by reverse peristalsis into the coprodeum. Here the protein is reabsorbed and recycled. Hydrogen ions are excreted into the urinary bladder, facilitating the precipitation of uric acid, which forms a semisolid white paste that is excreted.[19]

Cilia are present in the bladder stalk, but not the body, of lizards and terrestrial chelonians.[9] The bladder stalk also contains acid mucopolysaccharide-secreting cells. The cilia beat to move material out of the bladder and are found in reptiles that excrete primarily uric acid and not in species that primarily excrete urea, such as freshwater chelonians. The cilia are believed to expel urates from the bladder, which can then function as an additional water reserve, a particularly useful function for desert-adapted reptiles, such as the Gila monster[42] and desert tortoise.[43]

Electrolyte Regulation

Although 60% to 80% of filtered sodium and chloride is absorbed in the proximal tubules of mammals, only 30% to 50% is absorbed in reptiles.[21] A greater proportion is absorbed in the distal tubules and collecting ducts. The tubules also contribute to the absorption and secretion of potassium, phosphate, magnesium, sulfate, and amino acids, as well as the absorption of calcium, lactate, and glucose.[21] The urinary bladder also is involved in the regulation of sodium, potassium, and magnesium.[44]

Additional Functions

As well as fulfilling water conservation and excretory roles, the reptilian kidney has a number of additional functions. Similar to mammals, reptile kidneys contain juxtaglomerular cells and a functioning renin angiotensin system that can regulate blood pressure.[45] The reptile kidney also produces a number of hormones and vitamins. The kidney is the site of erythropoietin production, a protein required for the synthesis of erythrocytes.[46] Unlike mammals, which synthesize vitamin C primarily in the liver, reptiles manufacture this vitamin in the kidney.[47] The kidney also plays an important role in vitamin D metabolism, converting 25-hydroxycholecalciferol to the active forms, 1α,25-dihydroxycholecalciferol or 24,25-dihydroxycholecalciferol.[48]

SUMMARY

The kidneys found in reptiles are not as highly developed as those found in birds and mammals. To compensate, the essential functions of water conservation, nitrogenous waste excretion, and electrolyte balance are not solely the responsibility of the kidneys. These tasks are shared with the cloaca and urinary bladder. Together, the evolution of these organs has enabled reptiles to be the first class of vertebrates to shed their aquatic ancestry and make a life for themselves on the land.

REFERENCES

1. Cianciolo RE, Mohr FC. Urinary system. In: Maxie MG, editor. Pathology of domestic animals. St Louis (MO): Elsevier; 2016. p. 376–464.
2. Fox H. The urogenital system of reptiles. In: Gans C, editor. Biology of the reptilia. New York: Academic Press; 1977. p. 1–157.
3. O'Malley B. General anatomy and physiology of reptiles. In: Clinical anatomy and physiology of exotic species. Philadelphia: Saunders Limited; 2005. p. 17–39.
4. Canny C. Gross anatomy and imaging of the avian and reptilian urinary system. Semin Avian Exot Pet Med 1998;7:72–80.
5. Anderson CV, Higham TE. Chameleon anatomy. In: Tolley KA, Herrel A, editors. The biology of chameleons. Berkeley (CA): University of California Press; 2014. p. 7–55.
6. Beuchat CA. Phylogenetic distribution of the urinary bladder in lizards. Copeia 1986;1986:512–7.
7. Bell CJ, Hollenshead MG, Mead JI, et al. Presence of a urinary bladder in *Egernia depressa* (Squamata: Scincidae) in Western Australia. Rec West Aust Mus 2010; 25:459–62.
8. Sánchez-Martínez PM, Ramírez-Pinilla MP, Miranda-Esquivel DR. Comparative histology of the vaginal–cloacal region in Squamata and its phylogenetic implications. Acta Zool 2007;88:289–307.

9. Bolton BM, Beuchat CA. Cilia in the urinary bladder of reptiles and amphibians: a correlate of urate production? Copeia 1991;1991:711–7.
10. Beuchat CA, Braun EJ, Vleck D. An ephemeral urinary bladder in neonatal lizards. Herpetologica 1985;41:282–6.
11. O'Shea JE, Bradshaw SD, Stewart T. Renal vasculature and excretory system of the agamid lizard, *Ctenophorus ornatus*. J Morphol 1993;217:287–99.
12. Holz PH. The reptilian renal portal system - a review. Bull Assoc Rept Amphib Vet 1999;9:4–9.
13. Benson KG, Forrest L. Characterization of the renal portal system of the common green iguana (*Iguana iguana*) by digital subtraction imaging. J Zoo Wildl Med 1999;30:235–41.
14. Guo M, Ditrich H, Splechtna H. Renal vasculature and uriniferous tubules in the common iguana. J Morphol 1996;229:97–104.
15. Kell R, Wissdorf H. Beiträge zur Organtopographie bei ungiftigen Schlangen der Familien Boidae (Boas und Pythons) und Colubridae (Nattern). Tierarztl Prax 1992;20:647–56.
16. McCracken H. Organ location in snakes for diagnostic and surgical evaluation. In: Fowler ME, Miller RE, editors. Zoo and wild animal medicine, current therapy, vol. 4. Philadelphia: W.B. Saunders Co; 1999. p. 243–8.
17. Beddard FE. Some additions to the knowledge of the anatomy, principally of the vascular system, of *Hatteria, Crocodilus*, and certain Lacertilia. Proc Zool Soc Lond 1905;461–89.
18. Dantzler WH. Renal function (with special emphasis on nitrogen excretion). In: Gans C, editor. Biology of the reptilia. New York: Academic Press; 1976. p. 447–503.
19. Braun EJ. Comparative renal function in reptiles, birds, and mammals. Semin Avian Exot Pet Med 1998;7:62–71.
20. Zwart P. Anatomy, histology and physiology of the normal reptilian kidney. In: Studies on renal pathology in reptiles. Utrecht (Netherlands): Stichting Pressa Trajectina; 1963. p. 8–25.
21. Dantzler WH. Comparative aspects of renal function. In: Seldin DW, Giebisch G, editors. The kidney: Physiology and pathophysiology. New York: Raven Press; 1985. p. 333–64.
22. Braysher ML. Water and electrolyte balance in the agamid lizard, *Amphibolurus maculosus* (Mitchell), and the structure and function of the nasal salt gland of the sleepy lizard, *Trachydosaurus rugosus* (Gray). Adelaide (Australia): University of Adelaide; 1972. p. 236.
23. King D, Green B. Water use. In: Goanna. 2nd edition. Sydney (Australia): New South Wales University Press; 1999. p. 66–80.
24. Brewer KJ, Ensor DM. Hormonal control of osmoregulation in the chelonia. I. The effects of prolactin and interrenal steroids in freshwater chelonians. Gen Comp Endocrinol 1980;42:304–9.
25. Schmidt-Nielsen B, Davis LE. Fluid transport and tubular intercellular spaces in reptilian kidneys. Science 1968;159:1105–8.
26. Dantzler WH, Schmidt-Nielsen B. Excretion in fresh-water turtle (*Pseudemys scripta*) and desert tortoise (*Gopherus agassizii*). Am J Physiol 1966;210:198–210.
27. Akester AR. Radiographic studies of the renal portal system in the domestic fowl (*Gallus domesticus*). J Anat 1964;98:365–76.
28. Holz P, Barker IK, Crawshaw GJ, et al. The anatomy and perfusion of the renal portal system in the red-eared slider (*Trachemys scripta elegans*). J Zoo Wildl Med 1997;28:378–85.

29. Rennick BR, Gandia H. Pharmacology of smooth muscle valve in renal portal circulation of birds. Proc Soc Exp Biol Med 1954;85:234–6.
30. Gibbons PM. Therapeutics. In: Mader DR, Divers SJ, editors. Current therapy in reptile medicine and surgery. St Louis (MO): Elsevier; 2014. p. 57–69.
31. Sykes JM, Greenacre CB. Techniques for drug delivery in reptiles and amphibians. J Exot Pet Med 2006;15:210–7.
32. Gauvin J. Drug therapy in reptiles. Semin Avian Exot Pet Med 1993;2:48–59.
33. Beck K, Loomis M, Lewbart G, et al. Preliminary comparison of plasma concentrations of gentamicin injected into the cranial and caudal limb musculature of the eastern box turtle (*Terrapene carolina carolina*). J Zoo Wildl Med 1995;26: 265–8.
34. Holz P, Barker IK, Burger JP, et al. The effect of the renal portal system on pharmacokinetic parameters in the red-eared slider (*Trachemys scripta elegans*). J Zoo Wildl Med 1997;28:386–93.
35. Holz PH, Burger JP, Pasloske K, et al. Effect of injection site on carbenicillin pharmacokinetics in the carpet python, *Morelia spilota*. J Herpetol Med Surg 2002; 12:12–6.
36. Stoskopf MK. Clinical pathology. In: Stoskopf MK, editor. Fish medicine. Philadelphia: W.B. Saunders Company; 1993. p. 113–31.
37. Coulson RA, Hernandez T. Kidney. In: Alligator metabolism studies on chemical reactions in vivo. Oxford (England): Pergamon; 1983. p. 143–75.
38. Schmidt-Nielsen B, Skadhauge E. Function of the excretory system of the crocodile (*Crocodylus acutus*). Am J Physiol 1967;212:973–80.
39. Dantzler WH. Transport of organic substances by renal tubules. In: Comparative physiology of the vertebrate kidney. 2nd edition. New York: Springer; 2016. p. 173–236.
40. Minnich JE. Excretion of urate salts by reptiles. Comp Biochem Physiol 1972;41A: 535–49.
41. Minnich JE, Piehl PA. Spherical precipitates in the urine of reptiles. Comp Biochem Physiol 1972;41A:551–4.
42. Davis JR, DeNardo DF. The urinary bladder as a physiological reservoir that moderates dehydration in a large desert lizard, the Gila monster *Heloderma suspectum*. J Exp Biol 2007;210:1472–80.
43. Minnich JE. The use of water. In: Gans C, editor. Biology of the reptilia. Oxford (England): Academic Press; 1982. p. 325–95.
44. Brewer KJ, Ensor DM. Hormonal control of osmoregulation in the chelonia. II. The effect of prolactin and corticosterone on *Testudo graeca*. Gen Comp Endocrinol 1980;42:310–4.
45. Wilson JX. The renin-angiotensin system in nonmammalian vertebrates. Endocr Rev 1984;5:45–61.
46. Wickramasinghe SN, Shiels S, Wickramasinghe PS. Immunoreactive erythropoietin in teleosts, amphibians, reptiles, birds. Evidence that the teleost kidney is both an erythropoietic and erythropoietin-producing organ. Ann N Y Acad Sci 1994;718:366–70.
47. Gillespie DS. Overview of species needing dietary vitamin C. J Zoo Anim Med 1980;11:88–91.
48. Ullrey DE, Bernard JB. Vitamin D: metabolism, sources, unique problems in zoo animals, meeting needs. In: Fowler ME, Miller RE, editors. Zoo and wild animal medicine: current therapy, vol. 4. Philadelphia: W.B. Saunders Co.; 1999. p. 63–78.

Diseases of the Reptile Renal System

James G. Johnson III, DVM, MS, CertAqV, DACZM[a,b,*], Megan K. Watson, DVM, MS, DACZM[c]

KEYWORDS

- Disease • Gout • Infectious • Kidney • Renal • Reptile • Urinary

KEY POINTS

- Reptile renal system anatomy and physiology is different than that of mammals, with variations among reptile taxa that should be considered during clinical evaluation of renal disease.
- Renal disease in reptiles can result from infectious agents, some of which may be zoonotic, and noninfectious diseases, including metabolic conditions from improper husbandry.
- Gout and soft tissue mineralization can be primary renal diseases; however, they are also common sequelae to other causes of renal dysfunction.
- Renal disease in reptiles may manifest with ambiguous or nonspecific clinical signs, such as anorexia, lethargy, and dehydration.

INTRODUCTION

Diseases of the renal system, whether primary or secondary to other systemic disorders, account for a considerable amount of morbidity and mortality in reptiles.[1] These diseases result from a variety of causes, including inadequate husbandry practices, infectious diseases, physiologic disturbances, dehydration, neoplasia, and toxicity. To maintain osmoregulatory balance and prevent accumulation of toxic levels of metabolic wastes, the kidneys and urinary tract rely heavily on vascular perfusion to adequately filter blood and provide nutrition and oxygen delivery to the renal parenchyma.

Reptiles with renal disease may display few and nonspecific signs of illness. Given the ambiguity of clinical signs, renal disease may go unnoticed, with affected animals more likely to have a protracted clinical history that may extend over weeks or months.

Disclosure Statement: The authors have nothing to disclose.
[a] Department of Animal Health, Saint Louis Zoo, One Government Drive, St Louis, MO 63110, USA; [b] Department of Veterinary Preventative Medicine, College of Veterinary Medicine, The Ohio State University, Columbus, OH, USA; [c] Department of Animal Health, Zoo New England, 1 Franklin Park Road, Boston, MA 02121, USA
* Corresponding author. Department of Animal Health, Saint Louis Zoo, One Government Drive, St Louis, MO 63110.
E-mail address: johnson.4013@gmail.com

Vet Clin Exot Anim 23 (2020) 115–129
https://doi.org/10.1016/j.cvex.2019.08.006
1094-9194/20/© 2019 Elsevier Inc. All rights reserved.

Often when clinical signs become apparent, disease has progressed to an advanced stage. As a result, most reptile patients with chronic renal disease present dehydrated and emaciated.[2] Clinical signs in advanced disease can also include variable or decreased appetite and decreased activity or lethargy. Caregivers rarely report polyuria or polydipsia.[2]

The clinical approach to renal disease in reptiles is multifaceted and relies on an understanding of reptile biology and proper husbandry, knowledge of common diseases affecting the urinary system and pathophysiology, and application of this information when creating diagnostic and treatment plans. The reptile practitioner should pay careful attention to the unique variations in the anatomy and physiology of each species when evaluating dysfunction and disease of the renal system. For example, only chelonians and certain lizards possess a urinary bladder.[1] This article aims to highlight urinary pathophysiology and summarize causes of renal disease in reptiles.

REPTILE RENAL PATHOPHYSIOLOGY

Nitrogenous waste production is a byproduct of nutrient consumption.[1] Excretion of these metabolic wastes is fundamental for life. Waste removal helps to maintain homeostasis and prevents pathologic accumulation of these products, which predominantly consist of inorganic salts and nitrogenous wastes.[1] The kidneys and urinary tract rely heavily on vascular perfusion both for filtration of metabolic wastes, as well as nutrition and oxygen delivery to the renal parenchyma. Vascular fluid volume is critical for maintaining renal perfusion for filtration of salts and metabolic waste, emphasizing the importance of animal hydration. During periods of decreased glomerular filtration, renal perfusion is decreased.

In addition to mitigating the accumulation of metabolic wastes, the renal system also functions in osmoregulation and water conservation. Unlike mammalian nephrons, reptilian nephrons lack a loop of Henle, rendering reptile kidneys unable to generate a concentration gradient greater than plasma osmolality in the renal medulla, which aids in reabsorption and conservation of fluid from the renal collecting ducts.[3] Hence, other water and fluid conservation strategies are important for reptiles.[3] Uric acid is excreted with minimal water loss through the renal tubules in most terrestrial reptiles. Fluid can also be reabsorbed through the colon after urine is refluxed from the cloaca. In species that possess a urinary bladder, sodium and water can also be reabsorbed.[3] Decreased glomerular perfusion occurs secondary to afferent renal vascular constriction in response to arginine vasotocin and the renin–angiotensin system. When afferent renal perfusion is decreased, the presence of a renal portal system allows perfusion of the renal tubules to be maintained, thereby preventing tubular necrosis.[4]

Although these physiologic adaptations allow reptiles to tolerate decreased water availability, prolonged or severe dehydration can overwhelm these mechanisms, leading to insult and dysfunction of the reptile kidney and lower urinary tract. Therefore, for reptiles in human care, the prevention of dehydration is key to maintaining adequate vascular volume and renal perfusion. Reptiles maintained in habitats with improper humidity, temperature, or without proper access to water may become subclinically dehydrated with decreased vascular fluid volume, and thus may be predisposed to renal compromise or an inability to recover from renal insult, such as infection or toxic exposure.

Renal insult from a variety of diseases can also lead to functional changes that disrupt the regulatory mechanisms of the kidneys, including failure to excrete toxic metabolic wastes and loss of important plasma proteins. For instance, loss of albumin, which maintains oncotic pressure in the vasculature, results in tissue edema.[5] Like other vertebrate species, reptiles may develop acute or chronic renal disease. Acute renal failure tends to be the result of infectious disease or a toxic insult, whereas dehydration, inadequate husbandry, poor nutrition, and secondary nutritional hyperparathyroidism are considered to be common predisposing factors for chronic renal disease. Degenerative nephroses are commonly encountered and are usually characterized by degeneration or necrosis of the glomeruli or tubules resulting in glomerulonephrosis or tubulonephrosis (**Fig. 1**).[4]

INFECTIOUS DISEASES
Bacterial Diseases

Bacterial causes of renal disease in reptiles are usually due to extension of systemic infection to the kidneys. Aggregates of bacterial organisms can form septic showers that occlude renal vasculature and glomerular capillaries, resulting in ischemia and inflammation of the renal tissue.[6]

Reptiles are most commonly infected with gram-negative bacteria. Common bacterial organisms encountered in reptiles include *Salmonella* spp., *Pseudomonas* spp., *Aeromonas* spp., and *Mycobacterium* spp. Mycobacteriosis can cause focal renal granulomas[7]; however, mycobacterial infections are usually systemic. Renal infections with *Mycobacterium chelonae* and *M avium* have been documented in sea turtles, and renal extension of systemic mycobacteriosis has been documented in crocodilians. *Mycobacterium szulgai* was detected in the kidney of a freshwater crocodile (*Crocodylus johnstoni*) with primary mycobacterial pneumonia.[6–8]

Although bacterial species with specific predilection for the reptile kidney are largely unknown, *Leptospira* spp., which are classically known to cause renal disease in mammals, have been documented in reptiles.[9] Multiple studies have documented seroprevalence of leptospiral antibodies in snakes, lizards, and turtles.[9] Pathogenic serovars found include Grippotyphosa, Tarassovi, Copenhageni, Pomona, Australis, Hardjo, Canicola, Autumnalis, Pyrogenes, Andamana, and

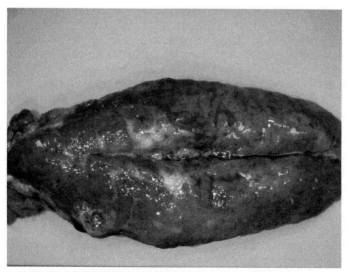

Fig. 1. Nephrosclerosis in an iguana (*Iguana* sp.) with the kidney appearing swollen and pale. (*Courtesy of* M. Garner, DVM, Dipl. ACVP, Monroe, WA.)

Javanica. Some species of reptiles were seropositive for one or more serovars.[9,10] Leptospiral DNA has also been detected in reptile gastric and cloacal washes independent of seropositivity, suggesting that reptiles could potentially shed the organism and be a cause for zoonotic concern.[9] Clinical renal disease from leptospirosis in reptiles is rare; however, interstitial nephritis has been documented in an experimentally inoculated common garter snake (*Thamnophis sirtalis*). In another study, crocodiles with the highest leptospiral titers presented underweight and in the poorest condition.[9,11,12]

Fungal Diseases

Similar to bacterial infection, fungal causes of renal disease in reptiles are usually due to extension of systemic infection to the kidneys. Pathologic changes in the urinary systemic owing to mycotic infection are variable and can consist of granulomatous nodules or cellular necrosis and inflammation.[7]

Geotrichum candidum is ubiquitous as resident microflora in the gastrointestinal tracts of giant tortoises (*Geochelone nigra*); however, it has been documented to be pathogenic. *Penicillium griseofulvum* has also been documented to cause renal disease in Seychelle's giant tortoises (*Megalochelys gigantea*).[7] In veiled chameleons (*Chamaeleo calyptratus*) suffering from systemic mycosis owing to *Chamaeleomyces granulomatis* and secondary bacterial septicemia, the most common postmortem finding was renal failure of different forms, such as gout or pigment nephrosis.[13]

Microsporidia are a group of unicellular acid-fast and variably gram-positive organisms that were previously thought to be protozoa but are now considered fungi.[6] Microsporidia that commonly infect reptiles include *Encephalitozoon* spp., *Pleistophora* spp., and *Nosema* spp. Disease often manifests as systemic infection with organisms detected in renal epithelial cells.[6,7] *Encephalitozoon pogonae* caused fatal disease in bearded dragons (*Pogona vittaceps*) that resulted in necrogranulomatous inflammation with intrahistocytic clusters of spores that expanded the renal and adrenal parenchyma.[14] Numerous *E pogonae* spores were found in the kidneys and intestinal tracts of affected bearded dragons, suggesting urinary and fecal shedding of the organism could lead to horizontal transmission by the fecal–oral route.[14]

Viral Diseases

Reptiles are susceptible to many viral infections and subsequent renal disease is usually secondary to systemic infection. The genus *Ranavirus* is an emerging pathogen in the family *Iridoviridae* that affects ectothermic animals, including reptiles, and is able to cross species and taxonomic groups. Frog virus 3-like viruses are the most common *Ranavirus* to affect reptiles in the United States, often causing disease in chelonians, such as box turtles (*Terrapene carolina*), red-eared slider turtles (*Trachemys scripta elegans*), and tortoise species. Clinically, affected animals often suffer severe systemic disease and present with oculonasal discharge, oral plaques and ulcerations, and swelling.[15] Renal insult in clinical cases is usually due to extension of systemic inflammation from viral infection to the kidneys resulting in necrosis of vascular endothelium and epithelial cells with heterophilic infiltration in fatal cases.[15]

Inclusion body disease (IBD) is a disease primarily of snakes in families Boidae and Pythonidae and an understanding of IBD is continually evolving. IBD was previously thought to be caused by retroviruses, but more recently arenaviruses have been detected in snakes with IBD. Clinical signs of IBD can be variable, ranging from subclinical infection to marked neurologic disease characterized by torticollis, opisthotonus, loss of righting reflex, regurgitation, and paralysis resulting in death.[16] Clinical signs can also include stomatitis and pneumonia, and often the duration of clinical disease can continue for weeks or longer.[16] IBD is histologically characterized by eosinophilic to amphophilic intracytoplasmic inclusions in a variety of tissues of infected animals, including renal tubular epithelial cells.[16] Although neurologic disease is the most prominent manifestation of IBD infection, glomerulonephritis can develop in IBD-infected snakes.[7]

Other viral infections can result in renal disease, although a thorough understanding of renal pathophysiology related to many viruses is still developing. Viruses in the genus *Topivirus* are picornaviruses, that were previously recognized as virus "X", are most commonly detected in spur-thighed tortoises (*Testudo graeca*), but can infect other species.[17] Clinical signs of picornavirus infection vary from inapparent infection to rhinitis, conjunctivitis, ascites, lethargy, and death, but one unique manifestation in juvenile tortoises is sudden softening of the carapace and plastron.[17] Tubulonephrosis and the lack of calcium uptake in the kidneys has been proposed as the primary cause for severe shell softening in affected animals.[18]

Adenoviruses have been documented to affect a variety of lizard species. Clinical signs of adenoviral infection consist of wasting, anorexia, and possibly neurologic signs.[19] Pathologic changes in affected organs typically consist of necrotic or proliferative changes and, although these often occur in the liver, they can occur in the kidney resulting in renal dysfunction.[19]

Herpesviruses are well-known and can infect a variety of reptiles, but are most notable in chelonians, including tortoises, box turtles, aquatic turtles, and sea turtles. Testudinid herpesvirus 1 and 3 are more commonly known and cause anorexia, oculonasal discharge, oral plaques and ulcerations, and liver lesions. Inflammatory infiltration and eosinophilic to amphophilic intranuclear inclusions were found in the kidneys of pancake tortoises (*Malacochersus tornieri*) and Horsfield's tortoises (*Testudo horsfieldii*) with herpes viral infection.[17,20] In map turtles (*Graptemys barbouri*), herpes virus-like infection resulted in renal tubular cell degeneration with intranuclear inclusions as well.[21] A unique clinical manifestation of herpes viral renal disease is seen in sea turtles with fibropapillomatosis. Herpes viral DNA was detected in the kidney of a green sea turtle (*Chelonia mydas*). Visceral fibropapillomatosis owing to chelonid herpesvirus 5 occurred as firm, white, multilobulated masses in the kidney with cystic nodules.[22]

Parasitic Diseases

Flagellated protozoa are common in reptiles. These parasites often initially infect the intestinal lumen, although they can ascend into the urinary tract and infect the kidneys. Flagellates pathogenic to the urinary tract typically belong to genus *Spironucleus* (synonymous with *Hexamita*). These organisms typically have a direct life cycle and infect the host through ingestion of contaminated feces or urine.[6] *Spironucleus* spp. can infect the renal tubules causing glomerular lesions and generalized tubulointerstitial nephritis with heterophilic inflammation (**Fig. 2**).[23,24] Clinical disease can be ambiguous and may manifest as lethargy, anorexia, and weight loss, and organisms can be detected in fresh urine or feces.[23,24] In 1 review of 29 cases of renal flagellate infection, chelonians and chameleons represented a majority of cases. Clinical renal disease in these cases was compounded by soft tissue mineralization and gout.[24] Vague clinical signs of anorexia and lethargy owing to renal flagellate infection with secondary gout has also been described in a black and white tegu (*Salvator merianae*). If detected early, treatment with metronidazole is generally effective. Disease can be prevented by maintaining a clean environment.[25]

Intranuclear coccidia have been sporadically reported to cause systemic disease in chelonians; however, organisms are commonly found in the urinary tract resulting in

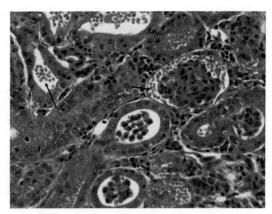

Fig. 2. Flagellate protozoa in the glomerulus (*right arrow*) and tubule (*left arrow*) in the kidney of a bearded dragon (*Pogona* sp.), with inflammatory infiltrates and cellular casts in the tubules also apparent. Hematoxylin and eosin stain; original magnification ×10. (*Courtesy of* M. Garner, DVM, Dipl. ACVP, Monroe, WA.)

inflammation of the kidneys and urinary bladder with opportunistic secondary bacterial infection (**Fig. 3**).[5] Other protozoa, such as *Entamoeba invadens*, *Cryptosporidium* sp., and *Eimeria* sp., can infect the kidney, usually as an extension of systemic disease. *E invadens* has a direct life cycle. The organism is typically a primary pathogen of the gastrointestinal system of snakes and some chelonians; however, organisms can be found in the glomeruli or renal tubules and can cause renal necrosis with secondary bacterial infection.[6,7] *Cryptosporidium* sp. generally infect the gastrointestinal tract as well; however, renal cryptosporidiosis has been reported in an iguana and a chameleon.[19]

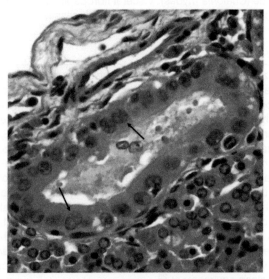

Fig. 3. Intranuclear coccidial organisms (*arrows*) in tubular epithelial cells of an Asian forest turtle (*Manouria emys*) kidney. Hematoxylin and eosin stain; original magnification ×10. (*Courtesy of* M. Garner, DVM, Dipl. ACVP, Monroe, WA.)

Klossiella is a genus of coccidia with a direct life cycle that infects the renal collecting ducts and ureters; *Klossiella boae* has been documented in boa constrictors (*Boa constrictor*).[7,23] *Klossiella* organisms can be detected in renal epithelial cells and within the lumens of renal tubules (**Fig. 4**). Although infected cells may become swollen and bulge, little pathology or clinical disease has been associated with *Klossiella* infection in reptiles.[7,23] *Klossiella* sporocysts can be detected in fresh urine or urates and prevention can be achieved with cleaning and disinfection.[23]

Myxosporidia are protozoa of class Myxosporea in the phylum Myxozoa. Although infrequently found in reptiles, genus *Myxidium* is best described in the renal system of chelonians.[6] *Myxidium* spores can be readily detected free in the urine, but the organism does not generally cause severe renal disease or pathology.[6,7] This parasite has been shown to be a cause of renal disease in Indo-Gangetic flap-shelled turtles (*Lissemys punctata andersonii*) and crowned river turtles (*Hardella thurjii*), causing renal tubular necrosis, tubular mineralization, and chronic interstitial nephritis coupled with membranoproliferative glomerulopathy.[6,26]

Trematodes may parasitize the kidneys of reptiles but rarely cause clinical disease or pathologic changes.[23] However, the trematodes *Styphlodora renalis* and *S horrida* can infect the ureters in boas and pythons, causing dilation and yellowish coloration of the ureter and accumulation of parasites, urates, mucus, small amounts of calcium, and cellular debris.[6,7] *S horrida* has also been found in the kidney of a boa constrictor.[6] Spirorchid flukes have also been found in the ureters of aquatic turtles with ureteroliths. Urolithiasis likely developed secondary to microgranuloma formation around the ova of the parasite within the vasculature.[6]

NONINFECTIOUS DISEASES

Chronic renal diseases include degenerative changes associated with fibrosis, gout, and mineralization, along with nonspecific inflammatory changes.[19] Glomerulonephrosis (degeneration or necrosis of the glomeruli) or tubulonephrosis

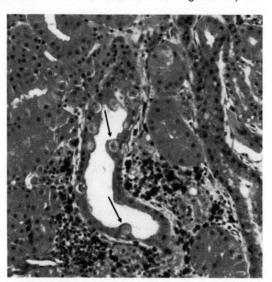

Fig. 4. Developing coccidia oocysts (*arrows*) in the cytoplasm of renal tubular epithelium of a boa constrictor (*Boa constrictor*). Hematoxylin and eosin stain; original magnification ×10. (*Courtesy of* M. Garner, DVM, Dipl. ACVP, Monroe, WA.)

(degeneration affecting the tubules) are some of the most common conditions encountered, particularly in older reptiles.[27]

Clinical signs of chronic renal disease are often vague and may include lethargy, dehydration, or anorexia. Renal disease is commonly described in the green iguana (*Iguana iguana*) with nephromegaly as a common sequelae. Nephromegaly can also cause physical obstruction of the distal intestine or colon owing to the intrapelvic location of the kidneys.[4,28] Clinically, these animals may be seen straining to defecate or are constipated.

Decreases in the calcium:phosphorous ratio may indicate renal dysfunction before any elevations in circulating uric acid. Increases in the calcium × phosphorous product or solubility index indicate an increased risk of dystrophic mineralization.[5] Green iguanas may also display electrolyte disturbances.

Metabolic Diseases

Important risk factors for chronic renal disease likely include chronic dehydration from decreased environmental humidity, reduced water intake or limited water availability, temperatures below an animal's preferred optimal temperature zone, inadequate exposure to ultraviolet B radiation, or inappropriate diet. Although some risk factors have been identified, it is likely that development of disease is multifaceted and there are still risk factors left to be identified.[2,4,29]

Renal secondary hyperparathyroidism

Renal secondary hyperparathyroidism is common in older animals with a gradual loss of kidney function.[30] As disease progresses, the kidneys are unable to convert calcidiol (25-hydroxycholecalciferol) to the active form, cholecalciferol or vitamin D_3, which leads to a lack of response to parathyroid hormone and hypertrophy of the parathyroid glands.[30] Decreased glomerular filtration will eventually lead to hyperphosphatemia. Increased phosphorus can lead to the binding of available calcium, decreasing serum calcium concentrations and stimulating production of parathyroid hormone.

Nutritional secondary hyperparathyroidism is also a predisposing condition for the development of renal disease. Chronic limited availability of calcium in the blood stimulates the production of parathyroid hormone and subsequent progressive resorption of calcium from the bones. Reptiles that recover from nutritional secondary hyperparathyroidism may also suffer from sustained renal damage owing to the cytotoxic effects of excess parathyroid hormone.[31] This should be considered when evaluating any animal with a history of nutritional secondary hyperparathyroidism or other metabolic bone disease.

Urolithiasis

Urinary calculi have been reported in lizards, turtles, and snakes.[2,32–34] In chelonians, uroliths are often found within the bladder. In female tortoises, an egg may be retropulsed into the urinary bladder and subsequently serve as a nidus for calculus formation because it cannot be passed in a normograde fashion.[6] The mean prevalence of urolithiasis in client-owned chelonians was approximately 5% in a recent retrospective study, occurring most commonly in desert tortoises (*Gopherus* sp.). In that study, all uroliths were composed of 100% urate.[35] In reptiles without urinary bladders, such as snakes, urine may pool at the distal ureters leading to urolith formation. In Lacertilia, cloacal uroliths may predispose to and manifest as cloacal prolapse.[19] Renal calculi have not yet been reported in reptiles.[5]

A major risk factor for urinary calculi formation is dehydration, which can occur from inappropriate environmental humidity or inadequate water sources. During chronic dehydration, the body attempts to conserve water. Many reptiles are uricotelic, meaning they excrete uric acid as their primary nitrogenous waste. Because reptiles lack a loop of Henle and are unable to concentrate their urine, insoluble urates may aggregate. Nutritional imbalances are also an important etiologic factor for the development of urolithiasis.

Nutritional Imbalances

Nutritional imbalances may include hypovitaminosis A, hypervitaminosis D, hypercalcemia, excess dietary protein, or excess dietary oxalates, as found in spinach or other dark leafy greens. Hypovitaminosis A is most commonly seen in chelonians, and in particular in turtles. Vitamin A deficiency causes the normal epithelium to be replaced by squamous metaplasia and hyperkeratosis. In many reptilian species, this may manifest predominantly as dry eye caused by blockages of the lacrimal glands or aural abscesses in Emydid turtles.[36] However, hypovitaminosis A can also affect other epithelial surfaces, such as the lining of the renal tubules. Squamous metaplasia of the renal tubules can ultimately lead to decreased renal clearance of urates. Hypovitaminosis A has also been implicated as the cause of renal tubular squamous metaplasia and subsequent gout in farm-raised saltwater and freshwater crocodiles.[37]

Mineralization of the renal tubules has been noted in chameleons fed diets lacking adequate levels of vitamins D, A, and calcium. Although dystrophic mineralization in the absence of excess supplementation is counterintuitive, a complex mechanism of action has been hypothesized in which the breakdown of inhibitors of soft tissue mineralization occurs secondary to hyperparathyroidism and hypovitaminosis D.[19,38] Hypovitaminosis D has also been associated with metastatic calcification in green iguanas and dystrophic mineralization in uromastyx (*Uromastyx aegyptia*).[19,38]

High-protein diets rich in purines, most commonly found in dog or cat food, can lead to significant hyperuricemia in herbivorous reptiles that can ultimately result in gout (described elsewhere in this article) and renal disease.[39,40]

Gout

Gout is a condition commonly found in reptile patients. Knowledge of the pathophysiology and treatment of this condition in birds and reptiles relies on extrapolation from human medical literature.[1,2] Uric acid formation is the result of protein breakdown into purines, primarily adenine and guanine, which are further degraded to xanthine then into uric acid by the enzyme xanthine oxidase.[2,41,42] Uric acid is poorly water soluble, precipitating at low concentrations. When uric acid concentrations are increased in the blood or body fluids, the uric acid precipitates into insoluble crystals of monosodium urate that are deposited in various tissues, including synovial fluid (articular gout), periarticular tissues (periarticular gout), and other internal organs (visceral gout) **(Fig. 5)**.[2,41]

Primary gout is related to the overproduction of uric acid. In humans, increased uric acid production can be the result of inherited enzyme defects or excessive intake of dietary protein diet. The latter can occur in a herbivorous reptile consuming a diet high in animal protein.[2,43] Alternatively, farmed crocodilians can develop gout when overfed without intervening fasts, suggesting that protein overload may contribute to the development of gout in carnivorous animals as well.[44,45] Conversely, when plant protein diets were fed to farmed American alligators (*Alligator mississippiensis*), there were no adverse effects to the liver or kidneys, or changes to the biochemistry profile.[46]

A   B

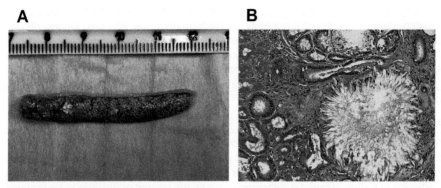

Fig. 5. Renal gout in an adult corn snake (*Pantherophis guttatus*). (*A*) Gross image of the kidney that is obscured by diffuse pale tan to white nodules of uric acid deposition. (*B*) Characteristic histologic lesion of renal tubular ectasia with intralumenal, acicular to stellate masses of crystalline material admixed with organic and cellular debris (tophi). Hematoxylin and eosin stain; original magnification ×10. (*Courtesy of* C. Rodriguez, DVM, DACVP, Lake Buena Vista, FL.)

Secondary gout occurs when hyperuricemia results from other disease processes or the administration of drugs that affect the excretion of uric acid.[2] Reptiles that form uric acid clear it from the blood through the renal tubules.[2] When the majority of renal function has been compromised, gout is a common sequela. Animals with a history of inappropriate temperature, inadequate humidity, poor nutrition, or reduced water availability may also be at higher risk for developing gout. Environmental factors, such as decreased temperatures and dehydration, have been implicated in hyperuricemia and secondary gout in reptiles owing to their effect in reducing renal perfusion and tubular excretion of uric acid.[2] In snakes, secondary gout associated with dehydration is most common and uric acid deposition in the kidneys often occurs before deposition in other tissues.[47]

In free-ranging reptiles, environmental factors may also contribute to decreased renal function. Iohexol clearance testing has been used to determine glomerular filtration rates for juvenile Kemp's ridley turtles (*Lepidochelys kempii*) that stranded owing to cold stunning.[48] The initial glomerular filtration rates were negatively correlated with initial plasma uric acid concentrations and 1 study showed evidence of reduced renal function in cold-stunned turtles.[48,49]

Inflammation

Amyloid is an insoluble pathologic proteinaceous substance deposited between cells in various tissues and organs of the body. Amyloid formation often occurs secondary to systemic inflammation and ultimately can result in renal failure from infiltration and pressure atrophy of adjacent cells.[50]

Overall, amyloid deposition is poorly documented in reptiles. Deposition of amyloid-like material that is Congo red positive has been reported in the kidneys of Komodo dragons (*Varanus komodoensis*).[51] Systemic amyloidosis in an African tiger snake (*Telescopus semiannulatus*) has also been described secondary to systemic inflammation with some aggregation and Congo red staining in the kidneys.[52]

In a recent study performed in Eastern box turtles (*Terrapene carolina carolina*), cyclo-oxygenase 1 (COX-1) and COX-2 were found in the liver, kidney, grossly normal muscle, and grossly traumatized (inflamed) muscle of all turtles.[53] In all cases, COX-1 and COX-2 proteins were increased in traumatized muscle over grossly normal nontraumatized muscle.[53] The highest levels of COX-1 and COX-2 proteins were found in the kidney and liver.[53]

Neoplasia

Renal adenocarcinomas are frequently diagnosed in snakes, with colubrids being overrepresented.[54–58] A caudal coelomic mass associated with the left kidney was resected by performing a left adrenalectomy and nephrectomy in a woma python (*Aspidites ramsayi*). Histopathologic examination identified an inter-renal (adrenocortical) cell adenocarcinoma. Eighteen months after the surgery an ultrasound examination of the snake revealed significant tumor regrowth.[59]

Renal adenocarcinomas have infrequently been reported in lizards.[60] Clinical signs may include reduced appetite, swelling at the tail base, and constipation. The diagnosis of a renal adenocarcinoma and subsequent resection and removal of 90% of the kidney has been described in a beaded lizard (*Heloderma horridum horridum*) with recurrence in the contralateral kidney 3 years later.[61]

Toxicities

The administration of aminoglycosides, such as gentamicin or amikacin, is the most common cause of nephrotoxicity in reptiles.[62,63] It is important that patients receiving these medications have an appropriate hydration status. Often fluids are administered in conjunction with these treatments. When possible, it may be wise to choose a different antibiotic option if available.

In mammals, amphotericin B is a known nephrotoxin that causes renal vasoconstriction and a decreased glomerular filtration rate; it also has direct toxic effects on the membranes of the renal tubule cells.[63] Toxicity has not yet been documented in birds or reptiles[64]; however, this drug should still be used with caution. It is recommended to monitor uric acid, urea nitrogen, and electrolytes in reptilian patients being treated with amphotericin B. This drug should not be used in animals with known clinical renal disease.

Hypervitaminosis D, likely secondary to oversupplementation of oral vitamin D_3, can result in nephrocalcinosis and subsequent impairment of renal function. Excess vitamin D consumption can also occur with accidental ingestion of some rodenticides containing cholecalciferol. Heavy metals, such as lead, may also accumulate in the kidney and potentially compromise function.[27]

Traditional nonsteroidal anti-inflammatory drugs that block both COX isoforms might be more efficacious than COX-2–selective drugs. However, when administering to reptile, effects on the kidneys should be considered.

SUMMARY

In reptiles with nonspecific signs of illness, a full evaluation of the patient should always be performed. Renal disease should always be considered in the differential diagnosis and fully investigated owing to the ambiguity and nonspecific nature of clinical signs and also potential for marked impact on systemic health. In addition, given the insidious nature of chronic renal disease in reptiles, early investigation and prevention may result in highest success for treatment. Because renal dysfunction is often a result of improper husbandry practices and chronic, subclinical dehydration, corrective changes can be made that may result in a positive outcome for the animal if initiated early. It is important to identify areas of husbandry that could be improved to treat or prevent renal disease in these patients. Understanding renal anatomy, physiology, and pathophysiology in reptiles, especially compared with their mammalian counterparts, in addition to knowledge of differential diagnoses summarized in this article are essential in clinical management of renal disease in reptiles.

REFERENCES

1. Johnson J, Brandão J, Perry S, et al. Urinary system. In: Mitchell M, Tully T, editors. Current therapy in exotic pet practice. St. Louis (MO): Elsevier; 2015. p. 494–548. https://doi.org/10.1111/j.1440-1827.1955.tb01760.x.
2. Hernandez-divers SJ, Innis CJ. Renal disease in reptiles: diagnosis and clinical management. 2nd edition. St. Louis (MO): Elsevier; 2006. https://doi.org/10.1016/B0-7216-9327-X/50070-5.
3. O'Malley B. Clinical anatomy and physiology of exotic species. Elsevier Saunders; 2005. %60.
4. Selleri P, Hernandez-Divers SJ. Renal diseases of reptiles. Vet Clin North Am Exot Anim Pract 2006;9(1):161–74.
5. Rodriguez CE, Duque AMH, Steinberg J, et al. Chelonia. In: Terio KA, McAloose D, Leger J St, editors. Pathology of wildlife and zoo animals. 1st edition. San Diego (CA): Academic Press/Elsevier; 2018. p. 825–54. https://doi.org/10.1016/B978-0-12-805306-5/00034-1.
6. Reavill DR, Schmidt RE. Urinary tract diseases of reptiles. J Exot Pet Med 2010; 19(4):280–9.
7. Zwart P. Renal pathology in reptiles. Vet Clin North Am Exot Anim Pract 2006;9(1): 129–59.
8. Roh Y-S, Park H, Cho A, et al. Granulomatous pneumonia in a captive freshwater crocodile (Crocodylus johnstoni) by Mycobacterium szulgai. J Zoo Wildl Med 2010;41(3):550–4.
9. Ebani VV. Domestic reptiles as source of zoonotic bacteria: a mini review. Asian Pac J Trop Med 2017;10(8):723–8.
10. Lindtner-Knific R, Vergles-Rataj A, Vlahović K, et al. Prevalence of antibodies against Leptospira sp. in snakes, lizards and turtles in Slovenia. Acta Vet Scand 2013;55:65.
11. Pérez-Flores J, Charruau P, Cedeño-Vázquez R, et al. Evidence for wild crocodiles as a risk for human leptospirosis, Mexico. Ecohealth 2017;14(1):58–68.
12. Abdulla P, Karstad L. Experimental infections with Leptospira pomona in snakes and turtles. Zoonoses Res 1962;1:295–306.
13. Schmidt V, Plenz B, Pfaff M, et al. Disseminated systemic mycosis in Veiled chameleons (Chamaeleo calyptratus) caused by Chamaeleomyces granulomatis. Vet Microbiol 2012;161(1–2):145–52.
14. Shibasaki K, Tokiwa T, Sukegawa A, et al. First report of fatal disseminated microsporidiosis in two inland bearded dragons Pogona vitticeps in Japan. JMM Case Rep 2017;4(4). https://doi.org/10.1099/jmmcr.0.005089.
15. Miller DL, Pessier AP, Hick P, et al. Comparative pathology of Ranaviruses and diagnostic techniques. In: Gray MJ, Chinchar GV, editors. Ranaviruses: lethal pathogens of ectothermic vertebrates. New York: Springer; 2015. p. 171–208.
16. Marschang RE. Clinical virology. In: Mader DR, Divers SJ, editors. Current Therapy in Reptile Medicine and Surgery. St. Louis (MO): Elsevier; 2014. p. 32–52.
17. Marschang RE. Viral diseases of reptiles. In Pract 2016;38(6):275–85.
18. Paries S, Funcke S, Kershaw O, et al. The role of Virus "X" (Tortoise Picornavirus) in kidney disease and shell weakness syndrome in European tortoise species determined by experimental infection. PLoS One 2019;14(2):1–18.

19. Origgi FC. Lacertilia. In: Terio KA, McAloose D, Leger J St, editors. Pathology of Wildlife and zoo animals. 1st edition. San Diego (CA): Elsevier Inc.; 2018. p. 871–95.
20. Une Y, Uemura K, Nakano Y, et al. Herpesvirus infection in tortoises (malacochersus torneri and testudo horsfieldii). Vet Pathol 1999;36(6):624–7.
21. Jacobson ER, Gaskin JM, Wahlquist H. Herpesvirus-like infection in map turtles. J Am Vet Med Assoc 1982;181(11):1322–4.
22. Page-Karjian A, Gottdenker NL, Whitfield J, et al. potential noncutaneous sites of chelonid herpesvirus 5 persistence and shedding in green sea turtles chelonia mydas. J Aquat Anim Health 2017;29(3):136–42.
23. Holz P. Diseases of the urinary tract. In: Doneley B, Monks D, Robert Johnson BC, editors. Reptile medicine and surgery in clinical practice. 1st edition. Hoboken (NJ): John Wiley & Sons; 2018. p. 323–30.
24. Juan-Sallés C, Garner MM, Nordhausen RW, et al. Renal flagellate infections in reptiles: 29 cases. J Zoo Wildl Med 2014;45(1):100–9.
25. Holz P. Diseases of the urinary tract. In: Doneley B, Monks D, Johnson R, et al, editors. Reptile medicine and surgery in clinical practice. Hoboken (NJ): Wiley-Blackwell; 2018. p. 323–30. https://doi.org/10.1055/s-2008-1064948.
26. Garner MM, Bartholomew JL, Whipps CM, et al. Renal myxozoanosis in crowned river turtles Hardella thurjii: description of the putative agent Myxidium hardella n. sp. by histopathology, electron microscopy, and DNA sequencing. Vet Pathol 2005;42(5):589–95.
27. Divers SJ, Innis CJ. Urology. In: Divers SJ, Stahl SJ, editors. Mader's reptile and amphibian medicine and surgery. 3rd edition. St Louis (MO): Elsevier Inc; 2019. p. 624–48.
28. Banzato T, Hellebuyck T, Van Caelenberg A, et al. A review of diagnostic imaging of snakes and lizards. Vet Rec 2013;173(2):43–9.
29. Antinoff N. Renal disase in the green iguana, Iguana iguana. Proceedings of the Annual Conference of the Association of Reptilian and Amphibian Veterinarians. Reno, NV, October 18-22, 2000. p. 61–3.
30. Klaphake E. A fresh look at metabolic bone diseases in reptiles and amphibians. Vet Clin North Am Exot Anim Pract 2010;13(3):375–92.
31. Massry SG, Fadda GZ. Chronic renal failure is a state of cellular calcium toxicity. Am J Kidney Dis 1993;21(1):81–6.
32. Mans C, Sladky KK. Endoscopically guided removal of cloacal calculi in 3 African spurred tortoises (Geochelone sulcata). J Am Vet Med Assoc 2012;240(7):869–75.
33. Wolf KN, Troan BV, Devoe R. Chronic urolithiasis and subsequent cystectomy in a San Esteban Island Chuckwalla, Sauromalus varius. J Herpetol Med Surg 2008;18(3–4):106–12.
34. Innis CJ, Kincaid AL. Bilateral Calcium phosphate ureteroliths and spirorchid trematode infection in red-eared slider turtle, Trachemys scipta elegans, with a review of the pathology of spirochiasis. Proceedings of the Association of Reptile and Amphibian Veterinarians 1999. Columbus, Ohio, October 5-9, 1999.
35. Keller K, Hawkins M, Weber E, et al. Diagnosis and treatment of urolithiasis in client-owned chelonians: 40 cases (1987-2012). J Am Vet Med Assoc 2015;247(6):650–8.
36. Boyer TH, Scott PW. Nutritional diseases. In: Divers SJ, Stahl SJ, editors. Mader's reptile and amphibian medicine and surgery. 3rd edition. St. Louis (MO): Scott J. Stahl; 2019. p. 932–50.

37. Ariel E, Ladds PW, Buenviaje GN. Concurrent gout and suspected hypo-vitaminosis A in crocodile hatchlings. Aust Vet J 1997;75(4):247–9.
38. Hoby S, Wenker C, Robert N, et al. Nutritional metabolic bone disease in juvenile veiled chameleons (Chamaeleo calyptratus) and its prevention. J Nutr 2010; 140(11):1923–31.
39. Gibbons PM, Avian P. Reptile and amphibian urinary tract medicine: diagnosis and therapy. In: Proceedings Association of Reptilian and Amphibian Veterinar-ians. New Orleans, Louisiana, April 15-18, 2007. p. 69–86.
40. McArthur S. Problem solving approach to common diseases of terrestrial and semi- aquatic chelonians. In: McArthur S, Wilkinson R, Meyer J, editors. Medicine and surgery of tortoises and turtles. Oxford (England): Blackwell Publishing Ltd.; 2004. p. 309–77.
41. Neogi T. Gout. N Engl J Med 2011;364:443–52.
42. Duncan M. Gout in exotic animals. In: Miller RE, Fowler ME, editors. Fowler's zoo and wild animal medicine. 8th edition. St Louis (MO): Elsevier Saunders; 2015. p. 667–70.
43. Harrold L. New developments in gout. Curr Opin Rheumatol 2013;25:304–9.
44. Conley KJ, Shilton CM. Crocodilia. In: Terio KA, McAloose D, Leger J St, editors. Pathology of wildlife and zoo animals. 1st edition. San Diego (CA): Elsevier Inc; 2018. p. 855–70.
45. Jacobson ER. Immobilization, blood sampling, necropsy techniques and dis-eases of crocodilians: a review. J Zoo Wildl Med 1984;15:38–45.
46. DiGeronimo P, Di Girolamo N, Crossland N, et al. Effects of plant protein diets on the health of farmed American alligators (Alligator mississipiensis). J Zoo Wildl Med 2017;48(1):131–5.
47. Ossiboff RJ. Serpentes. In: Terio KA, McAloose D, Leger J St, editors. Pathology of wildlife and zoo animals. 1st edition. San Diego (CA): Academic Press/Elsevier; 2018. p. 897–919. https://doi.org/10.1016/B978-0-12-805306-5/00037-7.
48. Kennedy A, Innis C, Rumbeiha W. Determination of glomerular filtration rate in ju-venile Kemp's Ridley Turtles (Lepidochelys kempii) using iohexol clearance, with preliminary comparison of clinically healthy turtles vs. those with renal disease. J Herpetol Med Surg 2012;22(1–2):25–9.
49. Innis CJ, Kennedy A, McGowan JP, et al. Glomerular filtration rates of naturally cold-Stunned Kemp's ridley turtles (Lepidochelys kempii): comparison of initial vs. convalescent values. J Herpetol Med Surg 2016;26(3–4):100–3.
50. Reavill DR, Schmidt RE. Urogenital tract diseases of reptiles and amphibians. In: Proceedings Association of Reptilian and Amphibian Veterinarians. New Orleans, Louisiana, April 15-18, 2007. p. 87–109.
51. Garner M, Gyimesi Z, Rasmussen J, et al. An amyloid-like deposition disorder in Komodo dragons. In: Proceedings of the Tenth Annual Conference of the Asso-ciation of Reptile and Amphibian Veterinarians. Minneapolis, Minnesota, October 4-9, 2003. p. 50.
52. Burns RE, Gaffney PM, Nilsson KPR, et al. Systemic Amyloidosis in an African Ti-ger Snake (Telescopus semiannulatus). J Comp Pathol 2017;157(2–3):136–40.
53. Royal LW, Lascelles BDX, Lewbart GA, et al. Evaluation of cyclooxygenase pro-tein expression in traumatized versus normal tissues from eastern box turtles (Ter-rapene carolina carolina). J Zoo Wildl Med 2012;43(2):289–95.
54. Belasco-Zeitz M, Pye G, Burns R, et al. Clinical challenge spitting cobra. J Zoo Wildl Med 2013;44(3):807–10.
55. Gravendyck M, Marschang RE, Schröder-Gravendyck AS, et al. Renal adenocar-cinoma in a reticulated python (Python reticulatus). Vet Rec 1997;140(14):374–5.

56. Jacobson E, Long P, Miller R, et al. Renal neoplasia of snakes. J Am Vet Med Assoc 1986;189(9):1134–6.
57. Kao CF, Chen JL, Tsao WT, et al. A renal adenocarcinoma in a corn snake (Pantherophis guttatus) resembling human collecting duct carcinoma. J Vet Diagn Invest 2016;28(5):599–603.
58. Keck M, Zimmerman DM, Dvm ECR, et al. Renal adenocarcinoma in Cape Coral Snakes (Aspide lap s lubneus lubricus). J Herpetol Med Surg 2011;21(1):5–9.
59. Kaye SW, Daverio H, Eddy R, et al. Surgical resection of an interrenal cell adenocarcinoma in a woma python (Aspidites ramsayi) with 18 month follow-up. J Herpetol Med Surg 2016;26(1–2):26–31.
60. Burt D, Chrisp C, Gillett C, et al. Two cases of renal neoplasia in a colony of desert iguanas. J Am Vet Med Assoc 1984;185(11):1423–5.
61. Savageau NR, Gamble KC. Clinical challenge: renal adenocarcinoma in a beaded lizard (Heloderma horridum horridum). J Zoo Wildl Med 2016;47(3):945–7.
62. Montali RJ, Bush M, Smeller JM. The pathology of nephrotoxicity of gentamicin in snakes. A model for reptilian gout. Vet Pathol 1979;16(1):108–15.
63. Fitzgerald KT, Newquist KL. Poisonings in reptiles. Vet Clin North Am Exot Anim Pract 2008;11(2):327–57.
64. Kirchgessner M. Amphotericin B. J Exot Pet Med 2008;17(1):54–6.

Diagnostic Imaging of the Reptile Urinary System

Lauren Schmidt, DVM[a], Nicola Di Girolamo, DMV, MSc, PhD, DECZM (Herpetology)[a,*],
Paolo Selleri, DMV, PhD, DECZM (Herpetology & Small Mammals)[b]

KEYWORDS

- Reptile • Computed tomography • Radiology • MRI • Ultrasonography

KEY POINTS

- Understanding of specific reptile urinary tract anatomy is mandatory to assess the urinary tract.
- Radiology is an important resource if proper positioning and horizontal beam views are obtained.
- Renal tissue is easily visualized on ultrasonography and the echotexture may indicate the status.
- Computed tomography is a powerful tool that facilitates the diagnosis of disorders of the urinary tract.
- Contrast media are recommended to enhance urinary tract structures when performing a computed tomography scan.

INTRODUCTION

Reptiles are commonly kept as pets and are popular as display animals in professional care settings such as zoos and aquariums. These animals can develop various diseases associated with the urinary tract, including, but not exclusively, urolithiasis, gout, acute and chronic kidney injury, and secondary renal hyperparathyroidism.[1,2] In a retrospective study on morbidity in bearded dragons, urogenital disease was reported in 9.5% of animals, and was the fourth most common illness.[2] Diagnostic imaging can be instrumental in differentiating and diagnosing these ailments. This article describes the current approach to diagnostic imaging in reptile medicine for evaluation of urinary tract disease. The use of radiographs, ultrasonography, computed tomography (CT), MRI, and endoscopy is discussed and compared for the evaluation of urinary tract disease in reptiles.

Disclosures: The authors have no relationship with a commercial company that has a direct financial interest in subject matter or materials discussed in this article or with a company making a competing product.
[a] Oklahoma State University, Center for Veterinary Health Sciences, Stillwater, OK 74078, USA;
[b] Clinica per Animali Esotici, Roma, Italy
* Corresponding author.
E-mail address: nicoladiggi@gmail.com

RADIOGRAPHY
Diagnostic Technique

Radiographs can be a simple and useful tool for diagnostic evaluation that is available in most veterinary practices. Radiographs are an efficient, but not necessarily sensitive, modality for visualizing internal structures, including the urinary tract. Radiographic images should be obtained in multiple opposing views to properly evaluate three-dimensional structures in a two-dimensional plane and maximize diagnostic accuracy.

To perform radiographs, reptiles can be sedated or otherwise restrained using radiolucent materials. In most instances, appropriate positioning can be achieved safely without anesthesia and without radiation exposure to the operators. Chelonian radiographs should be obtained in 3 views: a lateral (horizontal beam), dorsoventral (vertical beam), and a craniocaudal (horizontal beam) projection. For vertical beam radiographs, a dorsally open-faced box fitting the dimensions of the carapace helps prevent movement (**Fig. 1**A, B). For horizontal beam radiographs, positioning chelonians on an elevated cylindrical surface smaller than the plastron stimulates the animals to extend the limbs, and also prevents ambulation (**Fig. 1**C). Lizards should be radiographed in both lateral (horizontal beam) and dorsoventral (vertical beam) projections. Lateral radiographs obtained using vertical beam with animals in lateral recumbency may result in displacement of the loosely attached viscera, making diagnostic

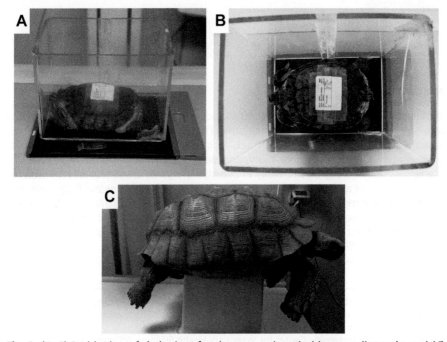

Fig. 1. (A, B) Positioning of chelonians for dorsoventral vertical beam radiographs and (C) for lateral and craniocaudal horizontal beam radiographs. Having radiotransparent boxes without tops and bottoms of various size helps confine chelonians for dorsoventral radiographs. For horizontal beam radiographs, using cylindrical or parallelepipedal structures that are roughly the same size as the plastron usually allows clinicians to position chelonians and in most cases the animals extend extremities. (*Courtesy of* N. Di Girolamo, DVM, MSc, PhD, Dipl ECZM (Herp), Stillwater, OK.)

interpretation more challenging. A horizontal beam should be used to maintain organs in normal anatomic position.[3]

Snakes should not be coiled for dorsoventral image acquisition because viscera can shift internally, making linear orthogonal projections challenging to compare. Furthermore, obtaining a coiled image may decrease the diagnostic accuracy of the radiograph.[4] To prevent coiling, snakes may be radiographed in plastic radiotransparent tubes small enough to allow the snake to enter the tube but not turn around. Snakes should be marked with radiopaque tags along the body to identify the location of the corresponding radiographic images. Tags should be used in both lateral and dorsoventral projections.

Urinary Tract Appearance

Snakes
Regardless of what radiographic technique is used, normal renal structures are usually not appreciable in snakes.[5] Alternatively, kidneys in snakes may be visualized when changes have occurred in their size or texture.[6]

Chelonians
In a study on live red-eared sliders (*Trachemys scripta elegans*) and on both live and deceased loggerhead sea turtles (*Caretta caretta*), renal structures were challenging to appreciate on radiographs, and could not be visualized without contrast. Contrast was only shown to outline the vasculature, and therefore it is unknown whether significant detail may be missed.[7,8] However, in chelonians with gout and nephromegaly, kidneys may become visible with increased radiopacity as ovoid structures cranial to the prefemoral fossae (**Fig. 2**).[9] The normal urinary bladder in chelonians is typically homogeneous to the remaining coelom and may also be challenging to appreciate radiographically (**Fig. 3**). Accumulation

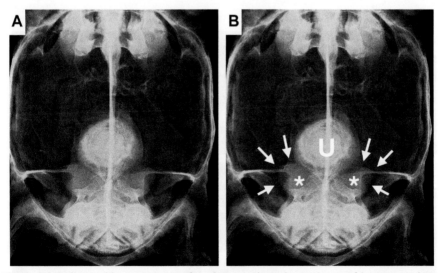

Fig. 2. (*A*) Radiographic appearance of nephromegaly and gout in an African spurred tortoise (*Geochelone sulcata*) with a urinary bladder urolith. In normal chelonians, the silhouette of the kidneys should not be visible during plain radiographs. (*B*) Notice the increased radiopacity of the kidneys (*asterisk*), and the increase in size of their silhouettes (*arrows*). U, urolith. (*Courtesy of* N. Di Girolamo, DVM, MSc, PhD, Dipl ECZM (Herp), Stillwater, OK.)

of urates in the dependent portion of the urinary bladder may help define its borders.[10]

Lizards

In lizards, the kidneys are usually located in the caudal dorsal coelom, lateral to the lumbar spine, except in monitor lizards, in which they are located in the midcaudal coelom.[1] Because of their location within or partially within the pelvic canal, radiographs of the kidneys are often unrewarding.[11] However, digital subtraction angiography, using a x-ray imaging intensifier, television camera, and image processor, has been successful in imaging the renal portal system of 6 common green iguanas (*Iguana iguana*).[12] In chameleons, the renal contour may be visible, especially in cases of nephromegaly or gout (**Fig. 4**).

Clinical Applications

Radiographs are often part of a multimodal diagnostic approach and can be beneficial in evaluating renal enlargement, urolithiasis, and displacement of soft tissues.[6,9,10]

In a case series on renal adenocarcinomas in cape coral snakes (*Aspidelaps lubricus*), 2 of 3 animals had evidence of a mass effect on radiographs around the region of the kidney. On coelomic exploration and necropsy, a renal mass was confirmed in both animals.[6] Although radiographs were not sensitive to renal disease specifically in this case, an accurate diagnosis was possible because of anatomic location and subsequent coelomic exploration.

Changes in the urinary bladder of chelonians visible on radiographs include changes in its repletion as well as the presence of uroliths or ectopic eggs (**Fig. 5**).[13] The presence of ectopic eggs in the urinary bladder must be confirmed via endoscopy or ultrasonography.

An overdistended urinary bladder can be noted as a soft tissue structure displacing the gastrointestinal tract cranially and compressing lung parenchyma dorsally.[10] An

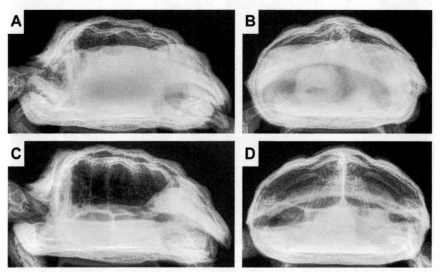

Fig. 3. (*A, B*) Radiographic (lateral and anteroposterior, horizontal beam) appearance of urinary bladder extremely distended and (*C, D*) after drainage. (*Courtesy of* N. Di Girolamo, DVM, MSc, PhD, Dipl ECZM (Herp), Stillwater, OK.)

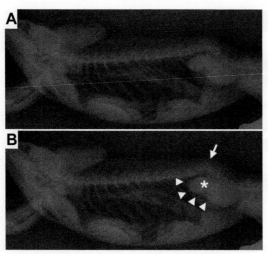

Fig. 4. (A) Radiographic appearance of nephromegaly and gout in a veiled chameleon (*Chamaeleo calyptratus*) with severe metabolic bone disease. (B) Notice the increased radiopacity of the kidney (*asterisk*), and the increase in size of its silhouette (*arrowheads*). The vertebral column is also altered (*arrow*). (*Courtesy of* N. Di Girolamo, DVM, MSc, PhD, Dipl ECZM (Herp), Stillwater, OK.)

empty urinary bladder may result in an increase of the lung/viscera ratio. When an empty urinary bladder is appreciated radiographically in chelonians with recent history of trauma, urinary bladder rupture should be suspected and further investigated by cystoscopy plus or minus contrast cystography (**Fig. 6**).

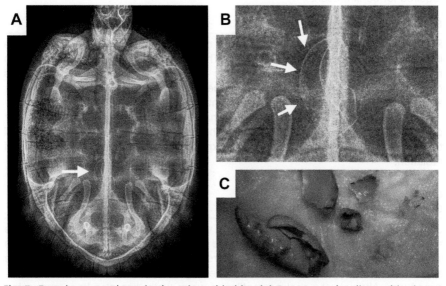

Fig. 5. Ectopic ruptured egg in the urinary bladder. (A) Dorsoventral radiographic view. A ruptured egg is visible in the midline (*arrow*). (B) Close-up of the ruptured egg (*arrows*). (C) Gross appearance of the egg after cystoscopic removal. (*Courtesy of* N. Di Girolamo, DVM, MSc, PhD, Dipl ECZM (Herp), Stillwater, OK.)

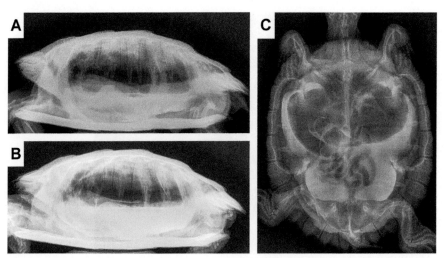

Fig. 6. Radiographic diagnosis of ruptured urinary bladder in a red-eared slider (*A*) before and (*B*) after contrast cystography. (*C*) Notice distribution of contrast media administered through cystoscopy in the entire coelom. (*Courtesy of* N. Di Girolamo, DVM, MSc, PhD, Dipl ECZM (Herp), Stillwater, OK.)

Radiographs are an optimal modality to screen tortoises for urolithiasis, because this technique is sensitive for identifying mineral opacities in contrast with surrounding soft tissue (see **Fig. 2**).[14,15] In the authors' experience, uroliths are often subclinical in tortoises and therefore a yearly screening program should be considered. Urolithiasis are not always distinguishable using radiographs alone,[16] and cystoscopy may be required for confirmation.

Benefits and Limitations

Radiographs are beneficial in that they are a noninvasive modality of appreciating the internal visceral and some overt changes. This diagnostic tool is readily available in most practices, offers rapid results, and is often affordable. Although radiographs require the patient to be still, this can frequently be achieved without anesthesia or sedation if the patient is kept in a radiolucent enclosure.

Radiographs are disadvantageous in that they are less sensitive than other diagnostic imaging modalities, in that there is significant superimposition of tissues. In addition, this technique also exposes the patient to small amounts of radiation.

ULTRASONOGRAPHY
Diagnostic Technique

Ultrasonography uses high-frequency sound waves to produce an image of soft tissue structures. In squamate reptiles, scales and the air between the scales can reduce imagine quality and make interpretation more challenging.[17,18] Coupling gel must be applied to create appropriate contact between the dermis and the ultrasonography transducer. Alternatively, soaking reptiles in warm water has also been suggested as a way of maintaining good surface contact with the probe.[17,18] Ultrasonography in most reptiles can be performed in conscious animals using manual restraint,[17,19–23] but exceptions are made for large, uncooperative chelonians. Sedation may facilitate ease of handling for ultrasonography.[18,24–26] Snakes and lizards may be held in dorsal, sternal, or lateral recumbency depending on body type and the organ system of interest.[19,20]

In snakes and lizards, application of the transducer on the caudal ventrum and dorsum is appropriate for visualizing urinary tract structures. In snakes, the kidneys can be easily identified in the caudal third of the body lateral to the intestinal tract[18,20] and caudal to the gonads. In bearded dragons and iguanas, the kidneys are best imaged from the dorsal region of the animal at the level of the pelvis (**Fig. 7**).[19] In water monitors (*Varanus salvator*) and savannah monitors (*Varanus exanthematicus*), the kidneys and urinary bladder were partially visualized from the ventrum.[17,22] Chelonian kidneys and urinary bladder are visualized through the prefemoral fossae, with animals held in sternal, lateral, or dorsal recumbency (**Fig. 8**).[21,23,25,27] In small chelonians, or in animals with severe calcium deficiency, transplastronal ultrasonography is feasible and allows visualization of the urinary bladder (**Fig. 9**).

Urinary Tract Appearance

Reptiles lack a distinct renal pelvis, cortex, and medulla; therefore, these structures appear uniformly echogenic on ultrasonography (**Figs. 10** and **11**).[22,23] The kidneys are hyperechoic compared with the liver and, depending on the species, may have a multilobulated surface. In a study evaluating 46 healthy snakes, renal structures

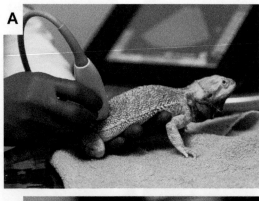

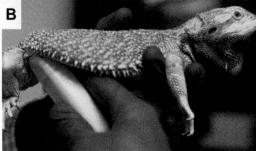

Fig. 7. Positioning of the ultrasonographic probe in a bearded dragon (*Pogona vitticeps*) for visualization of the intrapelvic kidneys. (*A*) Dorsal approach, (*B*) ventral coelomic approach. (*Courtesy of* N. Di Girolamo, DVM, MSc, PhD, Dipl ECZM (Herp), Stillwater, OK and L. Schmidt,)

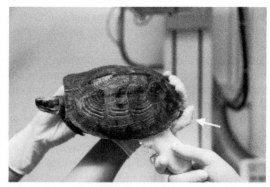

Fig. 8. Positioning of a Chinese 3-striped box turtle (*Cuora trifasciata*) for ultrasonography of the urinary tract through the prefemoral space. Notice that the operator holding the turtle is hyperextending the left hind limb (*arrow*). (*Courtesy of* N. Di Girolamo, DVM, MSc, PhD, Dipl ECZM (Herp), Stillwater, OK.)

were always appreciable sonographically, but were sometimes challenging to distinguish from adjacent fat bodies.[28] In a study involving 30 red-eared sliders, the kidneys were visible in all animals,[21] with a uniform echogenicity to surrounding structures and a mildly hyperechoic renal capsule.

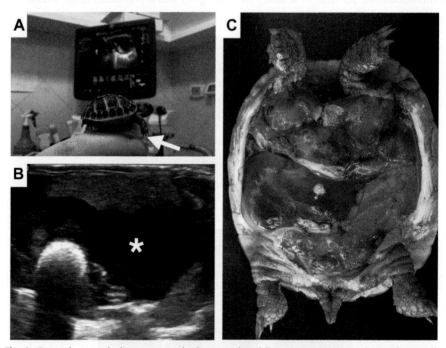

Fig. 9. Transplastronal ultrasonography in a posthatchling Hermann's tortoise with overdistended urinary bladder. (*A*) Positioning of the animal for transplastronal ultrasonography. Notice position of the linear transponder under the plastron (*arrow*). (*B*) Ultrasonographic view showing abundant fluid enclosed in the urinary bladder (*asterisk*). (*C*) Postmortem of the animal following natural death revealing overdistended urinary bladder and abundant urates (left urinary bladder lobe). (*Courtesy of* N. Di Girolamo, DVM, MSc, PhD, Dipl ECZM (Herp), Stillwater, OK.)

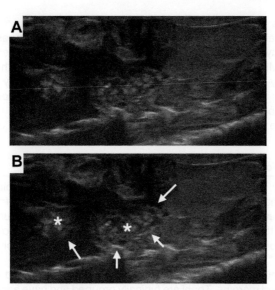

Fig. 10. Ultrasonographic visualization of normal renal tissue (*asterisks and arrows*) in a bearded dragon (*P vitticeps*). (*Courtesy of* N. Di Girolamo, DVM, MSc, PhD, Dipl ECZM (Herp), Stillwater, OK and L. Schmidt,)

In reptiles with a urinary bladder, the organ is visualized in the caudal coelom as a fluid-filled structure with a thin hyperechoic wall, often containing material of mixed echogenicity suggestive of liquid urine with urates (see **Fig. 9**).[21] In the aforementioned study examining 30 red-eared sliders, the urinary bladder was visible in all individuals.[21] Ureters with evident peristaltic activity were identified in 6 out of 16 snakes (2 ball pythons *Python regius* and 4 Indian rock pythons *Python molurus*), but only through transverse scans.[28]

Because of either size or interference from gas-filled loops of bowel, ultrasonic imaging of kidneys has been reported as challenging in some species, such as

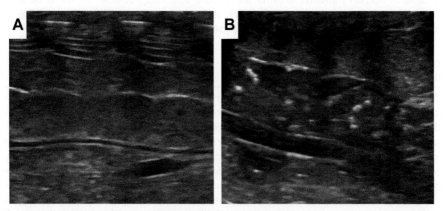

Fig. 11. Ultrasonographic visualization of (*A*) normal and (*B*) abnormal renal tissue in boa constrictors (*Boa constrictor*). Notice presence of disseminated hyperechoic spots in the kidney consistent with gout or mineral deposits. (*Courtesy of* P. Selleri DMV, PhD, Dipl ECZM (Herp & Small Mammals), Roma, Italy, and A. Nicoletti, Roma, Italy.)

leopard geckos (*Eublepharis macularius*) and green iguanas.[24,29] In a study involving 11 healthy adult female geckos, urinary tract structures could not be identified in any individuals on either ventral or dorsal projections using a 13-MHz to 18-MHz linear array transducer.[24] In green iguanas, the kidneys were identified in only 4 of 26 animals evaluated in dorsal recumbency using a 5-MHz to 12-MHz linear array transducer.[29] However, the availability of more advanced ultrasonography probes, such as high-frequency probes in the range of 15 to 18 MHz, has the potential to make ultrasonographic visualization of urinary structures easier.

Clinical Applications

Ultrasonography is routinely used for clinical purposes. Urinary bladder repletion, renal parenchyma evaluation, and visualization of urinary bladder for cystocentesis are some of the most common indications. Sonography has been used to diagnose ectopic eggs within the urinary bladder of a Florida cooter (*Pseudemys concinna*) and a leopard tortoise (*Stigmochelys pardalis*), following radiographs suggestive of egg retention.[13,30]

In humans, gout tophi have been described as hyperechoic and heterogeneous, with poorly defined margins. Tophi are typically grouped and have anechoic haloing.[31] Distinction between gout and other forms of mineralization is unlikely to be possible based solely on ultrasonography (see **Fig. 11**B).

Ultrasonography has also been used to evaluate urinary calculi. In dogs, urinary bladder calculi are described as having acoustic shadowing caused by mineral density.[32] This technique has also resulted in an overestimation of urolith size when measured in dogs.[33] Again, these findings may be similar when applied to reptiles, but there are limited reports on the subject.

Benefits and Limitations

Ultrasonography is a quick, readily available diagnostic tool that helps in diagnosing urinary tract disorders. The main clinical limitation of ultrasonography is that it can be challenging when interfacing gas or mineralized surfaces and is limited by chelonians' anatomy. In comparing diagnostic imaging modalities for the evaluation of urolithiasis in human patients, uroliths were more often appreciable on CT in 68% of patients compared with ultrasonography, with which they were identified in 52% of patients.[34] Similar comparisons have not been performed in reptiles.

COMPUTED TOMOGRAPHY
Diagnostic Technique

The increasing availability of CT in veterinary practices is revolutionizing reptile medicine. CT allows the rapid acquisition of internal structures with good three-dimensional differentiation between various organ systems. CT can be obtained under sedation, general anesthesia, or with appropriate restraint techniques that prevent movement.[3,35] In anesthetized chelonians, obtaining CT scans in sternal recumbency with legs extended allows viscera to remain in its normal anatomic location and reduces compression of the coelomic contents.[3]

CT scans have been successfully obtained in conscious reptiles, provided the animal is motionless throughout by either confining it within a box or with the assistance of foam wedges to restrict movement.[4,36,37] Appropriate positioning may be difficult to achieve in awake animals, resulting in artifacts with unknown effects on accurate interpretation. In 1 study of boas, animals without chemical restraint were measured as shorter in length when imaged in a straight tube, compared with when they were awake on physical examination. These animals measured even shorter in length when coiled. This difference was likely caused by the animals remaining tense; however, the effects of these differences on evaluating the urinary system are unknown.[4] To maximize the diagnostic information provided by CT scan, examinations should be obtained with and without intravenous nonionic iodinated contrast. Suggested doses of contrast vary from 2.2 mL/kg[38] to 2 mL/kg, or 800 mg/kg.[39] Intravenous contrast can be given via the jugular vein in chelonians, the abdominal or coccygeal vein in lizards, and the coccygeal vein in snakes.[38,39]

Urinary Tract Appearance

In chelonians, kidneys are easily identified in the retrocoelomic space in contrast-enhanced scans (**Fig. 12**). The kidneys appear homogeneous, without any gross distinction between cortex, medulla, and renal pelvis.[35] In red-eared sliders, good enhancement of the kidneys was present 20 seconds after injection; however, there was no contrast enhancement of the urinary bladder within 180 seconds after contrast.[39]

In lizards, using a soft tissue window, kidneys are visualized within the pelvic canal in bearded dragons and green iguanas, and are seen slightly more cranially in tegus. Renal tissues appear heterogeneous in tegus and green iguanas, and homogeneous in bearded dragons. The urinary bladder and ureters were not appreciable in tegus and green iguanas on CT.[38] Contrast media are recommended to enhance structures when performing a CT scan; however, the time between intravenous administration and uptake in the kidneys has not been reported in lizards.

To the authors' knowledge, there are no studies evaluating complete soft tissue CT anatomy, including urinary systems, in snakes. Existing CT studies in snakes primarily focus on pulmonary evaluation and general body positioning.[4,37]

Clinical Applications

CT scan has been successfully used to diagnose several disorders in reptiles, but only occasionally for identification of disease involving the urinary tract. In dogs, CT has

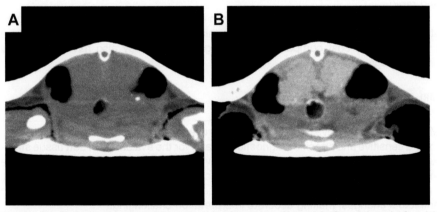

Fig. 12. CT of pelvic area in a red-eared slider (*T scripta elegans*) before (*A*) and after (*B*) administration of contrast (iohexol, 440 mg/kg). Notice the delineation of the renal parenchyma in the contrast-enhanced CT scan. In the plain CT, differentiation of renal parenchyma from surrounding tissue is difficult. (*Courtesy of* N. Di Girolamo, DVM, MSc, PhD, Dipl ECZM (Herp), Stillwater, OK.)

been suggested as a superior modality for assessing urolithiasis composition.[40] These mineralized structures are easily distinguishable from soft tissue on CT imaging, and CT has been suggested as a more sensitive mechanism for evaluating urolithiasis within the urinary tract system.[34]

In reptiles, uroliths primarily contain uric acid salts[15,16]; however, other compositions have been reported.[41] In a retrospective study on the evaluation of urolithiasis in chelonians, animals underwent coelomic CT. There was evidence of uroliths in the urinary bladder in all 13 animals.[16] CT was also successful in identifying urate calculi within either the coprodeum or urinary bladder of a leopard gecko. Using these findings, the gecko was successfully managed for the obstruction with focused treatment.[36]

No proper comparison between CT and other diagnostic techniques for the diagnosis of renal abnormalities in reptiles has been performed. However, CT imaging is also reportedly the most sensitive imaging modality for evaluating tophaceous gout, compared with MRI and ultrasonography in humans.[42] Without further investigation, it is unknown whether this would be translatable to reptile medicine for sensitive evaluation of changes to the renal parenchyma and subsequent renal and visceral gout. CT has been successfully used for the evaluation of soft tissue abnormalities in snakes. A woma python (*Aspidites ramsayi*) underwent CT to assess for recurrence and metastasis, several months after nephrectomy for an adenocarcinoma. Imaging revealed a soft tissue and fat attenuating mass at the previous excision site, consistent with evidence of either granulation tissue or recurrence.[43]

The use of CT imaging in diagnosis of urinary diseases in reptiles is likely an underreported or underused modality. However, with increasing accessibility, this tool may be more readily and efficiently used for guiding treatment in these species.

Benefits and Limitations

Considering the peculiar anatomy of reptiles, and in particular chelonians, CT is likely to offer a relevant improvement because of increased detail and contrast between tissue densities compared with radiographic imaging.[44] CT imaging is rewarding in reptiles, because superimposition of soft tissues with shell, osteoderms, and ribs does not occur.[44] This diagnostic technique is also noninvasive and rapid.

However, CT scanners are not common in general veterinary practices and trained staff are required to operate and maintain this specialized equipment. CT also has a greater financial cost compared with radiographs, but they also have significantly greater image quality.

MRI
Diagnostic Technique

MRI offers a noninvasive means of evaluating internal structures. MRI has been proved to be a sensitive and specific diagnostic modality for the evaluation of soft tissue structures. MRI is a slow process and can take several minutes to hours, depending on the machine used and the area evaluated. To acquire an appropriate image, the animal must be immobilized while MRI is performed,[45,46] because any motion results in artifactual changes, making accurate interpretation challenging.

Urinary Tract Appearance

Coronal, transverse, and sagittal slices can be obtained of the entire animal or a specific region. In chelonians, T1-weighted MRI provided the best visibility of internal anatomy, including the kidneys; however, Valente and colleagues[45] (2006) found that the kidneys of loggerhead sea turtles were best evaluated with T2-weighted images.[46]

Clinical Use

In mammals, MRI is the reference standard diagnostic for assessing subtle details in soft tissue structures. MRI in reptiles is not commonly used, although this modality has been successfully used to diagnose an expansive seminoma in a spur-thighed tortoise (*Testudo graeca*).[47]

MRI has also been used to evaluate the anatomic features of various chelonians under anesthesia. In loggerhead sea turtles, T1-weighted and T2-weighted images were performed on 5 live animals. The kidneys appeared hyperintense to the surrounding tissues on T2-weighted images. However, ureters were unappreciable, and no difference was evident between T1-weighted and T2-weighted images on evaluation of the urinary bladder.[45] In 63 turtles, including red-eared sliders, coastal plain cooters, hieroglyphic river cooters (*Pseudemys concinna hieroglyphica*), and yellow-bellied sliders (*Trachemys scripta scripta*), MRI was effective in evaluating kidney size. Tissue intensity and shape, as well as the appearance of other urinary tract structures, were not discussed.[46]

Benefits and Limitations

MRI is considered a sensitive tool for the evaluation of soft tissues; therefore, it may offer detailed information about the urinary structures and disease therein. However, MRI requires prolonged anesthesia or sedation to ensure the patient remains motionless throughout the scan.

ENDOSCOPY

Endoscopy is a valuable tool for the diagnosis of urinary tract disorders in reptiles. Two distinct approaches exist for evaluating urinary structures in reptiles: coelioscopy and cystoscopy. Valuable information can be acquired from either technique, depending on the disease entity and intended purpose of the procedure.

Coelioscopy

Diagnostic technique

For this approach, chemical immobilization is requisite and therefore the patient should be clinically stable and starved before the procedure.[48] A 2.7-mm scope has been suggested as having the most versatility for reptilian patients.[48–50] The patient is aseptically prepared and a small incision is made through the skin to the body wall. The body wall is then bluntly penetrated with a hemostat, or obturator and sheath, to access the coelomic cavity.[48,51] Once access has been achieved, insufflation of the coelomic cavity can be performed.[48,50]

Urinary tract appearance

Access point and anatomy varies with each species. Most lizards should be positioned in dorsal recumbency, except laterally compressed lizards, which can be positioned laterally.[48] In these species a paramedian or paralumbar approach is appropriate for visualizing visceral contents, with typically no difference in left versus right approach when evaluating urinary structures.[48,50] Described landmarks include the ribs cranially, the spine dorsally, and pelvic limb caudally.[48] The kidneys are located along the caudodorsal aspect of the coelom in lizards, with the exception of iguanas, in which they reside intrapelvically. Ventral to these structures, the urinary bladder can be appreciated, when present.[48] In snakes, lateral access, between or medial to the ribs, should be performed at the level of the kidney.[48] In chelonians, there are 2 distinct ways to visualize or biopsy the kidneys, both from the prefemoral space. One approach consists of entering the coelom, directing the endoscope caudally, making an incision in the retrocoelomic membrane and therefore gaining access to the kidney. A potentially simpler approach does not enter the coelom. Instead, the endoscope is directed dorsocaudally once it has entered the subcutaneous space of the prefemoral cavity. In either approach, the contralateral kidney is generally difficult to visualize and biopsy, and a bilateral approach is usually required.[49]

Clinical applications
Coelioscopy is a useful diagnostic tool in reptilian medicine. This method is often used to sex hatchling chelonians,[52,53] but it has also been used to evaluate viscera and obtain biopsy samples, including from the kidneys.[49]

Research applications
Research using endoscopic techniques has become increasing popular. In a study of 23 green iguanas, animals were anesthetized for coelioscopy using a right lateral approach to evaluate and biopsy the left kidney. Biopsies were easily harvested, and technique offered good visualization of the gross appearance of the kidneys.[50]

Benefits and limitations
Coelioscopy is a minimally invasive approach for gross evaluation and sampling of intracoelomic tissues. This approach allows the evaluation of the texture and color of tissues, which is not available through noninvasive diagnostic techniques. However, coelioscopy is a surgical procedure that requires access directly into the coelom, so it carries all the standard risks associated with such a procedure. There is also a risk of iatrogenic tissue trauma from the scope or obturator.

Cloacoscopy/Cystoscopy

Diagnostic technique
Cloacoscopy is performed by introducing an endoscope into the vent or cloacal sphincter. The scope may be further advanced through the cloaca and into the urethral orifice and urinary bladder when present.[53] The bladder is then distended by an infusion of warm crystalloid fluids.[53,54] A 2.7-mm 30° rigid scope is recommended for this procedure.[53,54] For this approach, chemical immobilization is often used[14,53] but is not always necessary.[55] When cystoscopy is performed in chelonians, the animals are usually positioned in ventral recumbency[53,56];however, dorsal recumbency has been described as well.[13]

Urinary tract appearance
Renal tissue can be visualized through the transparency of the urinary bladder or of the accessory urinary bladders (in aquatic turtles). In red-eared sliders, renal visualization was subjectively easier from accessory bladder cloacoscopy than from cystoscopy (**Fig. 13**).[57] Cystoscopy performed on 15 deceased Hermann's tortoises (*Testudo hermanni*) and 25 live animals was successful for evaluating viscera. The kidneys were visible in females through the thin urinary bladder wall, but, because of superimposition of testicles, the kidneys were challenging to evaluate in males.[53] Cloacoscopy was easily achieved in 32 anesthetized adult loggerhead sea turtles. However, on performing cystoscopy in these individuals, the wall of the urinary bladder was so thick

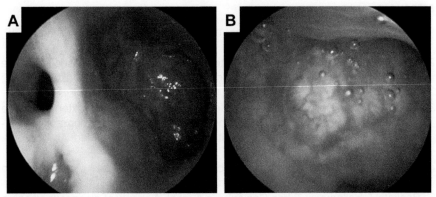

Fig. 13. Visualization of the lateral surface of a grossly altered right kidney through the right accessory bladder in a red-eared slider (*T scripta elegans*). (*A*) Entrance of the right accessory bladder. (*B*) Close-up of the altered kidney as visualized from the medial side of the right accessory bladder. The kidney is abnormally large and discolored. (*Courtesy of* N. Di Girolamo, DVM, MSc, PhD, Dipl ECZM (Herp), Stillwater, OK.)

that, even when distended with saline, visualization of coelomic organs was not possible.[58]

Cloacoscopy has also been performed in snakes, but with limited diagnostic value. Six apparently healthy adult horned vipers (*Vipera ammodytes*) were manually restrained for cloacoscopy. The urodeum was appreciable once the saline was flushed to distend the cloaca; however, further evaluation of urinary tract structures was not discussed and likely not achievable through this technique.[55]

Clinical applications
Most reports of clinical use of cystoscopy and cloacoscopy have been in chelonians. Cloacoscopy has been successful in evaluation and removal of cloacal calculi in African spurred tortoises (*Centrochelys sulcata*) initially identified on radiographs.[14] Similarly, cystoscopy has been successfully performed on 3 Florida river cooters and a leopard tortoise to evaluate and remove ectopic eggs identified in the urinary bladder on ultrasonography and radiographs.[13,56]

Benefits and limitations
Cloacoscopy and cystoscopy are efficient and minimally invasive techniques for evaluating internal organs and the contents of the urinary bladder; however, acquisition of biopsy samples from other organ systems is not possible. Potential risks include iatrogenic bladder rupture from crystalloid infusion into the urinary bladder,[54] and possibly cystitis if the tissue is compromised.[13]

SUMMARY

Diagnosis of disease in reptilian patients is often challenging, so the appropriate use of diagnostic imaging is critical. The modality used may be directed by examination findings or indications from other diagnostic tests. The increased availability of advanced diagnostic techniques in veterinary practice, such as CT scan, ultrasonography, and MRI, will increase the understanding of reptile diseases and significantly improve the chances of making a proper antemortem diagnosis.

REFERENCES

1. Reavill DR, Schmidt RE. Urinary tract diseases of reptiles. J Exot Pet Med 2010; 19(4):280–9.
2. Schmidt-Ukaj S, Hochleithner M, Richter B, et al. A survey of diseases in captive bearded dragons: a retrospective study of 529 patients. Vet Med (Praha) 2017; 62(9):508–15.
3. Mans C, Drees R, Sladky KK, et al. Effects of body position and extension of the neck and extremities on lung volume measured via computed tomography in red-eared slider turtles (Trachemys scripta elegans). J Am Vet Med Assoc 2013; 243(8):1190–6.
4. Hedley J, Eatwell K, Schwarz T. Computed tomography of ball pythons (Python regius) in curled recumbency. Vet Radiol Ultrasound 2014;55(4):380–6.
5. Banzato T, Hellebuyck T, Van Caelenberg A, et al. A review of diagnostic imaging of snakes and lizards. Vet Rec 2013;173(2):43–9.
6. Keck M, Zimmerman DM, Ramsay EC, et al. Renal adenocarcinoma in cape coral snakes (Aspidelaps lubricus lubricus). J Herpetol Med Surg 2011;21(1):5–9.
7. Holz P, Barker IK, Crawshaw GJ, et al. The anatomy and perfusion of the renal portal system in the red-eared slider (Trachemys scripta elegans). J Zoo Wildl Med 1997;26:378–85.
8. Valente AL, Cuenca R, Parga ML, et al. Cervical and coelomic radiologic features of the loggerhead sea turtle, Caretta caretta. Can J Vet Res 2006;70(4):285.
9. Che'Amat A, Gabriel B, Chee NW. Cystic calculi removal in African spurred tortoise (Geochelone sulcata) using transplstron coeliotomy. Vet World 2012;5(8).
10. Di Girolamo N, Selleri P. What is your diagnosis? J Am Vet Med Assoc 2016; 249(3):271–3.
11. Hernandez-Divers SJ. Green iguana nephrology: a review of diagnostic techniques. Vet Clin North Am Exot Anim Pract 2003;6(1):233–50.
12. Benson KG, Forrest L. Characterization of the renal portal system of the common green iguana (Iguana iguana) by digital subtraction imaging. J zoo Wildl Med 1999;30(2):235–41.
13. Mans C, Foster JD. Endoscopy-guided ectopic egg removal from the urinary bladder in a leopard tortoise (Stigmochelys pardalis). Can Vet J 2014;55(6):569.
14. Mans C, Sladky KK. Endoscopically guided removal of cloacal calculi in three African spurred tortoises (Geochelone sulcata). J Am Vet Med Assoc 2012;240(7): 869–75.
15. Wolf KN, Troan BV, DeVoe R. Chronic urolithiasis and subsequent cystectomy in a San Esteban Island Chuckwalla, Sauromalus varius. J Herpetol Med Surg 2008; 18(3):106–12.
16. Keller KA, Hawkins MG, Weber ES III, et al. Diagnosis and treatment of urolithiasis in client-owned chelonians: 40 cases (1987–2012). J Am Vet Med Assoc 2015; 247(6):650–8.
17. Prades RB, Lastica EA, Acorda JA. Ultrasound features of the kidneys, urinary bladder, ovarian follicles and vaginal sacs of female water monitor lizard (Varanus marmoratus, Weigmann, 1834). Philipp J Vet Anim Sci 2013;39(1):115–24.
18. Isaza R, Ackerman N, Jacobson ER. Ultrasound imaging of the coelomic structures in the Boa constrictor (Boa constrictor). Vet Radiol Ultrasound 1993;34(6): 445–50.
19. Bucy DS, Guzman DS-M, Zwingenberger AL. Ultrasonographic anatomy of bearded dragons (Pogona vitticeps). J Am Vet Med Assoc 2015;246(8):868–76.

20. Krishna SM, Rajkumar K, Karhik M, et al. Standardization of ultrasonographic anatomy of coelomic organs in Indian spectacled cobra (Naja naja) and Russell's viper (Daboia russelii) Paper presented at: American Association of Zoo Veterinarians. Salt Lake City, UT, September 26–October 2, 2003.

21. Martorell J, Espada Y, de Gopegui RR. Normal echoanatomy of the red-eared slider terrapin (Trachemys scripta elegans). Vet Rec 2004;155(14):417–20.

22. Sainsbury AW, Gili C. Ultrasonographic anatomy and scanning technique of the coelomic organs of the bosc monitor (Varanus exanthematicus). J Zoo Wildl Med 1991;22(4):421–33.

23. Penninck DG, Stewart JS, Paul-Murphy J, et al. Ultrasonography of the California desert tortoise (Xerobates agassizi): anatomy and application. Veterinary radiology 1991;32(3):112–6.

24. Cojean O, Vergneau-Grosset C, Masseau I. Ultrasonographic anatomy of reproductive female leopard geckos (Eublepharis macularius). Vet Radiol Ultrasound 2018;59(3):333–44.

25. Meireles YS, Shinike FS, Matte DR, et al. Ultrasound characterization of the coelomic cavity organs of the red-footed tortoise (Chelonoidis carbonaria). Cienc Rural 2016;46(10):1811–7.

26. Samaniego CAA, Lastica-Ternura EA, Acorda JA, et al. Ultrasonographic findings in the liver, gallbladder and kidneys of captive reticulated pythons (Python reticulatus) with pneumonia. Philipp J Vet Anim Sci 2016;41(2):119–26.

27. Pease A, Blanvillain G, Rostal D, et al. Ultrasound imaging of the inguinal region of adult male loggerhead sea turtles (Caretta caretta). J Zoo Wildl Med 2010;41(1):69–76.

28. Banzato T, Russo E, Finotti L, et al. Ultrasonographic anatomy of the coelomic organs of boid snakes (Boa constrictor imperator, Python regius, Python molurus molurus, and Python curtus). Am J Vet Res 2012;73(5):634–45.

29. Holland MF, Hernandez-Divers S, Frank PM. Ultrasonographic appearance of the coelomic cavity in healthy green iguanas. J Am Vet Med Assoc 2008;233(4):590–6.

30. Thomas HL, Wilier CJ, Wosar MA, et al. Egg-retention in the urinary bladder of a Florida cooter turtle, Pseudemys floridana floridana. J Herpetol Med Surg 2002;12(1):4–6.

31. Thiele R, Schlesinger N. Diagnosis of gout by ultrasound. Rheumatology 2007;46(7):1116–21.

32. Hecht S. Diagnostic imaging of lower urinary tract disease. Vet Clin North Am Small Anim Pract 2015;45(4):639–63.

33. Byl KM, Kruger JM, Kinns J, et al. In vitro comparison of plain radiography, double-contrast cystography, ultrasonography, and computed tomography for estimation of cystolith size. Am J Vet Res 2010;71(3):374–80.

34. Passerotti C, Chow JS, Silva A, et al. Ultrasound versus computerized tomography for evaluating urolithiasis. J Urol 2009;182(4S):1829–34.

35. Valente A, Cuenca R, Zamora M, et al. Computed tomography of the vertebral column and coelomic structures in the normal loggerhead sea turtle (Caretta caretta). Vet J 2007;174(2):362–70.

36. DeCourcy K, Hostnik ET, Lorbach J, et al. Unsedated computed tomography for diagnosis of pelvic canal obstruction in a leopard gecko (Eublepharis macularius). J zoo Wildl Med 2016;47(4):1073–6.

37. de Souza JCS, Fernandes THT, de Albuquerque Bonelli M, et al. Quantitative computed tomography of healthy adult boas (Boa constrictor). J Zoo Wildl Med 2018;49(4):1012–5.

38. Banzato T, Selleri P, Veladiano I, et al. Comparative evaluation of the cadaveric and computed tomographic features of the coelomic cavity in the green iguana (*Iguana iguana*), black and white tegu (*Tupinambis merianae*) and bearded dragon (*Pogona vitticeps*). Anat Histol Embryol 2013;42(6):453–60.

39. Sochorcova V, Proks P, Cermakova E, et al. Contrast-enhanced computed tomography of the liver, gall bladder and urogenital tract in female red-eared terrapins (Trachemys scripta elegans). Vet Med (Praha) 2017;62(12):674–80.

40. Pressler BM, Mohammadian LA, Li E, et al. In vitro prediction of canine urolith mineral composition using computed tomographic mean beam attenuation measurements. Vet Radiol Ultrasound 2004;45(3):189–97.

41. McKown RD. A cystic calculus from a wild western spiny softshell turtle (Apalone [Trionyx] spiniferus hartwegi). J Zoo Wildl Med 1998;29(3):347.

42. Gerster J, Landry M, Dufresne L, et al. Imaging of tophaceous gout: computed tomography provides specific images compared with magnetic resonance imaging and ultrasonography. Ann Rheum Dis 2002;61(1):52–4.

43. Kaye SW, Daverio H, Eddy R, et al. Surgical resection of an interrenal cell adenocarcinoma in a woma python (Aspidites ramsayi) with 18 month follow-up. J Herpetol Med Surg 2016;26(1–2):26–31.

44. Mackey EB, Hernandez-Divers SJ, Holland M, et al. Clinical technique: application of computed tomography in zoological medicine. J Exot Pet Med 2008;17(3):198–209.

45. Valente ALS, Cuenca R, Zamora MA, et al. Sectional anatomic and magnetic resonance imaging features of coelomic structures of loggerhead sea turtles. Am J Vet Res 2006;67(8):1347–53.

46. Mathes KA, Schnack M, Rohn K, et al. Magnetic resonance imaging measurements of organs within the coelomic cavity of red-eared sliders (Trachemys scripta elegans), yellow-bellied sliders (Trachemys scripta scripta), Coastal plain cooters (Pseudemys concinna floridana), and hieroglyphic river cooters (Pseudemys concinna hieroglyphica). Am J Vet Res 2017;78(12):1387–99.

47. Pees M, Ludewig E, Plenz B, et al. Imaging diagnosis–seminoma causing liver compression in a spur-thighed tortoise (testudo graeca). Vet Radiol Ultrasound 2015;56(2):E21–4.

48. Divers SJ. Reptile diagnostic endoscopy and endosurgery. Vet Clin North Am Exot Anim Pract 2010;13(2):217–42.

49. Divers SJ, Stahl SJ, Camus A. Evaluation of diagnostic coelioscopy including liver and kidney biopsy in freshwater turtles (Trachemys scripta). J Zoo Wildl Med 2010;41(4):677–87.

50. Hernandez-Divers SJ, Stahl SJ, Stedman NL, et al. Renal evaluation in the healthy green iguana (Iguana iguana): assessment of plasma biochemistry, glomerular filtration rate, and endoscopic biopsy. J Zoo Wildl Med 2005;36(2):155–69.

51. Hernandez-Divers S. Endoscopic renal evaluation and biopsy of chelonia. Vet Rec 2004;154(3):73–80.

52. Hernandez-Divers SJ, Stahl SJ, Farrell R. An endoscopic method for identifying sex of hatchling Chinese box turtles and comparison of general versus local anesthesia for coelioscopy. J Am Vet Med Assoc 2009;234(6):800–4.

53. Selleri P, Di Girolamo N, Melidone R. Cystoscopic sex identification of posthatchling chelonians. J Am Vet Med Assoc 2013;242(12):1744–50.

54. Di Girolamo N, Selleri P. Clinical applications of cystoscopy in chelonians. Vet Clin North Am Exot Anim Pract 2015;18(3):507–26.

55. Oliveri M, Morici M, Novotný R, et al. Cloacoscopy in the horned viper (Vipera ammodytes). Acta Vet 2016;85(3):251–3.

56. Minter LJ, Wood MW, Hill TL, et al. Cystoscopic guided removal of ectopic eggs from the urinary bladder of the Florida cooter turtle (Pseudemys floridana floridana). J Zoo Wildl Med 2010;41(3):503–9.

57. Di Girolamo N, Spadola F, Selleri P, Insacco G. Comparison of urinary and accessory bladder approach during cloacoscopy of chelonians. Paper presented at: Association of Reptilian and Amphibian Veterinarians. Oakland, CA, October 21–26, 2012.

58. Spadola F, Morici M, Oliveri M, et al. Description of cloacoscopy in the loggerhead sea turtle (Caretta caretta). Acta Vet 2017;85(4):367–70.

Clinical Management of Reptile Renal Disease

Stacey Leonatti Wilkinson, DVM, DABVP (Reptile and Amphibian)[a,*],
Stephen J. Divers, BVetMed, DZooMed, DECZM (Zoo Health Management, Herpetology), DACZM, FRCVS[b]

KEYWORDS

- Reptile • Renal • Kidney • Gout • Kidney disease • Treatment • Uric acid

KEY POINTS

- Renal disease is one of the most common medical conditions of captive reptiles, but often signs of disease are nonspecific and not present until the condition is life threatening.
- Acute and chronic renal disease can develop in reptiles, and differentiating the 2 is critical in terms of treatment and prognosis.
- Many factors can contribute to the development of renal disease, including chronic subclinical dehydration, improper diet and supplementation, other inadequate husbandry practices, infection, trauma, toxin ingestion, neoplasia, and urinary calculi.
- Diagnosis can be difficult and often requires multiple tests, such as clinical pathology, radiology, ultrasonography, endoscopy, computed tomography/magnetic resonance imaging, scintigraphy, iohexol clearance studies, and renal biopsy.
- Treatment is multimodal and renal disease can sometimes be managed, but long-term prognosis is poor, especially for chronic renal disease.

INTRODUCTION

Renal disease is one of the most common medical conditions encountered in captive reptiles. Many factors contribute to the development of renal disease, and the etiology often is multifactorial. Unfortunately, in most cases, signs of disease are nonspecific and often are not present until the condition is life threatening. Therefore, prevention is greatly preferred to treatment. Understanding the pathophysiology, potential causes, and treatment options is essential for the reptile veterinarian to manage this condition. A primary goal of the veterinarian is to differentiate between the end-stage presentation of chronic renal disease, which carries a poor to hopeless prognosis, and acute renal failure (guarded prognosis). A more complete review of reptile

Disclosure Statement: The authors have nothing to disclose.

[a] Avian and Exotic Animal Hospital of Georgia, 118 Pipemakers Circle, Suite 110, Pooler, GA 31322, USA; [b] Department of Small Animal Medicine and Surgery, College of Veterinary Medicine, University of Georgia, 501 D.W. Brooks Drive, Athens, GA 30602, USA

* Corresponding author.

E-mail address: drw@avianexotichospital.com

renal disease has recently been published in *Mader's Reptile and Amphibian Medicine and Surgery*, third edition.[1]

ANATOMY AND PHYSIOLOGY

The urinary system of reptiles includes the kidneys, ureters, and urinary bladder, if present. The kidneys are located in the caudal coelom in most species and within the pelvic canal of many lizards (**Fig. 1**). Glomeruli in reptilian kidneys are poorly developed compared with those in birds, and they contain far fewer nephrons (**Fig. 2**).[1] The distal convoluted tubules of many squamates undergo hypertrophy (sexual segment proliferation of mucous-secreting cells) during the breeding season; the precise function of this segment is poorly understood but seems to assist with sperm carriage.[1–3] Reptiles also lack a loop of Henle, so urine cannot be concentrated above that of plasma at the time the urine is produced. Reptiles possess a renal portal system whereby blood flow from the caudal end of the body may supply the renal tubules (but not the glomeruli) before reaching systemic circulation. This can potentially affect the renal excretion of certain medications and increase harmful side effects of others.[1,4] Although such phenomena have proved statistically significant in various pharmacokinetic studies, they are not considered clinically significant, but it remains common practice to avoid injections in the caudal half of the body for medications with possible renal side effects (eg, amino-glycosides).[1,4,5] The ureters empty into the urodeum of the cloaca.

Chelonians and most lizards possess a urinary bladder, but snakes and crocodilians do not. The bladder empties into the urodeum of the cloaca; as such, the contents of the bladder are never sterile. The bladder also functions as a site of fluid storage and reabsorption in times of low water availability, and the bladder, colon, and cloaca can

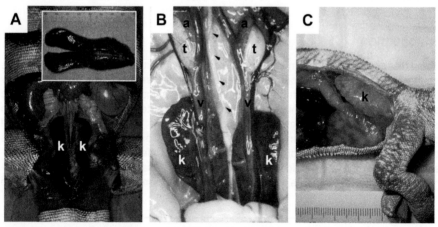

Fig. 1. Saurian kidneys. (*A*) The pelvis has been removed to reveal the ventral view of the normal intrapelvic kidneys (k) in a female iguana (*Iguana* sp). (*Inset*) Note how the caudal poles of the kidneys are fused. (*B*) Ventral view of the caudal coelomic healthy kidneys (k) in a monitor lizard (*Varanus* sp). Note the close association with the renal veins (v), dorsal aorta (*arrows*), testes (t) and adrenal glands (a). (*C*) Left lateral view of the caudal coelomic left kidney (k) in a chameleon (*Chamaeleo* sp). This kidney is not normal and demonstrates renomegaly and pallor due to glomerulonephrosis, renal calcification, and gout. (*Courtesy of* S. Divers, BVetMed, DZooMed, DECZM (Zoo Health Management, Herpetology), DACZM, FRCVS, Athens, GA.)

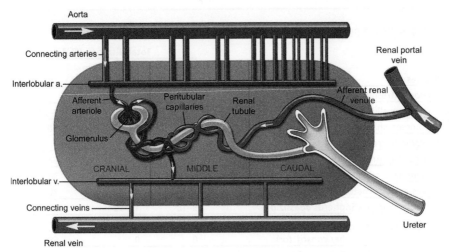

Fig. 2. Schematic illustration of the nephron and associated vasculature in a green iguana (*Iguana iguana*) kidney. a, artery; v, vein. (*Courtesy of* K. Carter, AA, BFA, Athens, GA.)

be important sites of sodium excretion and water resorption.[1,2] Some species (eg, iguanids and sea turtles) possess extrarenal salt excreting glands as well.

The kidneys eliminate nitrogenous wastes resulting from protein metabolism. Protein metabolism results in ammonia, which must be filtered from the blood into the urine to prevent toxic levels that cannot be tolerated by the brain (a process that requires large amounts of water) or converted to a less toxic compound that can remain in the bloodstream.[1] Reptiles vary in their excretion of different nitrogenous waste products (**Table 1**). Reptiles that live in fresh water eliminate a large portion of their waste as ammonia because they are in no danger of becoming dehydrated and do not need to waste energy on water conservation.[1] Reptiles that have intermittent access to fresh water need to conserve some water, so they convert some of their waste to urea, which is water soluble and less toxic than ammonia.[1] Reptiles with minimal access to fresh water place a premium on water conservation. They convert urea to uric acid, which has low toxicity but is water insoluble; it requires much less water to be actively secreted from proximal tubules and excreted.[1] The disadvantage is during dehydration, ultrafiltrate flow through the kidneys may be severely reduced or even absent, allowing uric acid to precipitate or crystallize in kidney tubules or glomeruli.[1] If this occurs in tissues, gout develops. Many reptiles can shift the balance of how much ammonia to uric acid is produced in urine depending on the water available, although there are limits to this shift.[1]

HISTORY, SIGNALMENT, AND CONTRIBUTING FACTORS

Renal disease can occur in any reptile species, although it seems to occur more frequently in lizards and chelonians. A variety of diseases have been reported, including renal cysts, interstitial nephritis, glomerulonephritis, pyelonephritis, tubulonephrosis, renal edema, and amyloidosis, along with gout and dystrophic mineralization.[1,6] Infectious causes, such as bacterial, fungal, or parasitic (especially *Hexamita* spp) infections, also can cause renal damage.[1,3,6] Trauma or toxin ingestion also is possible.[3,6] Renal neoplasia has also been reported, most often in snakes and lizards.[1,3,6,7] Renal, ureteral, cystic, and urethral calculi also have been reported.[1,3,6,8]

Table 1
Nitrogenous end-products excreted by reptiles

Species	Total Nitrogen (%)[a]		
	Ammonia	Urea (Serum Urea Nitrogen)	Uric Acid
Chelonia (freshwater aquatic)			
Common slider (*Trachemys scripta*)	4–44	45–95	1–24
Common snapping turtle (*Chelydra serpentine*)	11	80	10
Chelonia (terrestrial)			
African spurred tortoise (*Centrochelys sulcata*)	3	20	55
Kleinmann tortoise (*Testudo kleinmanni*)	4	49	34
Western or ornate box turtle (*Terrapene ornata*)	23	47	30
Desert tortoise (Gopherus *agassizii*)	3–18	15–50	20–50
Squamata			
Eastern racer (*Coluber constrictor*)	0	0	58
Kenyan sand boa (*Gongylophis colubrinus*)	6	0	63
Cuban rock iguana (*Cyclura nubila*)	<1	1	98–99
Carolina anole (*Anolis carolinensis*)	13	13	73
Crocodilia			
Nile crocodile (*Crocodylus niloticus*)	66	5	21
Spectacled caiman (*Caiman crocodilus*)	53	6	27
Salt water crocodile (*Crocodylus porosus*)	77	21	2

[a] Calculated as percent sum of the ammonia, urea, and uric acid when total nitrogen data were not available. Molecular weights of 18, 60.1, and 168.1 and percentages N of 83%, 46.7% and 33.3% were used, respectively, in calculations.

From Divers SJ and Innis CJ (2019). Urology In: Divers SJ, Stahl SJ, eds. *Maders Reptile and Amphibian Medicine and Surgery.* 3rd ed: Elsevier, St. Louis. 2019. pp. 624-648; with permission.

Chronic subclinical dehydration is suspected to be a major contributing factor in the development of chronic renal disease.[1,2] Water must be provided in the appropriate manner for the species; many do not drink from standing water. Proper humidity is vital for reducing insensible water loss.[1,2] Clients often misjudge water needs of desert animals and fail to account for microclimates in the habitat. Providing structures, such as humid hide boxes, often is beneficial.

Improper diet and supplementation are large contributors to the development of chronic renal disease. High-protein diets are a common cause of renal disease in herbivorous species.[1] Excessive vitamin D_3 supplementation can lead to soft tissue mineralization and renal disease.[1] Patients who have had nutritional secondary hyperparathyroidism when young, even if the condition was recognized and husbandry deficiencies corrected, also are predisposed to renal disease because of the cytotoxic effects of parathyroid hormone.[9] Hypovitaminosis A may contribute by causing squamous metaplasia of renal epithelium, restricting the lumen of the renal tubules and decreasing the functional capacity of the nephrons.[1,3,6] Improper temperatures can predispose to renal disease because if the reptile cannot reach its preferred optimum temperature zone, renal metabolism may be slower than needed to actively secrete uric acid from the proximal renal tubules to the ureters.[1,2]

In recent years, there seems to be an increased incidence of young bearded dragons less than 2 years old with articular gout. Anecdotal reports suggest a possible association with feeding Dubia roaches (*Blaptica dubia*) that have themselves been fed high-protein dog or cat food. As such, these feeder insects are gaining a reputation, which is likely undeserved, of contributing to gout. It is more likely that protein enrichment, rather than the roach itself, is the main problem. More commonly, many adult bearded dragons continue to be fed a largely insectivorous diet with little to no plant material. This certainly can result in excessive dietary protein and increased demands on uric acid excretion. Certain sources of lineages also appear to be more commonly affected, and a genetic predisposition is also possible. Further research is required, and clinicians are advised to continue to recommend necropsy on affected animals despite the ease of diagnosing gout antemortem.

CLINICAL SIGNS

Clinical signs of chronic renal disease are vague or even absent until the condition is advanced. Most clinical signs are nonspecific, including lethargy, reduced appetite, weight loss, and signs of dehydration, such as sunken eyes and thick, ropy saliva (**Fig. 3**).[1] Often animals are weak and recumbent rather than sitting up in a normal posture. Although polyuria and polydipsia are not as common as in mammals, reptiles can exhibit these signs, especially with acute renal failure.

A common sign is tenesmus or constipation, especially in lizards. The kidneys lie within the pelvic canal of many species, so if renomegaly is present, the kidneys can compress the distal colon, making it difficult to pass feces. The kidneys should be palpated via digital cloacal examination in large lizards. Enlarged kidneys sometimes are palpable cranial to the pelvic rim within the coelomic cavity. The kidneys cannot be palpated in chelonians and are difficult to palpate in snakes.

Diseases that result in urinary or gastrointestinal loss of protein may result in hypoalbuminemia and edema, especially in the pharyngeal area.[1,10] A foul odor to the oral cavity, difficulty swallowing, and/or gulping motions may be seen as well.[1] Regurgitation often is seen late in disease.[1] The eyes may appear swollen with enlarged scleral or iridial blood vessels that may be associated with hypertension.[1]

The presence of multiple swollen joints often is indicative of articular gout. If renal secondary hyperparathyroidism is present, signs of hypocalcemia are seen, including weakness, tremors, or seizures and soft bowed long bones and softening of or fibrous osteodystrophy of the mandible.[11] These signs must be differentiated from hyperparathyroidism of nutritional origin, which typically is seen in younger, growing animals.[11]

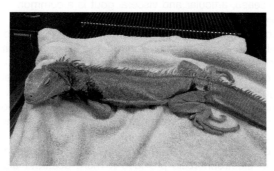

Fig. 3. Typical appearance of a lizard (*Iguana iguana*) with chronic renal disease. (*Courtesy of* S. Leonatti Wilkinson, DVM, DABVP (Reptile and Amphibian), Pooler, GA.)

MINIMUM DATABASE

A complete blood cell count and chemistry panel are the initial diagnostic tests of choice. In reptiles, however, diagnosis of renal disease based on bloodwork parameters can sometimes be challenging. Bloodwork parameters often are unreliable markers of renal disease because they can be affected by other factors and often only rise late in the course of disease. It also is not unusual for reptiles that are severely ill to have unremarkable results compared with published ranges, leaving the veterinarian unsure how to interpret these results unless previous, healthy values from the same patient are on file. Other factors, such as age, gender, season, reproductive status, laboratory used, and where and how the sample was collected, all can influence results.[1,12]

Hematology

Elevations in packed cell volume (PCV) usually indicate dehydration.[1,12] Nonregenerative anemia secondary to chronic renal disease and lack of erythropoietin occurs as well, just as in mammalian species.[1,12] When both anemia and dehydration are present, the PCV may be normal and mask hemoconcentration.[1]

An elevated white blood cell count may indicate infection or inflammation (eg, pyelonephritis), but the absence of a leukocytosis, or leukopenia, does not rule infection in or out.[1] The white blood cell count may be elevated in acute cases, but leukocyte changes often are reduced and more subtle in chronic cases.[1] Eosinophilia may be present when the kidneys are affected by parasitic diseases.[1] If a reptile is not kept at its preferred optimum temperature zone, immunocompromise may occur and the reptile may fail to demonstrate an appropriate leukocyte response.[1]

Biochemistry

Renal function in reptiles cannot be evaluated by standard blood parameters alone, but several analytes may be useful in the diagnosis of renal disease. Uric acid is the main nitrogenous waste product in most squamates. Reduction in the secretion of uric acid by renal tubules leads to hyperuricemia. Significant damage to the kidneys must occur before levels start to rise.[13] Persistent or high elevations of uric acid are often indicative of severe renal insufficiency, acute or chronic.[1,13] Hyperuricemia can also be secondary to severe dehydration and a reduction in renal blood flow.[13] Elevations in uric acid are normal adaptations for some desert species or after a meal in carnivorous reptiles, so interpretation must be done with caution in these species, especially in cases of protracted anorexia.[1,13] If hyperuricemia is present secondary to severe renal disease, articular and visceral gout is a common sequela once uric acid levels exceed 25 mg/dL.[1,14]

Creatinine is not produced in high enough quantities in reptiles to be useful in the diagnosis of renal disease.[1,13] Serum urea nitrogen is a significant nitrogenous waste product in most chelonians and is of greater importance than uric acid in aquatic species, and trends can be more helpful than a single value.[1,5,9] Furthermore, ammonia also can be a significant metabolite in many aquatic reptiles.[1,13] Given the variability and relative importance of uric acid, serum urea nitrogen, and ammonia, the reliance on uric acid in anything other than squamates represents a deficiency in many commercial reptile profiles.

Chronic renal disease can cause protein loss, leading to hypoalbuminemia and edema.[1,10] Protein electrophoresis provides a more accurate albumin level than most in-house analyzers, because bromocresol green determinations have been shown to be inaccurate in lizards and chelonians.[1,13]

Calcium and phosphorus are important parameters for evaluating renal function, particularly in lizards, but they may be influenced by many factors. Most analyzers measure total calcium, but ionized calcium may be more appropriate because it allows the clinician to determine biologically active calcium.[1,13,15] Gravid females often have an extreme hypercalcemia, but a normal ionized calcium.[1,13] Animals suffering from nutritional secondary hyperparathyroidism may have a normal total calcium and/or low ionized calcium until near terminal, and it is important to be able to differentiate these patients from those with renal disease.[11,13] Hypoalbuminemia can affect calcium levels because most calcium is protein bound.[1,13] The optimum calcium phosphorus ratio is typically 1.5:1 to 2:1; a reduction or inversion of this ratio can be indicative of renal disease, particularly if the phosphorus level is elevated.[1,16] If the calcium phosphorus product, or solubility index, is elevated (>55–70 mg/dL), mineralization of the tissues can occur.[1]

Aspartate aminotransferase, creatine phosphokinase, lactate dehydrogenase, and γ-glutamyl transferase are present in small amount in the reptilian kidney.[1,13,17] Because these enzymes are found in many tissue types, however, they are nonspecific markers of renal disease.[1,13,17] These enzymes also tend to be elevated more acutely, and, because reptiles tend to present late in the course of disease, elevations in these enzymes are often missed.

Changes in sodium, potassium, and chloride can occur as well. Hyponatremia and hyperkalemia may be present from renal disease or dysfunction of the cloaca, colon, or bladder[1,13]; 90% of potassium excretion is via the kidney, so any decrease in function can lead to decreased potassium excretion, hyperkalemia, and a metabolic acidosis.[13] Hyperchloremia is associated with dehydration, possible renal tubular disease, or disorders of the salt glands.[1,13]

Urinalysis

Urinalysis may be helpful, but there are many limitations in reptiles. Reptiles lack a loop of Henle so they are unable to concentrate urine above the concentration of plasma. In species with a bladder, it serves as a site for fluid storage along with fluid and electrolyte exchange.[1,2] Postrenal modification of urine can occur in the cloaca, colon, or bladder depending on species, potentially changing the composition of ureteral urine.[1,2] Urine passes through the urodeum of the cloaca and typically is not sterile. Samples can be obtained via cystocentesis in species with a bladder. Ultrasonography makes this much easier, however, because of the thin, fragile nature of the bladder wall, danger of urine leakage into the coelom postsampling is a valid concern.[1] A urine sample also can be obtained through catheterization of the bladder assisted by cloacoscopy.[1]

Despite these limitations, urinalysis can still be helpful. Although few studies are available, urine pH in herbivorous tortoises is typically alkaline,[1,18] whereas the pH of omnivorous or carnivorous species is more acidic.[1,19] Thus suspicion of an abnormality may be appropriate with a carnivorous reptile producing alkaline urine or an herbivorous reptile producing acidic urine. Acidic urine has been observed in herbivorous tortoises during drought, with high-protein diets, near the end of hibernation, or during prolonged periods of anorexia from illness.[1,18] In box turtles and tortoises, zero to trace protein levels seem normal.[1] Glucose is not normally present in significant amounts.[1] Blood may be positive in samples obtained by cystocentesis or expression.[1] Ketones, nitrite, and leukocytes have not been evaluated in reptiles, and bilirubin and urobilinogen are not useful in reptiles because they are produced in extremely small amounts, if any.[1]

Urine sediment evaluation is the most useful test in evaluating reptile urine. Erythrocytes, leukocytes, epithelial cells, microorganisms, spermatozoa, crystals, and casts may be identified.[1] Evaluation of normal tortoise and box turtle urine indicates small numbers of leukocytes and epithelial cells can be normal, but urine is mostly acellular.[1] The presence of erythrocytes, leukocytes, epithelial cells, casts, and certain pathogens (fungal elements, parasites, pure bacterial growth, and so forth) can have significance and indicate infection.[1] The presence of *Hexamita* should always be of concern, because this protozoa can ascend and infect the kidneys.[1,20] The significance of casts and crystals is still unclear, but in 1 study they were seen in tortoises with renal disease and not in healthy tortoises.[1]

DIAGNOSTIC IMAGING
Radiography

The kidneys and urinary bladder in most reptiles cannot normally be seen on plain radiography. In lizards, however, renomegaly may be identified as a soft tissue mass extending cranially from the pelvic canal (**Fig. 4**).[21] Enlarged kidneys may decrease the diameter of the pelvic canal, leading to obstruction of the colon and constipation or obstructive dystocia.[1,21] The presence of uroliths and soft tissue mineralization also can be identified. The most common locations for soft tissue mineralization are the

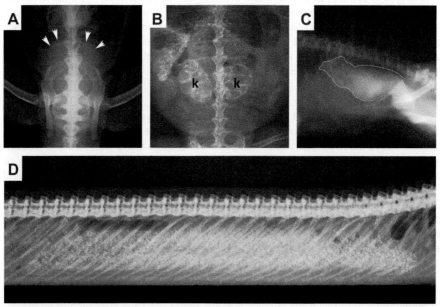

Fig. 4. (*A*) Dorsoventral radiograph of the caudal coelom of a green iguana (*Iguana iguana*) demonstrating protrusion of the renal silhouettes (*arrows*) cranial to the pelvic rim, suggestive of renal enlargement. (*B*) Dorsoventral radiograph of the caudal coelom of a spiny-tailed lizard (*Uromastyx aegyptius*) demonstrating mineralization of both kidneys (k). (*C*) Lateral radiograph (excretory urogram) of a Chinese water dragon (*Physignathus cocincinus*) demonstrating an irregular and enlarged kidney (*dotted line*) after intravenous iohexol administration. (*D*) Lateral radiograph of a boa constrictor with renal gout demonstrating a characteristic starburst pattern along the length of the kidney due to dilation and impaction of the renal tubules. (*Courtesy of* S. Divers, BVetMed, DZooMed, DECZM (Zoo Health Management, Herpetology), DACZM, FRCVS, Athens, GA.)

great vessels and the lining of the stomach.[7] If renal secondary hyperparathyroidism is present, there may be decreased bone density.[1,21] Conventional radiography requires significant loss of bone density before changes are noticed; dual-energy x-ray absorptiometry is the technique of choice for measuring bone density in iguanas.[22]

Contrast can be used to differentiate the kidneys from other soft tissue structures.[1] Intravenous (IV) urography can be used to further evaluate the kidneys and ureters. A cranial IV catheter (placed in the jugular or cephalic vein) is used to administer an aqueous iodinated contrast medium before serial radiographs are taken.[1] Iodine contrast media (eg, iopamidole and iohexol) is given at a dose of 800 mg/kg to 1000 mg/kg, and dorsoventral and lateral radiographs are taken at 0 minutes, 0.5 minutes, 2 minutes, 5 minutes, 15 minutes, 30 minutes, and 60 minutes (see **Fig. 4**C).[1,21] Contrast can be administered via the ventral coccygeal vein, but, due to the presence of the renal portal system, uptake can be affected and images differ based on whether contrast is given in the cranial or caudal half of the body.[1]

Ultrasonography

Ultrasonography can also be used to evaluate the kidneys in many species. A probe with a frequency of 5 MHz to 20 MHz is recommended, depending on patient size.[1,23] The animal is placed in ventral recumbency and manual restraint often is adequate. Water can be used as a conducting medium, or alcohol can be applied to the scales before the ultrasound gel. Either technique helps fill the spaces between the scales to allow for better contact of the probe. Conditions, such as mineralization, crystallization, urolithiasis, abscesses, and/or neoplasia, should be readily apparent. Ultrasound guidance also can be used to obtain urine samples by cystocentesis and renal biopsy samples, although significant risks of trauma and hemorrhage certainly exist.[1] Ultrasound-guided renal aspirates are safer.

In large lizards, the probe can be placed cranial to the rear leg and angled caudally or between the tail base and rear limb angled cranially. The normal renal parenchyma is uniform because no cortex and medulla are distinguishable.[1,23] In chelonians, the leg is pulled caudally and the probe is placed in the prefemoral fossa. In large chelonians sedation may be needed so that the ultrasound probe does not become trapped and damaged by the powerful rear leg. A transcloacal approach to the kidneys often is more rewarding in large chelonians. The thin-walled bladder may contain a large amount of fluid and fill the coelom, making urine difficult to differentiate from coelomic effusion.[23] The kidney is imaged by directing the probe dorsally. The medulla often appears hypoechoic and triangular to oval in shape.[23]

Advanced Imaging

Computed tomography and magnetic resonance imaging can also be useful to provide images of the kidneys, especially in large chelonians.[24,25] Computed tomography is rapidly becoming the radiographic technique of choice because there are many advantages over conventional radiographs, but standardization of technique and interpretation is important. Precontrast and postcontrast image series in both soft tissue and bone algorithms should be acquired. Nuclear scintigraphy is also available and normal images have been developed for the green iguana (*Iguana iguana*) at the University of Tennessee.[26]

Advanced imaging can be used to measure renal blood flow or renal clearance of various compounds; however, these techniques require expensive equipment, serial blood sampling, or catheterization for urine collection. Catheterization of the ureters is required because of postrenal urine modification in the cloaca, colon, or bladder.[1,2]

RENAL FUNCTION TESTING

Iohexol clearance studies have been shown in the green iguana to be a safe and effective method for estimating glomerular filtration rate (GFR) and renal function.[18] This technique has been extrapolated to Kemp's ridley sea turtles (*Lepidochelys kempii*) as well.[27,28] Iohexol is excreted exclusively by glomerular filtration.[29] The plasma clearance of iohexol can be calculated by analyzing the plasma iohexol concentration over time after a single IV injection.[16] This technique has the advantages of not requiring any special equipment and relying on blood rather than urine sampling. The patient should be fasted for 24 hours and well hydrated before iohexol is administered.[16] Iohexol is administered IV at 75 mg/kg, and blood samples are collected at 4 hours, 8 hours, and 24 hours postinjection.[16] These samples are submitted to Michigan State University for iohexol assays and GFR calculation.[16] Normal GFR for green iguanas is reported to be 16.56 mL/kg/h ± 3.90 mL/kg/h (14.78–18.34 mL/kg/h).[16] Normal GFR for Kemp's ridley turtles are reported to be 12.6 mL/kg/h ± 2.17 mL/kg/h (9–17.4 mL/kg/h).[27]

ENDOSCOPY

Endoscopy is an invaluable tool in the evaluation of renal disease. Blood tests often are inconclusive in reptiles even with advanced disease, and endoscopy allows visualization of the external surface, borders, and colors of the kidneys. Endoscopy also typically is rapid to perform so anesthesia can be brief.[1,16] Small rigid endoscopes (typically 2.7 mm) are commonly available with a variety of instruments that can be inserted through an operating sheath in order to collect samples to make a diagnosis and potentially administer therapy.

For coelioscopy in lizards, the animal is placed in lateral recumbency and prepared for surgery (**Fig. 5**). A left lateral approach is preferred because it allows visualization of

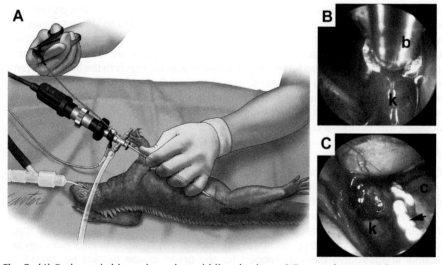

Fig. 5. (*A*) Endoscopic biopsy in an iguanid lizard using a 2.7-mm telescope, 4.8-mm operating sheath, and 1.7-mm biopsy forceps. (*B*) Endoscopic view of the biopsy forceps (b) being advanced onto the kidney (k). (*C*) Postbiopsy view of the kidney (k) demonstrating minor hemorrhage. Note the lack of trauma to the closely associated epididymis (*arrow*) and colon (c). (*Courtesy of* S. Divers, BVetMed, DZooMed, DECZM (Zoo Health Management, Herpetology), DACZM, FRCVS, Athens, GA.)

most other organs as well.[30] A paralumbar incision is made and the coelomic cavity is insufflated with carbon dioxide. The cranial pole of the kidney is visible as the endoscope is angled caudally toward the pelvic canal but can be difficult to visualize due to the fat bodies, urinary bladder, and colon.[30]

In chelonians, the kidneys can be visualized through a transcoelomic or extracoelomic approach.[1,30,31] The patient is positioned in lateral recumbency with the rear leg pulled caudally. For the transcoelomic approach, an incision is made in the prefemoral fossa and the coelom entered bluntly using hemostats.[30,31] The endoscope is inserted, the coelom insufflated, and the endoscope directed cranially and dorsally to visualize the kidneys.[30,31] For the extracoelomic approach, the endoscope does not enter the coelomic cavity but is generally restricted to those species with a flatter, less domed carapace. Once the tip of the endoscope has passed the skin incision, it is oriented in a caudodorsal direction and between the coelomic aponeurosis and the iliacus muscle.[30,31] Insufflation and lateral movements of the endoscope help advance the scope and visualize the caudal pole of the kidney.[30,31]

The elongated shape of snakes limits the usefulness of coelioscopy. Several entries are required to perform a complete survey, and this is complicated by the extensive nature of the fat bodies in the caudal coelom and the difficulty of insufflation.[30] When a targeted evaluation of just the kidneys is required, however, then a focal coelioscopy, often at 75% to 95% snout-to-vent length, can be used for evaluation and biopsy.[1,30]

RENAL BIOPSY

Renal biopsy is the gold standard for diagnosis, because often the clinician may suspect that renal disease is present but not be able to determine a definitive diagnosis or accurate prognosis. A definitive diagnosis can allow more specific treatment and improved treatment success, while determining long-term prognosis. It is not uncommon for a reptile to present with nonspecific signs of illness and have unremarkable clinicopathologic or imaging results. In those cases, direct visualization of the kidneys (and other organs) and biopsy via exploratory coeliotomy or endoscopy is the next step.

Endoscopy is ideal because it is minimally invasive and can be performed rapidly to both visualize and biopsy affected organs.[1,30,31] It is ideal to use scissors to incise the coelomic and renal membrane before collecting the biopsy sample to avoid crushing it. In snakes a renal biopsy can be obtained by making an incision in the caudal fourth of the coelomic cavity at the second row of lateral scales.[1] Even if the practitioner does not have access to endoscopy, however, coeliotomy can still be performed for collection of samples, although more readily in lizards and snakes than chelonians. In lizards, only the cranial pole of the kidneys is visible with both techniques. Unfortunately, cost, patient condition, anesthetic risk, and turnaround time for results may limit the practical usefulness of surgical biopsy by coelioscopy or coeliotomy.

An alternative technique for renal biopsy has been described in lizards (specifically iguanas). A cut-down procedure can be performed between the rear leg and base of the tail to access the caudal pole of the kidney and obtain a biopsy. This procedure often can be performed with sedation and a local anesthetic. An incision is made parallel to the tail beginning a few millimeters caudal to the angle of the hind limb and tail, and the kidney is identified by bluntly dissecting between the coccygeal muscles.[1]

Ultrasound-guided biopsy can be useful as well but requires a skilled operator and good-quality equipment.[1] This technique allows evaluation of the tissue and helps localize lesions so that biopsy samples can be obtained from affected areas. It is most useful in larger species where the kidneys are easily identified. There is a greater risk of hemorrhage and damaging other structures, such as the thin-walled urinary bladder.

OTHER DIAGNOSTICS

Articular and visceral gout are common sequelae of renal disease. Gout occurs when the uric acid level in the bloodstream rises high enough that crystals begin to precipitate. Visceral gout can be visualized as a gray to white sheen or discreet tophi within the oral mucosa or on the serosal surfaces of the heart or other organs. If joint swelling is present, an aspirate can be obtained and examined cytologically for uric acid crystals (**Fig. 6**).[1] A thick, white, gritty material expressed from a joint can be due to gout or pseudogout (calcium pyrophosphate deposition disease). Uric acid crystals are nonstaining, linear, needle-like crystals that can be confirmed and differentiated from other crystals using a polarizing filter.[1]

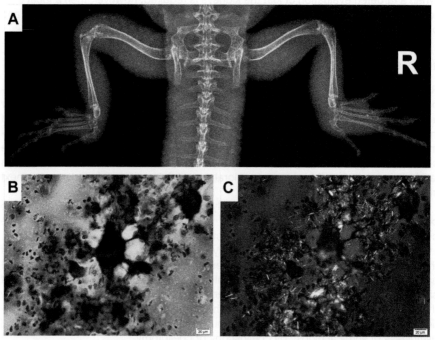

Fig. 6. (A) Dorsoventral radiograph of the pelvic limbs of a 2-year-old, male bearded dragon (*Pogona vitticeps*) with pronounced soft tissue swelling and joint effusion of the right tarsometatarsus. There is no evidence of abnormal mineralization or osteolysis. (B) Fine-needle aspirate of the same right tarsometatarsus viewed with nonpolarized light. Nonstaining crystal aggregates are visible but it is not possible to differentiate between uric acid (gout) and calcium-pyrophosphate (pseudogout) (modified Wright-Giemsa stain, ×50 objective, 20-μm bar). (C) The same microscopic field viewed with polarized light clearly demonstrates the negative birefringence of uric acid crystals confirming articular gout. (*Courtesy of* S. Divers, BVetMed, DZooMed, DECZM (Zoo Health Management, Herpetology), DACZM, FRCVS, Athens, GA.)

TREATMENT
Supportive Care

Management of renal disease is aimed first at stabilization of the critical patient (**Fig. 7**). For debilitated patients with severe signs of chronic disease and marked changes on bloodwork, the prognosis is poor. The animal should be warmed to its preferred optimum temperature zone and fluid therapy begun. Evaluate hydration status by measuring PCV and total protein. Fluids can be given orally, subcutaneously, intracoelomically (IC), IV, or intraosseously (IO). In emergency and critical cases, IV and IO fluids should be prioritized. Fluids are given at a rate of approximately 1 mL/kg/h to 1.5 mL/kg/h, although that rate can be increased up to 3 mL/kg/h to 5 mL/kg/h for the first 3 hours to 4 hours.[1] For larger reptiles, the placement of an IV catheter or central line is recommended. IC and SC routes may be the only practical options in smaller reptiles, whereas oral fluids should be used for maintenance. SC fluids (20 mL/kg every 12–24 hours) are preferred to IC due to poor absorption in some debilitated animals. Measurement of urine output is also valuable, especially in cases of acute renal failure. If the patient can tolerate it, shallow warm water soaks often are beneficial. More research has been done in recent years on plasma osmolality in reptiles. Although they do have differences from mammals, balanced electrolyte solutions clinically work well for reptiles and the use of Reptile Ringers has fallen out of favor.[32,33] For anuric patients, diuretics, such as mannitol 20% (2 mL/kg IV every 24 hours) or furosemide (2–5 mg/kg IV or IM every 24 hours), can be given to stimulate urine production.[1] Diuretic use in reptiles has also been controversial, because theoretically, loop diuretics, such as furosemide, should not work because reptiles lack a

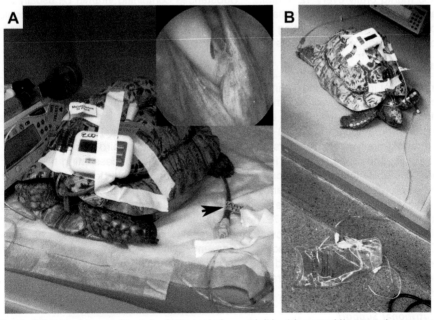

Fig. 7. (*A*) Critical leopard tortoise (*Stigmochelys pardalis*) with central line, esophagostomy tube, and indwelling bladder catheter (*arrow*). (*Inset*) Endoscopic view of the red rubber catheter being directed through the urodeal fold and into the urethra. (*B*) Same patient with collection bag containing urine. (*Courtesy of* S. Divers, BVetMed, DZooMed, DECZM (Zoo Health Management, Herpetology), DACZM, FRCVS, Athens, GA.)

loop of Henle and the ability to concentrate urine. Clinically, however, loop diuretics seem to help, and recent research suggests there are other mechanisms of action by which furosemide works to produce a diuretic effect in reptiles.[34]

Management of Hyperuricemia

Significant elevations in nitrogenous waste products can indicate severe renal compromise, either acute or chronic failure. If plasma uric acid levels are greater than 25 mg/dL, gout may develop.[1] Allopurinol at 20 mg/kg orally every 24 hours decreases the hepatic production of uric acid. If additional medications are needed to help decrease uric acid levels, medications that help prevent the tubular reabsorption of uric acid, such as probenecid or sulphapyrazole (1–3 mg/kg orally every 24 hours), also can be added. There is significantly less experience with these 2 medications in reptiles; thus, doses are extrapolated from other species and their clinical usefulness has not been determined. Varying doses of probenecid have been reported, from 2 mg/kg to 4 mg/kg orally every 24 hours[1] to 250 mg/kg orally every 12 hours.[35]

Management of Calcium and/or Phosphorus Levels

Alterations in calcium, phosphorus, and vitamin D_3 levels also can occur with chronic renal disease, leading to hyperphosphatemia and potentially significant hypocalcemia. Phosphate binders, such as aluminum hydroxide at 100 mg/kg orally every 12 hours to 24 hours, are useful to reduce the intestinal absorption of phosphorus. If hypocalcemia is present, calcium gluconate should be given IV or IO and carefully titrated to effect. An alternative route is 100 mg/kg IM every 6 hours to 12 hours. Once the animal improves, oral calcium can be continued (calcium glubionate, 50–360 mg/kg orally every 12 hours).[1,35] Substances containing vitamin D_3 usually are avoided because of the potential for soft tissue mineralization. Instead, reptiles should be provided with UV-B lighting at the proper distance or unfiltered natural sunlight in order to produce vitamin D_3 as needed.

Antimicrobials

In cases of infection, ideally, antibiotic use is prescribed based on renal biopsy and culture results; however, Gram-stained aspirates can help guide initial drug selection pending cultures. While awaiting culture results, first-tier antibiotic choices include trimethoprim-sulfa (10–30 mg/kg orally every 24 hours) or doxycycline (5–10 mg/kg orally every 24 hours).[35,36] Fluoroquinolones and third-generation cephalosporins should be reserved for cases of culture results necessitating their use.[35] Metronidazole (20–50 mg/kg orally every 24–48 hours) should be used if *Hexamita*, other protozoal infection, or anaerobic bacteria are suspected. If articular gout is present, analgesics should be prescribed, such as tramadol, 5 mg/kg to 10 mg/kg orally every 24 hours to 72 hours. Nothing reduces the joint swelling other than physical removal of the crystalline material, which itself causes joint damage. Other therapies currently used in canine and feline medicine, such as calcitriol, erythropoietin for anemia, and appetite stimulants, have not been investigated in reptiles, although anecdotal reports of their use exist. Further investigation into these therapies is warranted.

Nutritional Support

Nutritional therapy is an important component of management of renal disease in both acute and chronic cases. Most reptiles are able to go without food for prolonged periods of time, so in acute cases fluid therapy and other treatments are prioritized. Nutritional support, however, in the form of syringe feeding or tube feeding may be

Table 2
Selected nutritional compositions of various food items that deserve consideration in reptiles with renal disease

Invertebrates

	Cricket (*Acheta domesticus*)		Mealworm (*Tenebrio molitor*)	Superworm (*Zophobas morio*)	Silkworm (*Bombyx mori*)	Waxworm (*Galleria mellonella*)	Earthworm (*Lumbricus terrestris*)
	Adult	Juvenile					
Protein (% dry matter)	40–68	40–50	35–55	40–50	65	27–41	73

Vertebrates

	Mouse (*Mus musculus*)		Rat (*Rattus norvegicus*)	Meadow Vole (*Microtus pennsylvanicus*)	Smelt (*Sprinchus lanceolatus*)	Herring (*Clupea harengus*)	Chicken (*Gallus gallus domesticus*)	
	Adults	Pups					Adult	Day-old
Protein (% kcal)	48	29	55	63	63	39	47	52

Plants

	Romaine Lettuce	Iceberg Lettuce	Alfalfa Sprouts	Cabbage	Mushrooms	Sweet Potato	Squash	Forage & Hays		Apple	Cantaloupe
								Prickly Pear	Clover		
Protein (% dry matter)	36	13	37	37	30	17	16	5	19	1	8

	Lettuce	Cabbage	Cauliflower	Endive	Mushrooms	Sweet Potato	Prickly Pear	Raisons	Kale	Apple	Cantaloupe
Total purine load (mg uric acid/100 g)	13	37	51	17	5	16	15–17	107	48	14	33

	Romaine Lettuce	Iceberg Lettuce	Mustard Greens	Collards	Broccoli	Kale	Spinach
Na (mg/100 g)	8	9	25	18	18	27	79
K (mg/100 g)	290	158	358	169	325	447	558

From Divers SJ and Innis CJ (2019). Urology. In: Divers SJ, Stahl SJ, eds. Maders Reptile and Amphibian Medicine and Surgery, 3rd ed. St. Louis: Elsevier; 2019. pp. 624–648; with permission.

implemented according to species requirements in order to support the sick or malnourished reptile.

Diet is a major long-term control strategy of renal disease in humans and domesticated animals, and there are choices the reptile clinician can make to manage patients with chronic renal disease. The mainstays of dietary management include a reduction in protein (specifically purine) levels and phosphorus along with increasing water intake.[1] **Table 2** provides nutritional composition of various food items that may be considered in dietary management of renal disease.[1] To increase water intake, plant materials can be soaked and fed wet, mammal prey can be injected with water, and some herbivores can be fed watery fruits, such as melons[1] (see **Table 2**).

SUMMARY

In general, by the time most reptiles are presented for clinical signs of chronic renal disease, the prognosis is poor to hopeless. It may take at least 3 days to 5 days, sometimes longer, to see improvement from fluid therapy and medications. Syringe feeding may be needed initially until the animal is able to eat on its own. The diet should be modified (if possible) to be lower in protein and phosphorus. If no change in condition is seen within 3 days despite aggressive care, then euthanasia should be considered unless a definitive diagnosis indicates persistence is warranted. Patients with chronic renal disease often improve with supportive care, only to deteriorate when supportive measures are withdrawn. Long-term prognosis remains poor to hopeless, and 6 months or less is typical. Young bearded dragons with articular gout that are eating and active and either normouricemic or responsive to allopurinol often do well for a year or more.

Acute renal failure, although rare and typically associated with an infectious or inflammatory etiology, warrants an aggressive diagnostic investigation and therapeutic regime centered on fluid therapy, correction of metabolic disturbances, and reestablishment of urine flow. If successful, lost renal function can be reclaimed and the prognosis is improved.

REFERENCES

1. Divers SJ, Innis CJ. Urology. In: Divers SJ, Stahl SJ, editors. Mader's reptile and amphibian medicine and surgery. 3rd edition. St Louis (MO): Elsevier; 2019. p. 624–48.

2. Dantzler WH. Renal function (with special emphasis on nitrogen excretion). In: Gans C, Dawson WR, editors. Biology of the reptilia, vol 5, Physiology A. London: Academic Press; 1976. p. 447–503.

3. Reavill DR, Schmidt RE. Urinary tract disease of reptiles. J Exot Pet Med 2010;19: 280–9.

4. Perry SM, Mitchell MA. Routes of administration. In: Divers SJ, Stahl SJ, editors. Mader's reptile and amphibian medicine and surgery. 3rd edition. St Louis (MO): Elsevier; 2019. p. 1130–8.

5. Holz P, Barker IK, Burger JP, et al. The effect of the renal portal system on pharmacokinetic parameters in the red-eared slider (*Trachemys scripta elegans*). J Zoo Wildl Med 1997;28:386–93.

6. Zwart P. Renal pathology in reptiles. Vet Clin North Am Exot Anim Pract 2006;9: 129–59.

7. Garner MM, Hernandez-Divers SM, Raymond JT. Reptile neoplasia: a retrospective study of case submissions to a specialty diagnostic service. Vet Clin North Am Exot Anim Pract 2004;7:653–71.

8. Keller KA. Urolithiasis (cystic calculi and cloacal uroliths). In: Divers SJ, Stahl SJ, editors. Mader's reptile and amphibian medicine and surgery. 3rd edition. St Louis (MO): Elsevier; 2019. p. 1355–6.

9. Massry SG, Fadda GZ. Chronic renal failure is a state of cellular calcium toxicity. Am J Kidney Dis 1993;21:81–6.

10. Miller HA. Urinary diseases of reptiles: pathophysiology and diagnosis. Semin Avian Exot Pet Med 1998;7:93–103.

11. Boyer TH, Scott PW. Nutritional diseases. In: Divers SJ, Stahl SJ, editors. Mader's reptile and amphibian medicine and surgery. 3rd edition. St Louis (MO): Elsevier; 2019. p. 932–50.

12. Heatley JJ, Russell KE. Hematology. In: Divers SJ, Stahl SJ, editors. Mader's reptile and amphibian medicine and surgery. 3rd edition. St Louis (MO): Elsevier; 2019. p. 301–18.

13. Heatley JJ, Russell KE. Clinical chemistry. In: Divers SJ, Stahl SJ, editors. Mader's reptile and amphibian medicine and surgery. 3rd edition. St Louis (MO): Elsevier; 2019. p. 319–32.

14. Minnich JE. The use of water. In: Gans C, Harvey Pough F, editors. Biology of the reptilia, vol 12. Physiological ecology. London: Academic Press; 1982. p. 325–95.

15. Dennis PM, Bennett RA, Harr KE, et al. Plasma concentration of ionized calcium in healthy iguanas. J Am Vet Med Assoc 2001;219:326–8.

16. Hernandez-Divers SJ. Renal evaluation in the green iguana (*Iguana iguana*): assessment of plasma biochemistry, glomerular filtration rate, and endoscopic biopsy. J Zoo Wildl Med 2005;36:155–68.

17. Wagner RA, Wetzel R. Tissue and plasma enzyme activities in juvenile green iguanas. Am J Vet Res 1999;60:201–3.

18. Christopher MM, Brigmon R, Jacobsen E. Seasonal alterations in plasma β-hydroxybutyrate and related biochemical parameters in the desert tortoise (*Gopherus agassizii*). Comp Biochem Physiol 1994;108A:303.

19. Dantzler WH, Schmidt-Nielsen B. Excretion in the freshwater turtle (*Pseudemys scripta*) and desert tortoise (*Gopherus agassizii*). Am J Physiol 1965;210:198.

20. Juan-Salles C, Garner MM, Nordhausen RW, et al. Renal flagellate infections in reptiles: 29 cases. J Zoo Wildl Med 2014;45:100–9.

21. Holmes SP, Divers SJ. Radiography - lizards. In: Divers SJ, Stahl SJ, editors. Mader's reptile and amphibian medicine and surgery. 3rd edition. St Louis (MO): Elsevier; 2019. p. 491–502.

22. Grier SJ. The use of dual-energy X-ray absorptiometry in animals. Invest Radiol 1996;31:50–62.

23. Hochleithner C, Sharma A. Ultrasonography. In: Divers SJ, Stahl SJ, editors. Mader's reptile and amphibian medicine and surgery. 3rd edition. St Louis (MO): Elsevier; 2019. p. 543–59.

24. Sharma A, Wyneken J. Computed tomography. In: Divers SJ, Stahl SJ, editors. Mader's reptile and amphibian medicine and surgery. 3rd edition. St Louis (MO): Elsevier; 2019. p. 560–70.

25. Holmes SP, Wyneken J. Magnetic resonance imaging. In: Divers SJ, Stahl SJ, editors. Mader's reptile and amphibian medicine and surgery. 3rd edition. St Louis (MO): Elsevier; 2019. p. 571–85.

26. Greer LL, Daniel GB, Shearn-Bochsler VI, et al. Evaluation of the use of technetium Tc99m diethylenetriamine pentaacetic acid and technetium Tc99m

dimercaptosuccinic acid for scintigraphy imaging of the kidneys in green iguanas (*Iguana iguana*). Am J Vet Res 2005;66:87–92.

27. Kennedy A, Innis C, Rumbeiha W. Determination of glomerular filtration rate in juvenile Kemp's ridley turtles (*Lepidochelys kempii*) using Iohexol clearance, with preliminary comparison of clinically healthy turtles vs. those with renal disease. J Herpetol Med Surg 2012;22:25–9.

28. Innis C, Kennedy A, McGowan JP, et al. Glomerular filtration rates of naturally cold-stunned Kemp's ridley turtles (*Lepidochelys kempii*): comparison of initial vs. convalescent values. J Herpetol Med Surg 2016;26:100–3.

29. Nilsson-Ehle P, Grubb A. New markers for the determination of GFR: iohexol clearance and cystatin C serum concentration. Kidney Int Suppl 1994;47:17–9.

30. Divers SJ. Diagnostic endoscopy. In: Divers SJ, Stahl SJ, editors. Mader's reptile and amphibian medicine and surgery. 3rd edition. St Louis (MO): Elsevier; 2019. p. 604–14.

31. Hernandez-Divers SJ. Endoscopic renal evaluation and biopsy in chelonia. Vet Rec 2004;154:73–80.

32. Dallwig RK, Mitchell MA, Acierno MJ. Determination of plasma osmolality and agreement between measured and calculated values in healthy adult bearded dragons (*Pogona vitticeps*). J Herpetol Med Surg 2010;20:69–73.

33. Guzman DS-M, Mitchell MA, Acierno M. Determination of plasma osmolality and agreement between measured and calculated values in captive male corn snakes (*Pantherophis [Elaphe] guttatus guttatus*). J Herpetol Med Surg 2011; 21:16–9.

34. Parkinson LA, Mans C. Effects of furosemide administration to water-deprived inland bearded dragons (Pogona vitticeps). Am J Vet Res 2018;79:1204–8.

35. Klaphake E, Gibbons PM, Sladky K, et al. Reptiles. In: Carpenter JW, editor. Exotic animal formulary. 5th edition. St Louis (MO): Elsevier; 2018. p. 81–166.

36. Tang PK, Divers SJ, Sanchez S. Clinical bacterial isolates and antimicrobial susceptibility patterns from reptiles (2005–2016). J Am Vet Med Assoc, in press.

Disease Overview of the Urinary Tract in Exotic Companion Mammals and Tips on Clinical Management

Drury R. Reavill, DVM, DABVP (Avian Practice, Reptile & Amphibian Practice), DACVP[a],*,

Angela M. Lennox, DVM, DABVP (Avian Practice, Exotic Companion Mammal Practice), DECZM (Small Mammal)[b]

KEYWORDS

- Small mammals • Pathology • Kidney • Urinary bladder • Tumors • Renal • Uroliths
- Viral infections

KEY POINTS

- There are some species-specific disease conditions and anatomic structures of the urinary tract, including the composition of uroliths, an open inguinal ring in male rabbits and rodents, a cloaca in sugar gliders, and the presence of a baculum.
- Hematuria is a common clinical sign for various urinary tract diseases.
- Therapy for most urinary tract diseases is based on procedures common to domestic species (dogs and cats).

INTRODUCTION

The anatomy of the kidney is conserved among mammals. The kidneys are located within the sublumbar peritoneal space, with the right kidney positioned cranially to the left. In female rodents, there is a separate external orifice for the urinary tract and the reproductive tract. In male and female sugar gliders (*Petaurus breviceps*), the urinary tract terminates into a cloaca.[1] Male chinchillas (*Chinchilla lanigera*), guinea pigs (*Cavia porcellus*), rats (*Rattus norvegicus*), mice (*Mus musculus*), hamsters, gerbils, and ferrets (*Mustela putorius furo*) have an os penis or baculum.

Disclosure: The authors have no commercial or financial conflicts of interest nor any funding sources.

[a] Zoo/Exotic Pathology Service, 6020 Rutland Drive #14, Carmichael, CA 95608-0515, USA;
[b] Avian and Exotic Animal Clinic of Indianapolis, 9330 Waldemar Road, Indianapolis, IN 46268, USA
* Corresponding author.
E-mail address: DReavill@zooexotic.com

There are a few histologic differences of the kidney, including the number of papilla and length of the nephrons. Most differences are related to the natural environment of the animal. These differences are noted between desert-dwelling species requiring optimal ability to concentrate urine, and other species in which water deprivation is not common. Of clinical significance is the specific gravity of urine in desert-dwelling species, which is generally higher.[2]

FERRET
Common Problems

The most common problems affecting the ferret urinary system described in the literature are Aleutian disease of the kidney, renal tumors, renal cysts, urolithiasis, and bacterial cystitis. In one author's database (DRR), hydronephrosis, nephritis (all causes), and renal mineralization are the most common lesions of submitted kidneys.

Infectious/inflammatory

Aleutian disease is caused by a parvovirus.[3] The lesions are immune mediated and vary in severity. Gross lesions may be minimal and nonspecific. Emaciation and organ enlargement can be seen. In the kidney, membranous glomerulonephritis is common and a lymphocytic-plasmacytic inflammatory infiltrate is seen in the interstitium. This infection is uncommon in ferrets and the mortality is generally low.

Systemic coronavirus can also affect the kidneys, and the primary lesion is granulomatous inflammation.[4] In a study showing ultrasonography results in ferrets with systemic coronavirus, nephromegaly was found in 4 out of 11 patients.[5]

Canine distemper is essentially 100% fatal. Affected ferrets present with neurologic clinical signs, bronchopneumonia, hyperkeratosis of the planum nasale and footpads, and a papular rash starting on the chin. However, the most productive tissues to evaluate for viral inclusions are the urinary bladder, renal pelvis, and biliary epithelium, and in suspected cases these tissues should be submitted (**Fig. 1**). Immunohistochemistry can be applied for confirmation.

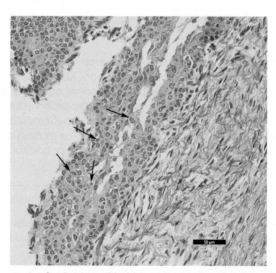

Fig. 1. Ferret (*M putorius furo*) urinary bladder with intracytoplasmic inclusions of a canine distemper infection. Confirmed with immunohistochemistry. Black arrows indicate a few of the intracytoplasmic eosinophilic viral inclusions (HE stain, 20× magnification). (*Courtesy of* D. R. Reavill, DVM, DABVP (Avian and Reptile & Amphibian Practice), DACVP, Carmichael, CA).

Bacterial nephritis and pyelonephritis occur in ferrets and can be severe. These conditions are thought to be caused by ascending infections of the lower urinary tract. A variety of organisms can be the cause. Grossly, the kidney may be abscessed and histologically there is necrosis and a neutrophilic infiltrate. Organisms may be seen but culture is necessary for a definitive diagnosis. Bacterial infection of the kidney, prostate, or urinary bladder can result in inflammatory cells (often undergoing degeneration) and bacteria in the urine.

Degenerative/congenital

Nephrosis is considered a degenerative disease of geriatric ferrets, and is often an incidental finding.[6] Nephrosis is characterized by damage of tubular epithelial cells. It is a nonspecific lesion that can have many causes, including ischemia, toxic exposure, and shock.

Nephrocalcinosis is reported more frequently in European pet ferrets than laboratory ferrets, and lesions include calcium deposition in the renal tubules.[7] The cause of renal mineralization is usually not determined. Soft tissue mineralization is usually considered dystrophic (secondary to tissue injury) or metastatic (associated with excessive calcium in the blood), but neither cause is obvious in most cases seen at necropsy. The lesion is usually in the renal papilla. Rare cases of lymphoma-associated hypercalcemia have also resulted in renal dystrophic mineralization. The mechanism is most likely azotemia and the nephrotoxic effects of prolonged hypercalcemia.[8]

Renal cysts are a common and usually incidental finding in the ferret (**Fig. 2**). A 17-year retrospective analysis of 54 ferrets with cystic kidney disease noted that 69% had renal cysts, and 26% primary polycystic disease.[9] Cysts may be single or multiple and may be present in the cortex of 1 or both kidneys. It is speculated that acquired cysts arise from gradual distention of the nephron, caused by obstruction by exudates or fibrosis tissue, although the cause is seldom determined. Rare cases of true polycystic disease have been reported in the ferret. This congenital lesion may result in markedly enlarged cystic kidneys that fill the posterior abdomen. Many small cysts throughout the cortex and medulla characterize polycystic kidneys.

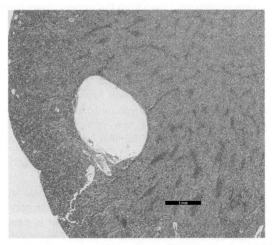

Fig. 2. Renal cysts within the cortex of the ferret (*M putorius furo*) kidney (HE stain, 1× magnification). (*Courtesy of* D. R. Reavill, DVM, DABVP (Avian and Reptile & Amphibian Practice), DACVP, Carmichael, CA).

Another rare congenital lesion is an extramural ectopic ureter. This condition is the most common congenital cause of urinary incontinence in domestic canines. Young ferrets present with urinary incontinence and urine scalding around perineal and inguinal areas. The ectopic ureter can be visualized via excretory urography. In 1 case, nephroureterectomy was chosen instead of ureteral transplant. The ureter progressed extramurally to enter the distal urethra, caudal to the urethral sphincter, or vagina (on contrast).[10]

Neoplastic

The most common renal neoplasm is malignant lymphoma. Lymphoma usually involves multiple organs and can be severe in the kidney. Grossly, there is variable replacement and distortion of the kidney. Histology is typical, with a diffuse monomorphic sheet of lymphoid cells. Impression smears can often provide a diagnosis. Other neoplasms have been reported, although primary tumors of the urinary tract system are uncommon.[11] From 1 study of 574 ferret tumors, only 6 urinary tumors were recognized. There were 3 renal carcinomas and 3 unspecified renal tumors.[11] Another study evaluating 856 ferret tumors identified only 1 renal tumor listed as a sarcoma, not otherwise specified, and lymphoma involving the kidney.[12] One renal adenocarcinoma is described in detail collected from an adult neutered female. This pleomorphic renal adenocarcinoma had multiple metastases to the lung, liver, greater omentum, right renal pelvis, and systemic lymph nodes. The tumor cells were pleomorphic with a large number of giant cells and arranged in tubular and cystic patterns. It was confirmed of renal origin by immunohistochemistry with strong positive CD10 and cytokeratin.[13] Two cases of transitional cell carcinoma arising from the renal pelvis, with 1 completely replacing the kidney, have been reported. The presenting complaint was hematuria.[14,15]

Obstructive disorders

Urolithiasis The clinical signs of urolithiasis include stranguria and dysuria. Uroliths in ferrets commonly consist of sterile struvite or magnesium ammonium phosphate. Based on 1 study evaluating 272 cases, neutered males have a significantly increased risk of developing sterile struvite urolithiasis.[16] These uroliths are more likely to be retrieved from the lower urinary tract than from the upper urinary tract.[16] Stone formation is suspected to be caused by a vegetable-based protein diet that increases urine pH, leading to struvite stone formation.[17]

Cystine uroliths are uncommon, with a reported incidence of 16% in 1 study evaluating 70 cases.[18] Again, males are predisposed to urolithiasis, possibly because the distal portion of the urethra has a J-shaped bend with a decreased diameter of the urethra. All cystine uroliths have been found in the lower urinary tract.[18] The uroliths are ovoid and smooth, light yellow to tan, and range in number from 1 to more than 100. Cystine uroliths are composed of nonessential sulfur-containing amino acid; there may be a familial cause based on studies in other mammals.[18]

Calcium oxalates are the next most common type of urolith.[19]

Prostatic disease Other causes of urinary obstruction in the male ferret are abnormalities of the prostate caused by adrenocortical disease. Males can develop prostatic hyperplasia, cysts, and abscesses. Prostatic enlargement is caused by increased levels of the hormones estradiol, testosterone, and 17-hydroxyprogesterone produced by the neoplastic adrenal cortex from an adrenal gland tumor. Some animals develop concurrent urinary tract infection, including small urethral or cystic calculi. Urethral blockages can also be caused by sloughed proteinaceous debris from squamous metaplasia of prostatic tissue and by small struvite calculi, which develop from the increase in pH caused by bacterial cystitis.[20]

Preputial tumors in male ferrets can also result in urethral obstruction. These aggressive tumors are poorly responsive to both surgery and radiation therapy. Nevertheless, wide surgical resection has been recommended, although the procedure may necessitate partial or total penile resection (**Fig. 3**).[21]

Treatment

Any disease of the kidneys can result in renal insufficiency or failure. Symptoms may include polyuria/polydipsia (PU/PD), weight loss, weakness, nausea, and decreased appetite, as can be seen in other traditional pet species. Physical examination findings are also consistent and often include dehydration, although hydration status can be challenging to determine by testing skin turgor in patients experiencing rapid weight loss. Some clinicians have anecdotally reported halitosis and oral ulcers in association with renal failure, but this is poorly documented.

Treatment protocols are based on those for traditional pet species, and include fluid diuresis for renal insufficiency and failure, antibiotic therapy for bacterial nephritis, and basic surgical approaches to the kidney.

Treatment of urinary tract disease follows guidelines established for traditional pet species, such as treatment of bacterial disease based on results of culture and sensitivity. General principles for treatment of renal insufficiency and renal failure are described later in this article. Treatment of adrenocortical disease is well described in any current literature about ferret endocrine diseases. Large associated prostatic cysts have been managed with marsupialization or omentalization of the cyst.[20]

Successful nephrotomy for removal of unilateral renoliths has been reported in the ferret.[22]

RABBIT
Common Problems

The most common causes of renal disease reported in the literature are *Encephalitozoon cuniculi*, chronic renal failure in older rabbits (*Oryctolagus cuniculus*), and urolithiasis. Other renal conditions seen in rabbits include bacterial nephritis, hydronephrosis, and papillary necrosis with renal mineralization.

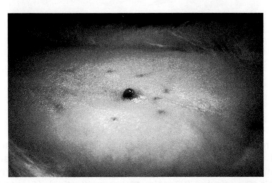

Fig. 3. Preputial tumor on a ferret (*M putorius furo*), prepped for surgical removal. (*Courtesy of* S. A. Kelleher, DVM, Deerfield Beach, FL).

Infectious/inflammatory

The most common renal disease of rabbits is infection caused by *E cuniculi*.[23–25] Although disease is often occult, rabbits with severe *E cuniculi*–associated renal disease may present with PU/PD and a host of other nonspecific signs, such as decreased appetite and weight loss, dehydration, and lethargy. In some rabbits, only renal changes are seen at necropsy. Grossly, there may be no lesions or the kidneys may be pitted. On histology, there is a chronic active lesion, which may be granulomatous or pyogranulomatous. Aggregates of organisms are found rarely in or around tubules as small, basophilic structures (**Fig. 4**).

Rare cases of polypoid cystitis and urethritis have been described in rabbits. The masses are white to transparent, spheroidal masses protruding into the lumen. On histology, the polyps are lined by variably hyperplastic to attenuated transitional epithelium over cores of edematous inflamed fibrovascular stroma. There may be transitional epithelium lining cysts within the stroma. These polyps are suspected to arise from a combination of inflammation and a hyperplastic reaction to chronic irritation of the urinary mucosa. Bacterial isolates have included *Proteus* and *Enterococcus* spp. The clinical signs associated with polypoid cystitis include perineal scalding, urinary sludge, and possibly hematuria.[26] Hematuria is frequently described as a clinical sign with obstructive urolithiasis, cystitis, bladder polyps, and pyelonephritis.[27] Red urine in rabbits may not necessarily be hematuria but may be the more common, and normal, porphyrin pigments. Urine dipstick is an easy method to differentiate porphyrinuria from hematuria.

Degenerative/congenital

Chronic renal disease or end-stage kidney disease seem to be common in older rabbits. Rabbits with renal failure can have lesions similar to those seen in old rats. The

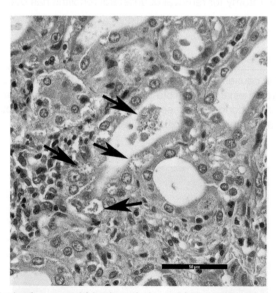

Fig. 4. *E cuniculi* microbes are within the tubular epithelial cells and these are sloughing into the lumen of the tubules. The black arrows indicate intratubular and intraepithelial densely packed microbes, which are small round/oval amphophilic structures. Samples from a dwarf rabbit (*O cuniculus*) (HE stain, 40× magnification). (*Courtesy of* D. R. Reavill, DVM, DABVP (Avian and Reptile & Amphibian Practice), DACVP, Carmichael, CA).

kidneys are grossly scarred and histologically there is marked interstitial fibrosis and glomerulosclerosis. This condition may be a sequela of encephalitozoon infection, but the cause is usually not determined.

Renal cysts are uncommon in rabbits. In a few reports, some cases were speculated to be inherited and to resemble human polycystic kidney disease.[28,29] In experimental studies, methylprednisolone acetate has been injected into newborn rabbits to induce polycystic kidneys.[30] The few cases of renal cysts (7 out of 796 rabbit renal submissions) in 1 author's database (DRR) have been in older rabbits (>5 years) and associated with lesions of chronic renal disease.

Neoplasia
Tumors of the urinary tract are rare in rabbits, with most involving the kidney. These tumors include benign embryonal nephroma, renal carcinoma,[31] renal adenocarcinoma, nephroblastoma (**Fig. 5**), and kidney hamartoma. A case of renal and ureteral transitional cell carcinoma produced hydronephrosis.[32] A urinary bladder transitional cell carcinoma in a female rabbit presented with acute hematuria, partial vaginal prolapse, and inappropriate urination. The gross appearance was a nodular cystic mass at the cranial central apex of the urinary bladder.[33]

Obstructive disorders
Urolithiasis and urinary sludge Uroliths are described in the kidney and urinary bladder of rabbits. Renoliths can be mild with few stones, or severe and produce renomegaly and complete destruction the kidney (**Fig. 6**).

Uroliths and urinary sludge in rabbits are usually composed of various calcium salts, predominately calcium carbonate. From a study evaluating more than 100 rabbit uroliths, the most common were calcium carbonate (69.4%), compound (23%), and mixed (3.3%).[19] Radiographs are usually confirmatory because calcium carbonate is radiopaque (**Fig. 7**). The predominance of calcium-based uroliths is most likely caused by the unique calcium metabolism of rabbits. Excess dietary calcium is absorbed unregulated, resulting in increased plasma calcium concentrations and excretion of excess calcium in the urine. Therefore, serum and urinary calcium levels are related to dietary intake. Urinary calcium can bind with other constituents when conditions are met for crystallization, such as dehydration, changes in pH, and urine

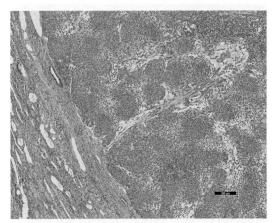

Fig. 5. Rabbit (*O cuniculus*) nephroblastoma is effacing the kidney (HE stain, 10× magnification). (*Courtesy of* D. R. Reavill, DVM, DABVP (Avian and Reptile & Amphibian Practice), DACVP, Carmichael, CA).

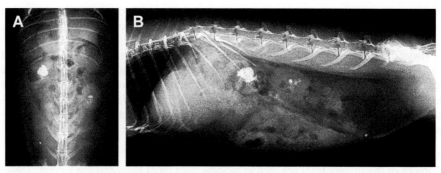

Fig. 6. (*A*) Bilateral nephrolithiasis in a rabbit (*O cuniculus*). The radiographs highlight the radiodense materials within the pelvis of the both kidneys. (*B*) Lateral view. (*Courtesy of* A. Lennox, DVM, DABVP (Avian Practice, Exotic Companion Mammal Practice), Diplomate ECZM (Small Mammal), Indianapolis, IN).

retention, to form both the sludge (which can appear as thick white to yellow material) and uroliths. Abnormal accumulations of calcium (sludge) are more common in older rabbits, possibly because of decreased mobility or water consumption.[34] There are rare reports of uroliths composed of silica, struvite, and calcium sulfate dehydrate or gypsum.[35] The gypsum urolith was associated with the rabbit eating gypsum-based plaster that was covered by a white paint containing barium sulfate.

Hernia Hernias can be classified by their anatomic location (body cavities or external, such as inguinal or femoral), cause (true hernia [through an anatomic structure and surrounded by peritoneum] or false hernia [traumatic through induced defects]), and contents.

Inguinal or scrotal hernias develop when abdominal contents, such as the urinary bladder, enter the inguinal canal or scrotum through a wide or defective inguinal canal. In male rabbits, the inguinal rings are open throughout life, increasing the risk of herniation. The typical appearance of bladder herniation is a fluid-filled mass in the scrotum and no bladder palpable in the abdomen. Some cases have concurrent

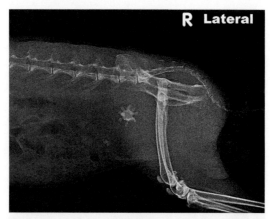

Fig. 7. Uroliths in the bladder can be of variable size and shape; although many are smooth, this urolith contained sharp points. The rabbit (*O cuniculus*) presented with anorexia and hunched posture, suggesting discomfort. (*Courtesy of* A. Lennox, DVM, DABVP (Avian Practice, Exotic Companion Mammal Practice), Diplomate ECZM (Small Mammal), Indianapolis, IN).

lesions of urinary sediment and multiple uroliths; 1 case featured a testicular tumor on the opposite side.[36] Inguinal herniation of the bladder seems uncommon in female rabbits (**Fig. 8**). Trauma was suspected to be the cause in 1 case of a female rabbit presenting with hematuria.[37]

Female rabbits may also evert the urinary bladder through the urethra. Recent kindling or a history of multiple litters is common. Rabbits present with a vaginal mass, which is the mucosal surface of the everted bladder.[38] Rarely, males may evert and prolapse the urinary bladder. This finding seems more likely in castrated males because penis length is reduced after castration.[39]

Another unusual presentation is diaphragmatic herniation of retroperitoneal fat and a kidney.[40] A case of kidney herniation occurred in conjunction with a diaphragmatic lipoma.[41]

Treatment
General management of renal insufficiency and renal failure is described later.

Encephalitozoonosis Treatment of *E cuniculi* is problematic because there is a lack of well-controlled scientific studies linking various treatment protocols with documented clearing of organisms. The problem relates to difficulties in establishing a diagnosis, and the observation that many affected rabbits recover spontaneously without treatment.[42] Rabbits with severe renal disease secondary to *E cuniculi* may not harbor renal organisms, and treatment is focused on managing acute or chronic renal failure. Treatment of *E cuniculi* has relied on benzimidazoles, such as fenbendazole,[42] but recently severe disease and deaths have been reported in rabbits treated with this class of drugs.[43] Benzimidazoles are radiomimetic and toxicity has been observed in many species; Graham and colleagues[43] recently reported deaths in 13 rabbits treated with various dosages of several drugs, including fenbendazole, albendazole, and oxibendazole. Clinical signs in rabbits were nonspecific and histopathology showed depletion of all bone marrow cell lines. For this reason, treatment should not be approached lightly, and serial monitoring of the complete blood count may be beneficial.

Surgical management of renal disease Various surgical approaches to the kidney have been described. Martorell and colleagues[44] described a lateral flank approach

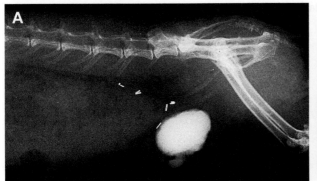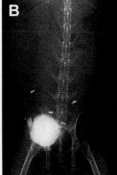

Fig. 8. Inguinal herniation of the bladder in a female rabbit (*O cuniculus*). The bladder is filled with microuroliths (bladder sludge), which are acting as natural contrast. Surgery to replace the bladder and correct the herniation was successful. (*A*) Lateral and (*B*) frontal view. (*Courtesy of* A. Lennox, DVM, DABVP (Avian Practice, Exotic Companion Mammal Practice), Diplomate ECZM (Small Mammal), Indianapolis, IN).

for access to the kidney for removal of uroliths; 1 author (AML) also found this approach simple and straightforward compared with a traditional midline abdominal approach (**Fig. 9**). Nephrectomy, performed through a ventral abdominal approach, was reported to manage hydronephrosis in a pet rabbit[45] and to remove a renal carcinoma.[32] Cases of diaphragmatic herniation were successfully treated by replacing the herniated kidney and fat followed by diaphragmatic herniorrhaphy,[40] and use of polypropylene mesh.[41]

Management of bladder sludge Strategies for managing urinary sludge include encouraging water consumption and exercise paired with dietary modification as needed. Accumulation of sludge can be temporarily managed by bladder catheterization and flushing, or sometimes by gently agitating the bladder to manually resuspend the mineral, followed by repeated expression of urine.

GUINEA PIG
Common Problems

Urolithiasis is commonly reported in the guinea pig. This condition usually involves the lower urinary tract. Inflammatory, degenerative, and other conditions are also reported.

Infectious/inflammatory
Chronic nephritis, interstitial nephritis, and pyelonephritis have been reported.[46,47] In these conditions the kidneys may be irregular grossly and the ureters may be dilated in pyelonephritis. On histology, the inflammation depends on the cause and the duration of the disease.

Cystitis in guinea pigs is common. Guinea pigs, like chinchillas and degus, have adapted to a semiarid habitat with varying, species-specific adaptations to water deprivation. However, several diseases have been linked to insufficient water intake, such as cystitis, urolithiasis, or obstipation. A decrease in urination frequency may favor bacterial infection and formation of uroliths.[48] The clinical signs of bacterial cystitis include dysuria, polyuria, hematuria, lethargy, or urethral discharge. The urinary bladder may be painful on palpation, small, firm, with a thickened wall. The most common isolate in a review series of adult female guinea pigs was *Escherichia coli*. Relapses were common. Two guinea pigs were diagnosed with encrusted cystitis (further description in relation to hedgehogs later).[49]

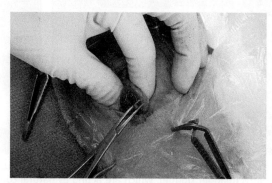

Fig. 9. Unilateral flank approach nephrotomy allowed removal of uroliths from the right kidney. (*Courtesy of* A. Lennox, DVM, DABVP (Avian Practice, Exotic Companion Mammal Practice), Diplomate ECZM (Small Mammal), Indianapolis, IN).

Degenerative/congenital

Renal cysts are a rarely reported and usually incidental finding.[50] Given the few reports of renal cysts in guinea pigs, it seems most cases are acquired cysts associated with chronic renal disease. One author (DRR) has seen 21 cases in adult guinea pigs (3–7 years of age), all with chronic renal lesions (fibrosing interstitial nephritis) out of 430 case submissions with kidneys (4.8%).

Chronic (segmental) nephrosclerosis is renal scarring of undetermined cause, which may be the result of vascular disease, infection, or immune-mediated disease. Grossly, the renal cortex is irregularly pitted and histologically there is interstitial fibrosis, variable glomerulosclerosis, tubular dilatation, and variable mononuclear inflammation (**Fig. 10**).

Renal mineralization can be incidental or associated with renal failure, resulting in uremia and soft tissue mineralization. The mechanism is complex but involves tissue death and secondary mineralization. In guinea pigs, exposure to excessive vitamin D is a common mechanism if renal failure is not present. Such exposure occurs when feeding guinea pigs a commercial diet with errors in formulation or commercial rodent diets. Commercial rodent diets are formulated with more vitamin D than is safe for guinea pigs.[51,52]

Neoplasia

Primary tumors are rare. Lymphoma occasionally involves the kidneys. Grossly, there is a diffuse white-gray infiltrate that replaces normal parenchyma. On histology, this is composed of immature lymphoid cells.

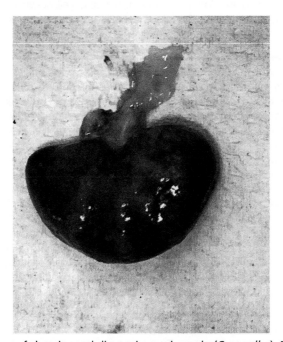

Fig. 10. Gross view of chronic renal disease in a guinea pig (*C porcellus*). Bands of blotchy white areas radiate out from the pelvis. The histology findings were of severe diffuse fibrosing lymphoplasmacytic interstitial nephritis with periglomerular sclerosis. (*Courtesy of* S. Brenner, MS, DVM, San Mateo, CA).

Obstructive disorders

Uroliths may be present from the renal pelvis to the urinary bladder. If in the ureter or bladder, there may be ureteral dilatation and renal swelling or shrinkage. The most common urolith is calcium carbonate, which is radiopaque.[19] Similar to rabbits and other hindgut-fermenting herbivores, guinea pigs excrete excess calcium[53] and they can eliminate up to 75% of their absorbed calcium via urine. Urine specific gravity and pH highly influence crystallization. Herbivore urine is commonly alkaline, which complicates dietary modification efforts to change urine pH and reduce urolith formation.[54]

Treatment

Strategies for treatment of acute and chronic renal failure are described later. Surgery of the kidney has not been described in pet guinea pigs.

The urethra of the female guinea pig is short and wide. Uroliths in the urethra and in the vaginal vestibulum can be visualized and removed manually with the aid of the Lone Star retractor.[55]

HAMSTER
Common Problems

Primary renal disease is uncommonly reported in pet hamsters, and mostly includes infectious and degenerative causes.

Infectious/inflammatory

Sporadic cases of bacterial cystitis and pyelonephritis are seen. Gross changes include thickening and exudation in the bladder and yellow-white foci of necrosis and inflammation in the kidney. Culture is usually necessary to establish a definitive cause.

Degenerative/congenital

The most common problem seen in the kidneys is amyloidosis, which has been reported in more than 50% of hamster necropsies in some colonies.[56,57] Amyloid is an insoluble pathologic proteinaceous substance, deposited between cells in various tissues and organs of the body. Systemic amyloidosis can be classified as primary (amyloid light chain), secondary (amyloid associated), or familial. Secondary amyloidosis is most commonly described in animals and has been described as a reaction to diverse inflammatory stimuli. Amyloid deposits are more common in female hamsters more than 18 months of age. Deposits can also be seen in almost any other organ. Amyloidosis can be associated with nephritic syndrome.[58] Grossly, the kidneys are pale and irregular. Microscopically, amyloid is eosinophilic to amphophilic and can be seen in glomeruli, interstitium, or both.

Glomerulonephropathy occurs in hamsters as well as other rodents.[59] Progressive nephropathy can result in renal failure. Grossly, kidneys are pitted and variably shrunken, and histologically there may be variable stages of mesangial and glomerular capillary thickening, periglomerular sclerosis, and variable interstitial nephritis. This condition has been described in both Chinese (Cricetulus griseus) and Siberian hamsters (Phodopus sungorus).[60]

Neoplasia

Primary tumors are rare in hamsters. Two cases of renal adenoma have been reported in aged Siberian hamsters.[59,61] One author (DRR) has seen 2 cases of lymphoma involving the kidney as well as 1 case of a renal adenoma out of 60 submissions that included the kidney.

Obstructive disorders

Uroliths are also uncommon in hamsters. From 1 study evaluating only 14 samples, the most common uroliths were calcium phosphate (28.6%), compound (28.6%), and calcium oxalate (21.4%).[19]

Treatment

Strategies for treatment of acute and chronic renal failure are described later. Surgery of the kidney has not been described in pet hamsters.

MOUSE
Common Problems

Renal disease is common in mice. Some conditions are strain related, and determining the genetic heritage of a pet mouse (if possible) may be of value in diagnosis. Amyloidosis is seen primarily in older animals.

Degenerative/congenital

Chronic progressive nephropathy or chronic nephritis in mice is similar to the condition in rats and other rodents.[62,63] Pathogenesis is unknown. Interstitial nephritis and pyelonephritis are also reported.[64,65] *Klossiella muris* infection is seen primarily in wild mice.[66]

Grossly, kidneys affected by these conditions have an irregular pitted cortex. Microscopically, there is glomerular sclerosis, tubular dilatation and degeneration, interstitial inflammation, and fibrosis. Lesions vary in severity according to their duration. In cases of klossiellosis, organisms can usually be seen on histology and may not be associated with significant inflammation. This organism is a parasitic protozoa of the phylum Apicomplexa. Species in this genus infect the renal tract of mammals and intestinal tract of snakes. This genus of the phylum Apicomplexa is unusual in having only a single host in its life cycle.

Polycystic kidneys occur in BALB/c mice, which are used as a model for human disease. Cysts vary in size and number, but the condition is progressive and results in loss of renal function and early mortality. The renal surface is irregular and fluid-filled cysts are visible. Cysts are also obvious in cut sections. Dilated tubules are seen histologically.

Neoplasia

Renal neoplasia occurs sporadically. Malignant lymphoma can efface the kidney and carcinomas are occasionally seen. Gross lesions are not specific. On histology, lymphoma is typical and carcinomas are usually composed of poorly differentiated cells with a loss of organized structure.

Obstructive disorders

Hydronephrosis can be unilateral or bilateral. Unilateral hydronephrosis is often an incidental necropsy finding and may be strain related or secondary to obstruction or inflammation of the renal pelvis. It is usually progressive and grossly there is variable dilatation of the renal pelvis with loss of renal parenchyma. One cause of obstructive hydronephrosis in male mice, as well as in rats and guinea pigs, is the retrograde movement of seminal plugs in the urethra (**Fig. 11**). These seminal vesicle secretions may coagulate and become impacted in the urethra and urinary bladder.[67]

RAT
Common Problems

Common renal conditions reported include hydronephrosis, polycystic kidneys,[68] and pyelonephritis, as well as neoplasms.[69–71]

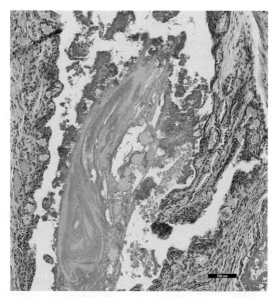

Fig. 11. Seminal plugs within the lumen of the urethra in a male guinea pig (*C porcellus*). The acellular coagulum is within the lumen. (HE stain, 20× magnification). (*Courtesy of* D. R. Reavill, DVM, DABVP (Avian and Reptile & Amphibian Practice), DACVP, Carmichael, CA).

Infectious/inflammatory

Trichosomoides crassicauda is a nematode that affects the urinary tract of rats. Adult worms can be seen in the renal pelvis and urinary bladder, but the condition is usually asymptomatic. Eggs are passed in the urine. Nematodes are present in the epithelium and there is variable inflammation (**Fig. 12**).[72]

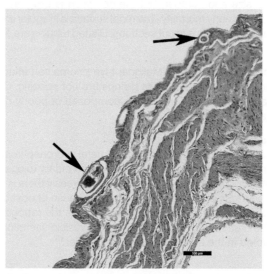

Fig. 12. *T crassicuada*, the rat (*R norvegicus*) urinary bladder nematode can be found in the lumen as well as in the mucosal epithelium (*black arrows*). (HE stain, 10× magnification). (*Courtesy of* D. R. Reavill, DVM, DABVP (Avian and Reptile & Amphibian Practice), DACVP, Carmichael, CA).

Degenerative/congenital

The most common renal disease in rats is chronic progressive nephropathy or old rat nephropathy.[73–75] The incidence can be up to 75% in affected strains. This disease affects older animals and is more common and severe in males, with a much higher incidence in S-D and Fischer 344 rats. High-protein diets are a factor in pathogenesis, as are immunologic factors, such as mesangial deposition of immunoglobulin M, and high levels of prolactin. Lesions of progressive nephropathy are characterized by irregular and pitted renal cortices. The cut surface is also irregular. Microscopic changes vary with duration. Glomeruli are thickened, tubules are dilated and may contain proteinaceous fluid, and there is interstitial fibrosis and inflammation.

Nephrocalcinosis is seen, usually as an incidental finding but also with diets low in magnesium and/or high in calcium and phosphorous. Mineral is deposited within the interstitium and tubules. Grossly, there are pale streaks and, histologically, basophilic mineral deposits are seen.

Neoplasia

Spontaneous tumors of the urinary tract are uncommon in rats. Tumors reported in the kidney include renal cell adenoma, lipoma/liposarcoma, renal cell carcinoma (with metastasis to the lung and liver), and a nephroblastoma with metastasis to the lung and local lymph nodes. Transitional cell carcinoma of the urinary bladder also occurs spontaneously and in 1 case there was metastasis to the lungs.[70,71,76]

Obstructive disorders

Uroliths in rats are generally struvite (80.4%) with fewer calcium phosphate (5.9%).[19]

CHINCHILLAS
Common Problems

Primary renal diseases are poorly described in chinchillas. Urolithiasis has been described, and, although rarely reported, suppurative nephritis is common in younger animals (**Fig. 13**). *E coli* has frequently been isolated based in 1 author's experience (DRR).

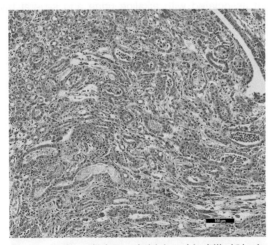

Fig. 13. Histology of a suppurative tubular nephritis in a chinchilla (*C lanigera*). A bacterial culture collected at the time of necropsy isolated *E coli*. (HE stain, 10× magnification). (*Courtesy of* D. R. Reavill, DVM, DABVP (Avian and Reptile & Amphibian Practice), DACVP, Carmichael, CA).

Obstructive disorders

Unlike rabbits and guinea pigs, chinchillas eliminate excessive calcium approximately 80% via feces and only 1% to 3% via urine. Nevertheless, their urine calcium concentration may show great individual variation. Urolithiasis is reported in chinchillas and most are calcium carbonate (87.7%) and miscellaneous (6.8%).[19] The clinical signs are as expected, with irritation around the preputial orifice, as well as hematuria, pollakiuria, and stranguria. Most uroliths are found in the urinary bladder, with fewer within the urethra. In males, most are in the proximal urethra near the pelvis and cranial to the os penis (**Fig. 14**). Prognosis is guarded with urethral stones and recurrence is common.[77] Within the urinary bladder there may be thickening of the bladder wall with an inflamed mucosa.[78]

Perineal hernias are described in 2 sexually intact males. The hernia contents were urinary bladder in 1 animal and lobules of fat in the other. In both cases, the testicles could be moved freely in and out of the inguinal canal.[79]

HEDGEHOGS
Common Problems

Hedgehogs (*Atelerix albiventris*) have been reported to have cystitis and uroliths, but the most common renal problem is chronic nephritis.[80] As in other species, chronic renal disease is likely to have a large number of causes, such as infections, immune-mediated disorders, and nephrotoxins. Renal disease may also be a part of a systemic condition. Grossly and histologically, the lesion is similar to others that have been previously described in other animals.

Inflammatory/infectious

Cystitis is uncommon in hedgehogs, with scarce descriptions in the literature. In females, uterine tumors are a much more common cause of hematuria. However, 1 author (DRR) has diagnosed cases of hemorrhagic acute to subacute cystitis. Lesions of the urinary system collected from the database of 1 author (DRR) are summarized in **Table 1**. One case was of encrusted cystitis. There was extensive mineralization of the urinary bladder with an ulcerative and/or necrotic cystitis. This type of lesion is uncommon and has been associated with alkaline urine and several bacteria, including *Staphylococcus pseudintermedius* and *Corynebacterium urealyticum* (**Fig. 15**).[81]

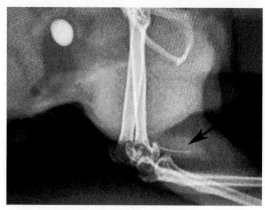

Fig. 14. A chinchilla (*C lanigera*) with a urinary stone and the os penis can be seen (*black arrow*). Lateral view. (*Courtesy of* C. Griffin, DVM, ABVP (avian practice), Kannapolis, NC).

Table 1 Data from Zoo/Exotic Pathology Service of 85 hedgehog (*Atelerix albiventris*) urinary lesions from 878 case submissions 1998 to 2019		
Lesion Category	Lesion	Number of Hedgehogs
Inflammatory	Nephritis, chronic fibrosing interstitial	46
	Cystitis	7
	Cortical infarct	6
	Nephritis, interstitial	5
	Glomerulitis	4
	Nephritis, suppurative	2
Neoplastic	Lymphoma	3
	Sarcoma, renal (not differentiated)	1
Miscellaneous	Renal mineralization	9
	Renal tubular necrosis (nephrosis)	8
	Nephrosis pigmentary	3
	Renal cysts	3

SUGAR GLIDERS
Common Problems

There are very few reports of urinary disease in sugar gliders.

Inflammatory/infectious

Renal klossiellosis has been described in pet sugar gliders. In affected sugar gliders there is tubular dilatation and interstitial nephritis. The various life cycle stages can be identified within the renal tubular epithelium. Based on morphologic evaluation, the name *Klossiella dulcis n.* sp was proposed. No treatment has been described.[82]

Obstructive disorders

Bilateral hydronephrosis in a male sugar glider developed secondarily to a functional obstruction suspected to be from hyperplasia and inflammation of the urinary bladder and ureteral epithelium. The animal presented with acute caudal abdominal swelling.[83]

One author (AML) has noted several cases of disease of the cloacal and paracloacal glands that resulted in apparent urinary obstruction; obstruction resolved with treatment of the primary cause. Both sexes have paracloacal glands (anterior, dorsal,

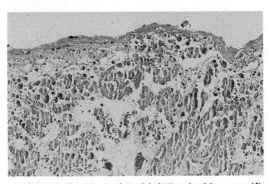

Fig. 15. Hedgehog (*A albiventris*) encrusted cystitis (HE stain, 20× magnification). (*Courtesy of* D. R. Reavill, DVM, DABVP (Avian and Reptile & Amphibian Practice), DACVP, Carmichael, CA).

and ventral), which are more developed in the male. Under the influence of testosterone, the dorsal paracloacal glands and testes increase in size.[1] Inflammation and neoplastic disease of these glands can result in functional obstruction of the digestive and urinary tract.[84] There are reports of a paracloacal cyst,[85] sebaceous nodular hyperplasia, and carcinomas in male sugar gliders. Self-mutilation, stranguria, and pericloacal swelling are the typical clinical signs. One case had a dorsal paracloacal gland carcinoma[84] and the other a transitional cell carcinoma with squamous differentiation.[86]

Toxic exposure

Copper toxicosis has been described in a sugar glider voiding red-brown urine and showing possible seizurelike activity. The kidneys were enlarged and dark red with marked, acute, multifocal renal tubular degeneration and necrosis with hemoglobin casts. Icterus was noted and the liver had marked, acute, centrilobular hepatocellular degeneration and necrosis with hepatocellular copper accumulation confirmed with rubeanic stain and a hepatic copper concentration of 709 parts per million (wet-weight basis). The provided mineral and vitamin supplement had 2.26 and 250 μg/mL respectively. It was unknown whether the vitamin supplement could have led to the toxicosis.[87]

In a review of sugar glider case submissions (DRR) from 1998 to 2019, out of 337 there were 86 urinary tract lesions. Interstitial nephritis was common, as was the nonspecific finding of renal tubular necrosis (nephritis). Other lesions included membranoglomerulopathy, renal cysts, and transitional cell carcinoma of the urinary bladder (**Fig. 16**). Lesions are summarized in **Table 2**.

TREATMENT OF RENAL INSUFFICIENCY AND FAILURE

Without benefit of evidence-based therapies for exotic mammals, treatment of renal insufficiency and failure is based on therapies considered most advantageous in traditional pet species.

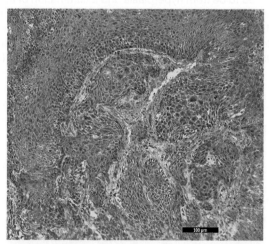

Fig. 16. Transitional cell carcinoma in the urinary bladder of a sugar glider (*P breviceps*) (HE stain, 10× magnification). (*Courtesy of* D. R. Reavill, DVM, DABVP (Avian and Reptile & Amphibian Practice), DACVP, Carmichael, CA).

Table 2
Data from Zoo/Exotic Pathology Service of 86 sugar glider (*Petaurus breviceps*) urinary lesions from 377 case submissions 1998-2019

Lesion Category	Lesion	Number of Sugar Gliders
Inflammatory	Nephritis, interstitial	43
	Membranoglomerulopathy	6
	Bacteremia	2
	Nephritis, tubular, bacteria	2
Neoplastic	Transitional cell carcinoma, urinary bladder	2
	Lymphoma	1
Miscellaneous	Renal tubular necrosis (nephrosis)	18
	Nephrosis pigmentary	4
	Hydronephrosis	1
	Renal cysts	1

Chronic Kidney Disease

The 2016 International Society of Feline Medicine guidelines for management of chronic kidney disease (CKD) may be useful. Even in cats, simple and accurate markers for renal function are currently unavailable; biomarkers such as blood urea nitrogen (BUN), creatinine, and urine specific gravity are useful, but interpretation can be difficult. The principles of treatment are supportive, and the overall goal is maintenance of quality of life. Even the goal of maintaining hydration has not been formally associated with increased longevity and improved quality of life in cats with CKD; however, the benefits of normohydration are considered obvious enough to continue recommendation of fluid therapy.[88]

Unstable or decompensated patients benefit from hospitalization and intravenous (IV) fluid therapy. Fluid rates are based on calculation of hydration deficit: body weight (kg) times estimated dehydration (%) times 1000. Hydration deficit is added to maintenance fluids (50 mL/kg/24 h in cats) and provided over 24 to 48 hours. Once normohydration is achieved, fluid therapy continues at maintenance rate, monitoring the patient carefully for evidence of fluid overload. Fluid therapy is tapered over several days once condition and appropriate biomarkers have improved.

For long-term maintenance of hydration, many recommendations for cats are appropriate in exotic mammals, and include free access to high-quality water using multiple water sources. In exotic pets, this means providing water in bowls along with traditional water bottles. Although moist canned food is not available for rabbits and rodents, moistening greens and hay may aid water intake, as well as supplementing with liquid foods designed for convalescing exotic pets; for example, Oxbow Critical Care or Carnivore Care depending on the nutritional needs of the species. In cats, placement of feeding tubes for oral hydration may be used long term; this approach is not useful for exotic species. However, subcutaneous fluid administration may have utility, because some owners can be taught to administer fluids to small patients at home. Commercial indwelling subcutaneous catheters have been used in cats, and 1 author (AML) has used one in a large rabbit with some success.

Acute Renal Failure

Acute renal failure (ARF) may be reversible if identified and treated early and aggressively. As in other species, ARF may be prerenal (shock, hypovolemia), renal (renal disease), or postrenal (obstruction). Urine specific gravity plus changes in BUN and creatinine levels can be helpful. ARF is treated by correcting perfusion deficits (discussed later) and dehydration, and diuresis, along with correction of an identified underlying cause. Once the patient is rehydrated and normotensive, continue fluid administration as maintenance (3–4 mL/kg/h) plus estimated losses (diarrhea/vomiting, if present, and estimated urine volume). Based on information in domestic species, patients with ARF may become 3% to 5% dehydrated each day because of ongoing losses. Fluid administration is decreased when the patient maintains hydration, begins to eat and drink, and BUN/creatinine levels normalize.[89]

IV catheterization is a standard procedure in rabbit medicine; IV access is also possible in large guinea pigs and some chinchillas. IV access may not be possible in any patient that is hypovolemic. For these cases, intraosseous (IO) catheterization is indicated. Placement sites in mammals include the proximal humerus, femur, and tibia.

Placement is best performed in a sedated patient with parenteral analgesia, and a local block (2–3 mg/kg lidocaine into the skin, subcutaneous tissue, and periosteum). Although short spinal needles are useful in rabbits and large rodents, most IO catheters are simple hypodermic needles, 25 to 18 gauge depending on the size of the bone cavity. Seat the needle into the proximal bone, and then orient the needle into the bone cavity. Cover with an IV catheter cap and secure to the limb with tape (**Fig. 17**).

Treatment of shock in rabbits and rodents has been described.[89] Management of fluid deficits is maintenance fluids estimated at 3 to 4 mL/kg/h in exotic mammals, or via allometric calculations of resting energy requirements (weight $[kg]^{75} \times 70$) plus hydration deficit, adjusting fluid rates for ongoing losses, such as polyuria in cases of renal insufficiency.

Other therapies include erythropoietin for treatment of anemia, analgesia as indicated, and support feeding.

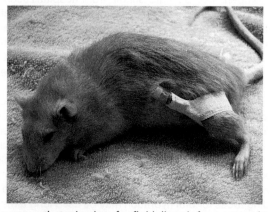

Fig. 17. An intraosseous catheter in place for fluid diuresis for a pet rat (*R norvegicus*). A 25-gauge needle was used for the catheter, which was taped into place and capped with an IV catheter cap. (*Courtesy of* A. Lennox, DVM, DABVP (Avian Practice, Exotic Companion Mammal Practice), Diplomate ECZM (Small Mammal), Indianapolis, IN).

ACKNOWLEDGMENTS

Histologic images were digitally processed by Animal Reference Pathology, Salt Lake City, UT.

REFERENCES

1. Bradley AJ, Stoddart DM. The dorsal paracloacal gland and its relationship with seasonal changes in cutaneous scent gland morphology and plasma androgen in the marsupial sugar glider (Petaurus breviceps; Marsupialia: Petauridae). J Zoology 1993;229(2):331–46.
2. Mbassa GK. Mammalian renal modifications in dry environments. Vet Res Commun 1988;12(1):1–18.
3. Welchman Dde B, Oxenham M, Done SH. Aleutian disease in domestic ferrets: diagnostic findings and survey results. Vet Rec 1993;132(19):479–84.
4. Lindemann DM, Eshar D, Schumacher LL, et al. Pyogranulomatous panophthalmitis with systemic coronavirus disease in a domestic ferret (Mustela putorius furo). Vet Ophthalmol 2016;19(2):167–71.
5. Dominguez E, Novellas R, Moya A, et al. Abdominal radiographic and ultrasonographic findings in ferrets (Mustela putorius furo) with systemic coronavirus infection. Vet Rec 2011;169(9):231.
6. Johnson-Delaney C. Applied clinical anatomy and physiology. In: Ferret medicine and surgery. Boca Raton (FL): CRC Press; 2017. p. 29.
7. Johnson-Delaney C. Disorders of the urogenital system. In: Johnson-Delaney C, editor. Ferret medicine and surgery. CRC Press; 2017. p. 366–70.
8. Bean AD, Fisher PG, Reavill DR, et al. Hypercalcemia associated with lymphomas in the ferret (Mustela putorius furo): four cases. J Exot Pet Med 2019; 29:147–53.
9. Jackson DN, Rogers AB, Maurer KJ, et al. Cystic renal disease in the domestic ferret. Comp Med 2008;58(2):161–7.
10. MacNab TA, Newcomb BT, Ketz-Riley C, et al. Extramural ectopic ureter in a domestic ferret (Mustela putorius furo). J Exot Pet Med 2010;19(4):313–6.
11. Li X, Fox JG, Padrid PA. Neoplastic disease in ferrets: 574 cases (1968–1997). J Am Vet Med Assoc 1998;212(9):1402–6.
12. Avallone G, Forlani A, Tecilla M, et al. Neoplastic diseases in the domestic ferret (Mustela putorius furo) in Italy: classification and tissue distribution of 856 cases (2000-2010). BMC Vet Res 2016;12(1):275–83.
13. Kawaguchi H, Miyoshi N, Souda M, et al. Renal adenocarcinoma in a ferret. Vet Pathol 2006;43(3):353–6.
14. Bell RC, Moeller RB. Transitional cell carcinoma of the renal pelvis in a ferret. Lab Anim Sci 1990;40(5):537–8.
15. Volgenaeu T, Greenacre CB, Smith J, et al. Challenging cases in internal medicine: what's your diagnosis? Vet Med 1998;9(93):797–804.
16. Nwaokorie EE, Osborne CA, Lulich JP, et al. Epidemiology of struvite uroliths in ferrets: 272 cases (1981-2007). J Am Vet Med Assoc 2011;239(10):1319–24.
17. Fox JG, Pearson RC, Bell JA. Diseases of the genitourinary system. In: Fox JG, editor. Biology and diseases of the ferret. 2nd edition. Baltimore (MD): Williams and Wilkens; 1998. p. 247–72.
18. Nwaokorie EE, Osborne CA, Lulich JP, et al. Epidemiological evaluation of cystine urolithiasis in domestic ferrets (Mustela putorius furo): 70 cases (1992-2009). J Am Vet Med Assoc 2013;242(8):1099–103.
19. Osborne CA, Albasan H, Lulich JP, et al. Quantitative analysis of 4468 uroliths retrieved from farm animals, exotic species, and wildlife submitted to the Minnesota Urolith Center: 1981 to 2007. Vet Clin North Am Small Anim Pract 2009;39(1):65–78.

20. Powers LV, Winkler K, Garner MM, et al. Omentalization of prostatic abscesses and large cysts in ferrets (*Mustela putorius furo*). J Exot Pet Med 2007;16(3): 186–94.

21. van Zeeland YRA, Lennox A, Quinton JF, et al. Prepuce and partial penile amputation for treatment of preputial gland neoplasia in two ferrets. J Small Anim Pract 2014;55(11):593–6.

22. Fisher P. Exotic mammal renal disease: diagnosis and treatment. Vet Clin North Am Exot Anim Pract 2006;9(10):69–96.

23. Hinton M. Kidney disease in the rabbit: a histological survey. Lab Anim 1981; 15(3):263–5.

24. Csokai J, Gruber A, Künzel F, et al. Encephalitozoonosis in pet rabbits (Oryctolagus cuniculus): pathohistological findings in animals with latent infection versus clinical manifestation. Parasitol Res 2009;104(3):629–35.

25. Leipig M, Matiasek K, Rinder H, et al. Value of histopathology, immunohistochemistry, and real-time polymerase chain reaction in the confirmatory diagnosis of Encephalitozoon cuniculi infection in rabbits. J Vet Diagn Invest 2013;25(1):16–26.

26. Di Girolamo N, Bongiovanni L, Ferro S, et al. Cystoscopic diagnosis of polypoid cystitis in two pet rabbits. J Am Vet Med Assoc 2017;251(1):84–9.

27. Garibaldi BA, Fox JG, Otto G, et al. Hematuria in rabbits. Lab Anim Sci 1987; 37(6):769–72.

28. Maurer KJ, Marini RP, Fox JG, et al. Polycystic kidney syndrome in New Zealand white rabbits resembling human polycystic kidney disease. Kidney Int 2004; 65(2):482–9.

29. Fox RR, Krinsky WL, Crary DD. Hereditary cortical renal cysts in the rabbit. J Hered 1971;62(2):105–9.

30. Ojeda JL, García-Porrero JA. Structure and development of parietal podocytes in renal glomerular cysts induced in rabbits with methylprednisolone acetate. Lab Invest 1982;47(2):167–76.

31. Durfee WJ, Masters WG, Montgomery CA, et al. Spontaneous renal cell carcinoma in a New Zealand white rabbit. Contemp Top Lab Anim Sci 1999;38(10): 89–91.

32. Rose JB, Vergneau-Grosset C, Steffey MA, et al. Adrenalectomy and nephrectomy in a rabbit (Oryctolagus cuniculus) with adrenocortical carcinoma and renal and ureteral transitional cell carcinoma. J Exot Pet Med 2016;25(4):332–41.

33. Cikanek SJ, Eshar D, Nau M, et al. Diagnosis and surgical treatment of a transitional cell carcinoma in the bladder apex of a pet rabbit (*Oryctolagus cuniculus*) (AEMV Forum). J Exot Pet Med 2018;27(2):113–7.

34. Clauss M, Burger B, Liesegang A, et al. Influence of diet on calcium metabolism, tissue calcification and urinary sludge in rabbits (*Oryctolagus cuniculus*). J Anim Physiol Anim Nutr 2012;96(5):798–807.

35. Kucera J, Koristkova T, Gottwaldova B, et al. Calcium sulfate dihydrate urolithiasis in a pet rabbit. J Am Vet Med Assoc 2017;250(5):534–7.

36. Thas I, Harcourt-Brown F. Six cases of inguinal urinary bladder herniation in entire male domestic rabbits. J Small Anim Pract 2013;54(12):662–6.

37. Grunkemeyer VL, Sura PA, Baron ML, et al. Surgical repair of an inguinal herniation of the urinary bladder in an intact female domestic rabbit (*Oryctolagus cuniculus*). J Exot Pet Med 2010;19(3):249–54.

38. Greenacre CB, Allen SW, Ritchie BW. Urinary bladder eversion in rabbit does. Comp Cont Educ Pract Vet 1999;21(6):524–8.

39. Szabó Z. Transurethral urinary bladder eversion and prolapse in a castrated male pet rabbit. Acta Vet Hung 2017;65(4):556–64.

40. Wu RS, Chu CC, Wang HC, et al. Clinical diagnosis and surgical management of diaphragmatic retroperitoneal perirenal fat and kidney herniation in a pet rabbit. J Am Vet Med Assoc 2016;248(12):1399–403.

41. Carrasco DC, Skarbek A, Lopez M. Surgical management of diaphragmatic lipoma and kidney herniation in a rabbit (Oryctolagus cuniculus) with a polypropylene mesh. Proceedings of the annual conference of the association of exotic mammal Veterinarians. Atlanta, 2018. p. 757.

42. Künzel F, Fisher P. Clinical signs, diagnosis, and treatment of Encephalitozoon cuniculi infection in rabbits. Vet Clin North Am Exot Anim Pract 2018;21(1):69–82.

43. Graham JE, Garner MM, Reavill DR. Benzimidazole toxicosis in rabbits: 13 cases (2003 to 2011). J Exot Pet Med 2014;23(2):188–95.

44. Martorell J, Bailon D, Majo N, et al. Lateral approach to nephrotomy in the management of unilateral renal calculi in a rabbit (Oryctolagus cuniculus). J Am Vet Med Assoc 2012;240(7):863–8.

45. Rhody JL. Unilateral nephrectomy for hydronephrosis in a pet rabbit. Vet Clin North Am Exot Anim Pract 2006;9(3):633–41.

46. Steblay RW, Rudofsky U. Spontaneous renal lesions and glomerular deposits of IgG and complement in guinea pigs. J Immunol 1997;107(4):1192–6.

47. Takeda T, Grollman A. Spontaneously occurring renal disease in the guinea pig. Am J Pathol 1970;60(1):103–18.

48. Wolf P, Schröder A, Wenger A, et al. The nutrition of the chinchilla as a companion animal – basic data, influences and dependences. J Anim Physiol Anim Nutr 2003;87(3–4):129–33.

49. Schuhmann B, Kück G, Cope I. Bacterial cystitis in four female guinea pigs (Cavia porcellus) resembling necrotising bacterial cystitis. Vet Rec Case Rep 2015;3(1):e000136.

50. Steele H. Subcutaneous fibrosarcoma in an aged guinea pig. Can Vet J 2001; 42(4):300–2.

51. Jensen JA, Brice AK, Bagel JH, et al. Hypervitaminosis D in guinea pigs with α-mannosidosis. Comp Med 2013;63(2):156–62.

52. Parsons JL. Feeding pocket pets: Nutritional physiology of rodents and lagomorphs. Proceedings of the annual conference of the American association of Zoo Veterinarians. Atlanta, 2016.

53. Clauss M, Hummel J. Getting it out of the (digestive) system: hindgut fermenters and calcium. Proceedings of the Annual Conference of the Comparative Nutrition Society, 2008. p. 30–36.

54. Jolánkai R, Guija de Arespacochaga A, Iben C. Urolithiasis in guinea pigs — Nutritional aspects. Cereal Res Commun 2006;34(1):743–6.

55. Lennox AM. A simple technique for removal of urethroliths in the female guinea pig. Proceedings of the Annual Conference of the association of exotic mammal Veterinarians. Orlando, 2014.

56. Hubbard GB, Schmidt RE. Noninfectious diseases. In: Van Hoosier GL Jr, McPherson CW, editors. Laboratory hamsters. Orlando (FL): Academic Press; 1987. p. 169–78.

57. Sobh M, Moustafa F, Hamed S, et al. Effect of colchicine on schistosoma-induced renal amyloidosis in Syrian golden hamsters. Nephron 1995;70(4):478–85.

58. Murphy JC, Fox JG, Niemi SM. Nephrotic syndrome associated with renal amyloidosis in a colony of Syrian hamsters. J Am Vet Med Assoc 1984;185: 1359–62.

59. McKeon GP, Nagamine CM, Ruby NF, et al. Hematologic, serologic, and histologic profile of aged Siberian hamsters (*Phodopus sungorus*). J Am Assoc Lab Anim Sci 2011;50(3):308–16.
60. Benjamin SA, Brooks AL. Spontaneous lesions in Chinese hamsters. Vet Pathol 1977;14(5):449–62.
61. Pour P, Mohr U, Althoff J, et al. Spontaneous tumors and common diseases in two colonies of 6. Syrian hamsters. III. Urogenital system and endocrine glands. J Natl Cancer Inst 1976;56(5):949–61.
62. Miyazawa S, Saiga K, Nemoto K, et al. A repeat biopsy study in spontaneous crescentic glomerulonephritis mice. Ren Fail 2002;24(5):557–66.
63. Imai H, Nakamoto Y, Asakura K, et al. Spontaneous glomerular IgA deposition in ddY mice: an animal model of IgA nephritis. Kidney Int 1985;27(5):756–61.
64. Montgomery CA. Interstitial nephritis, mouse. In: Jones TC, Hard GC, Mohr U, editors. Monographs on pathology of laboratory animals: urinary system. New York: Springer-Verlag; 1998. p. 238–43.
65. Montgomery CA. Suppurative nephritis, pyelonephritis, mouse. In: Jones TC, Hard GC, Mohr U, editors. Monographs on pathology of laboratory animals: urinary system. New York: Springer-Verlag; 1998. p. 244–8.
66. Barthold SW. Klossielosis, kidney, mouse, rat. In: Jones TC, Hard GC, Mohr U, editors. Monographs on pathology of laboratory animals: urinary system. New York: Springer-Verlag; 1986. p. 276–8.
67. Ninomiya H, Inomata T, Ogihara K. Obstructive uropathy and hydronephrosis in male KK-Ay mice: a report of cases. J Vet Med Sci 1999;61(1):53–7.
68. Shoieb A, Shirai N. Polycystic kidney disease in Sprague-Dawley rats. Exp Toxicol Pathol 2015;67(5–6):361–4.
69. Hard GC, Betz LJ, Seely JC. Association of advanced chronic progressive nephropathy (CPN) with renal tubule tumors and precursor hyperplasia in control F344 rats from two-year carcinogenicity studies. Toxicol Pathol 2012;40(3):473–81.
70. Dontas IA, Khaldi L. Urolithiasis and transitional cell carcinoma of the bladder in a Wistar rat. J Am Assoc Lab Anim Sci 2006;45(4):64–7.
71. Izumi K, Kitaura K, Chone Y, et al. Spontaneous renal cell tumors in Long-Evans Cinnamon rats. Jpn J Cancer Res 1994;85(6):563–6.
72. Bowman MR, Pare JA, Pinckney RD. Trichosomoides crassicauda infection in a pet hooded rat. Vet Rec 2004;154(12):374–5.
73. Burek JD, Duprat P, Owen R, et al. Spontaneous renal disease in laboratory animals. Int Rev Exp Pathol 1988;30:231–319.
74. Solleveld HA, Boorman GA. Spontaneous renal lesions in five rat strains. Toxicol Pathol 1986;14(2):168–74.
75. Kondo S, Yoshizawa N, Wakabayashi K. Natural history of renal lesions in spontaneously hypercholesterolemic (SHC) male rats. Nihon Jinzo Gakkai Shi 1995;37:91–9.
76. Chandra M, Riley MG, Johnson DE. Spontaneous renal neoplasms in rats. J Appl Toxicol 1993;13(2):109–16.
77. Martel-Arquette A, Mans C. Urolithiasis in chinchillas: 15 cases (2007 to 2011). J Small Anim Pract 2016;57(5):260–4.
78. Spence S, Skae K. Urolithiasis in a chinchilla. Vet Rec 1995;136(20):524.
79. Thöle M, Schuhmann B, Köstlinger S, et al. Treatment of unilateral perineal hernias in 2 male chinchillas (*Chinchilla lanigera*). J Exot Pet Med 2018;27(3):43–9.
80. Gardhouse S, Eshar D. Retrospective study of disease occurrence in captive African pygmy hedgehogs (Atelerix albiventris). Isr J Vet Med 2015;70(1):32–6.

81. Raab O, Béraud R, Tefft KM, et al. Successful treatment of Corynebacterium ure-alyticum encrusting cystitis with systemic and intravesical antimicrobial therapy. Can Vet J 2015;56(5):471–5.

82. Ardiaca M, Bennett MD, Montesinos A, et al. Klossiella dulcis n. sp. (Apicom-plexa: Klossiellidae) in the kidneys of Petaurus breviceps (Marsupialia: Petauri-dae). J Zoo Wildl Med 2016;47(2):622–7.

83. Cusack L, Schnellbacher R, Howerth EW, et al. Bilateral hydronephrosis in a sugar glider (Petaurus breviceps). J Zoo Wildl Med 2016;47(3):886–9.

84. Ju-Chi Chen, Pin-Huan Yu, Chen-Hsuan Liu, et al. Paracloacal gland carcinoma in a sugar glider (*Petaurus breviceps*). J Exot Pet Med 2018;27(1):36–40.

85. Thomas M, Parkinson L, Shaw G, et al. Paracloacal cyst in a sugar glider (*Petaurus breviceps*). J Exot Pet Med 2019;29(0):40–4.

86. Marrow JC, Carpenter JW, Lloyd A, et al. A transitional cell carcinoma with squa-mous differentiation in a pericloacal mass in a sugar glider (*Petaurus breviceps*). J Exot Pet Med 2010;19(1):92–5.

87. Kuroki K, DeBey BM, Pollock CG, et al. Pathology in practice. Copper toxicosis. J Am Vet Med Assoc 2011;239(12):1549–51.

88. Sparkes AH, Caney S, Chalhoub S, et al. ISFM consensus guidelines on the diag-nosis and management of feline chronic kidney disease. J Feline Med Surg 2016; 18(3):219–39.

89. Lennox AM, Gladden J. Emergency and critical care of small mammals. In: Ques-enberry K, Mans C, Orcutt C, editors. Ferrets, rabbits, and rodents, 4th edition Saunders, in press.

Diagnostic Imaging of the Renal System in Exotic Companion Mammals

Ruth Mackenzie Hallman, DVM, DACVR,
João Brandão, LMV, MS, DECZM (Avian)*

KEYWORDS

- Urinary tract • Radiography • Excretory urography • Ultrasonography
- Computed tomography • Small mammals • Rabbit • Ferret

KEY POINTS

- Radiographs can be used to easily visualize common types of urinary calculi in all parts of the urinary tract.
- Positive-contrast excretory urography and cystourethrography are sensitive to diseases within the ureters and urethra, most commonly obstruction.
- Ultrasound is widely available and noninvasive and can be used to evaluate renal architecture, ureteral dilation, urinary bladder wall disease, and urolithiasis.
- Computed tomography is increasing in availability and provides a large amount of cross-sectional information quickly and noninvasively.
- Multiple imaging modalities can be used to estimate or quantify glomerular filtration rate.

INTRODUCTION

Diagnostic imaging provides additional clinical information regarding structural changes to the kidneys and urinary tract, patency of the urinary tract, and the presence of calculi. Most imaging modalities are relatively noninvasive and easily available to the practitioner. Exotic companion mammal species are routinely imaged either under general anesthesia or injectable sedation; animals that are acclimated to handling or are obtunded or systemically ill may be imaged without any medication.

The mammalian kidney has a distinct cortex and medulla. Each nephron includes a loop of Henle that allows for water reabsorption, allowing mammals to concentrate urine for water conservation.[1] The ratio of medulla to cortex is directly related to the length of the loop of Henle and, therefore, to water-concentrating ability.[1] Most exotic

Disclosure: None.
Department of Veterinary Clinical Sciences, Center for Veterinary Health Sciences, Oklahoma State University, Stillwater, OK 74078, USA
* Corresponding author.
E-mail address: jbrandao@okstate.edu

pet mammalian species have a smoothly marginated kidney with a single renal papilla.[2]

Most exotic pet mammalian species have similar renal function and physiology, with rabbits showing some of the most significant variation among these species. Differences in calcium regulation and acid-base enzyme function result in a relatively higher urine alkalinity in this species, higher urine calcium excretion, and a higher susceptibility to acid-base imbalances.[3,4]

SURVEY RADIOGRAPHY

Abdominal radiographs using either film or a digital imaging system are commonly available and often are the first modality chosen to image the urinary system. Although traditional, slow-speed film systems provide the best resolution for small body parts, the widespread availability and improving resolution capabilities of digital radiography have made these systems equal to the task of abdominal imaging for the majority of exotic companion mammal patients. Additional benefits of digital imaging systems include the ability to annotate or manipulate the image after it is obtained and the ease of storage and transfer of these images for consultation. Radiographs are also sensitive to many types of urinary calculi and can be used to image extra-abdominal portions of the urethra or parts of the urinary system that may not be seen on ultrasound due to shadowing from gastrointestinal (GI) gas.

When abdominal radiography is performed in a patient with urinary disease, a minimum of 2 views (lateral and ventrodorsal) should be obtained; for complete evaluation of the abdomen, including the GI tract, 3 views, including left and right lateral projections, are recommended. A ventrodorsal view is preferred to the dorsoventral projection for increased contrast of the retroperitoneal structures. The entire urethra should be included in the lateral view; the perineal region soft tissues should be included at the caudal edge of the image. Depending on anatomy of the species, an additional lateral view with the hind legs flexed may be included to gain a complete view of the penile urethra and os penis. Fasting, to reduce the amount of ingesta within the stomach and large intestine, may increase the visibility of the urinary tract but often is not performed in clinical patients due to potential adverse side effects and other practical reasons. Radiographs often are performed under sedation or anesthesia, to ensure proper positioning without unnecessary stress to the patient and to limit the handler's exposure to radiation.[5]

The renal silhouette visible on survey radiographs is composed of the renal capsule, the cortex, medulla, and the pelvis or collecting system of the kidney. These parts cannot be distinguished on survey radiographs. Radiographs are sensitive to changes in the overall size and shape of the kidneys (**Fig. 1**) but often cannot determine a specific etiology for renomegaly. Some references for normal renal size are available (**Table 1**). The kidneys also may be compared with the length of the second lumbar spinal vertebra (L2) on the ventrodorsal image, with kidney:L2 ratios ranging from 2.1 to 4 in rats (*Rattus norvegicus*),[6] 2.1 to 2.3 in ferrets (*Mustela putorius furo*),[7] 1.9 to 2.28 in dwarf rabbits (*Oryctolagus cuniculus*),[8] and 2.3 to 2.6 in New Zealand white rabbits.[9] If established reference intervals or ratios are not available, kidney size can be compared with the contralateral organ (**Fig. 2**) or to other weight or sex-matched conspecific control subjects.

Radiographs are a sensitive test for the presence of calcium-based mineral accumulations within all parts of the urinary tract. Mineralization of the renal parenchyma or within the collecting system of the kidney can be identified on radiographs as well as calculi within the ureters, bladder, or urethra. Rabbits routinely have an

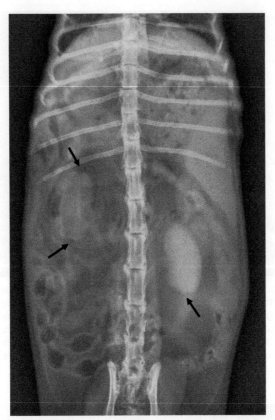

Fig. 1. Ventrodorsal radiograph of the abdomen of an adult ferret (*Mustela putorius furo*). Renal silhouettes are reduced in length and there is focal flattening of the cranial and caudal poles (*arrows*), consistent with chronic renal infarctions and/or degenerative nephrosis. (*Courtesy of* M. Hallman, DVM, DACVR, Stillwater, OK.)

increased concentration of calcium within the urinary bladder, which increases with a calcium-rich diet.[13] This mineral may accumulate within the bladder as a granular or amorphous sediment, or sludge (**Fig. 3**) or may form distinct calculi (**Fig. 4**).[14] Small amounts of sludge may be incidental in rabbits. Calculi and sludge are routinely

Table 1 Normal renal lengths of selected species	
Species	**Length (cm)**
Chinchilla	1.7–2.2
Ferret, male	2.2–2.7
Ferret, male	2.7–3.2
Gerbil, golden hamster	0.9–1.4
Guinea pig	1.4–2.5
Rabbit, small breed <2 kg	2.1–3.6
Rabbit, New Zealand white	4.0–4.8
Rat	1.4–2.7

Data from Refs.[6,9–12]

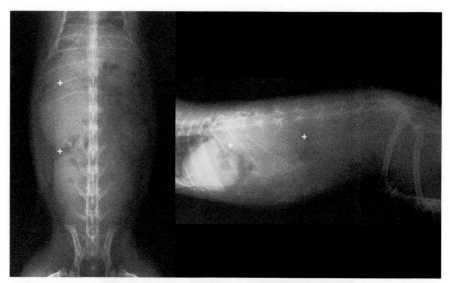

Fig. 2. Ventrodorsal (*left image*) and lateral (*right image*) radiographs of the abdomen of an adult rabbit (*Oryctolagus cuniculus*). The right kidney is significantly larger than the left, with irregular margination (calipers). Hydronephrosis due to pelvic and ureteral obstruction from transitional cell carcinoma was diagnosed via ultrasound and histopathology. (*From* Rose J, Vergneau-Grosset C, Steffey MA, et al, "Adrenalectomy and nephrectomy in a rabbit (Oryctolagus cuniculus) with adrenocortical carcinoma and renal and ureteral transitional cell carcinoma" J Exot Pet Med 2016;25:332–41; *with permission*.)

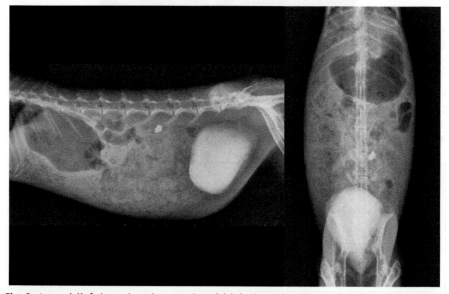

Fig. 3. Lateral (*left image*) and ventrodorsal (*right image*) radiographs of the abdomen of an adult rabbit (*Oryctolagus cuniculus*). A large amount of radiopaque sludge is present within the bladder. An irregular calculus is located caudal to the left kidney (not visible), presumably within the left ureter. (*Courtesy of* A. Le Roux DVM, DECVDI, DACVR, New York, NY.)

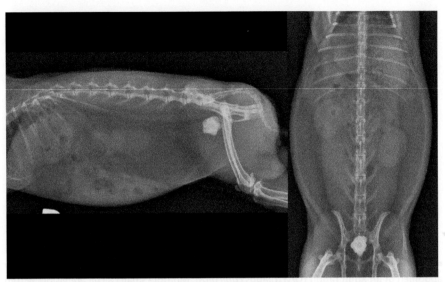

Fig. 4. Lateral (*left image*) and ventrodorsal (*right image*) radiographs of the caudal abdomen of an adult rabbit (*Oryctolagus cuniculus*). A large calculus is present within the urinary bladder. (*Image Courtesy of* S. Loeber, DVM, University of Wisconsin-Madison, Madison, WI.)

identified in other species as well, including guinea pigs (*Cavia porcellus*), ferrets, and less commonly chinchillas (*Chinchilla lanigera*).[14]

Struvite-based stones also are radiopaque and are seen in ferrets.[15,16] Calculi comprised mainly of cysteine or urate are radiolucent and may not be seen on survey radiographs.

Ureters are not visible on survey radiographs, but ureteral calculi may be identified within the retroperitoneal space caudal to the kidneys (see **Fig. 3**; **Fig. 5**). Ureteral obstruction from calculi may cause hydronephrosis, which appear as generalized renomegaly, usually unilateral, on survey radiographs.

The size of the urinary bladder on radiographs is variable, depending on how recently the patient has urinated. A distended urinary bladder that displaces small intestines cranially may be due to a urethral obstruction or can represent a functional atony. Urinary bladder wall thickness cannot be determined on radiographs without the aid of contrast.

The urethra is not distinguishable on survey radiographs, and disease in this region is not identified unless a radiopaque calculus is present (**Fig. 6**). Urethral calculi can occur in any both males and females of any species but are most commonly reported in males. The urethra, as well as the ureters, are best visualized when contrast media is applied to the urinary system, as described later.

CONTRAST EXCRETORY UROGRAPHY

The visibility of the urinary tract can be increased on radiography by applying a contrast agent, most commonly an iodine-based, nonionic agent, such as iohexol or iopamidol. These agents are freely filtered at the glomerulus and are quickly and completely excreted via the renal system. Nonionic contrast agents have an osmolality that is closer to plasma than previously available agents.

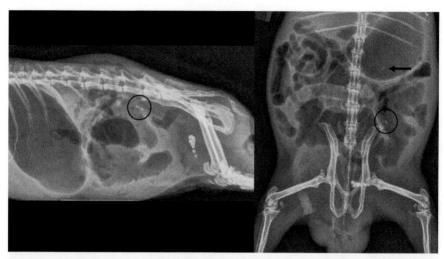

Fig. 5. Lateral (*left image*) and ventrodorsal (*right image*) radiographs of the caudal abdomen of an adult rabbit (*Oryctolagus cuniculus*). Multiple small calculi are visible within the urinary bladder, as well as within the left ureter (*circles*) and the pelvis of the left kidney ([*arrow*] ventrodorsal view). (*Courtesy of* D. Jimenez, DVM, DACVR, Athens, GA.)

Older contrast agents, such as diatrozoate, are ionic and hyperosmolar to plasma, have an increased incidence of negative side effects and are no longer recommended.

An excretory urogram (EU), also known as an intravenous pyelogram, can be accomplished by injecting contrast media intravenously and then obtaining 2-view radiographs or fluoroscopic images immediately and serially over the next several minutes (**Table 2**).[9,17–19] Image quality is optimized by evacuating the colon with enemas and instilling 5 mL/kg of air into the urinary bladder via a urethral catheter prior to the study. At least 2 views should be obtained immediately after injection, again at 2 minutes and 5 minutes postinjection, and again at 20 minutes and 40 minutes,[19] although the nephrogram phase may persist for several hours.[17]

Contrast doses for exotic companion mammals often are extrapolated from studies performed in cats and dogs. Recommended doses range from iodine, 600 mg/kg body weight to 850 mg/kg body weight.[5,17,18,20,21] Doses of iodine, 850 mg/kg, yielded

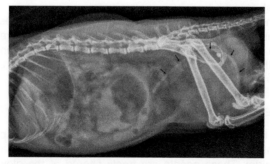

Fig. 6. Lateral radiograph of the abdomen of an adult chinchilla (*Chinchilla lanigera*). A small calculus is present within the pelvic urethra, immediately ventral to the urethral catheter (*arrows*). (*Courtesy of* D. Jimenez, DVM, DACVR, Athens, GA.)

Table 2
Phases of excretory urogram (radiographic or computed tomographic)

Phase	Time Postinjection	Imaging Findings
Vascular	Immediate to 30 s	Enhancement of aorta and renal vessels
Nephrogram	10–30 s, up to several hours	Corticomedullary and then medullary enhancement, steadily lessening over time
Pyelogram	1.5–2 min, up to several hours	Enhancement of the pelvis, ureters, and contrast accumulation in the bladder

Data from Vilalta L, Altuzarra R, Espada Y, et al. Description and comparison of excretory urography performed during radiography and computed tomography for evaluation of the urinary system in healthy New Zealand White rabbits *(Oryctolagus cuniculus)*. Am J Vet Res 2017;78:472-81; and Altuzarra R, Vilalta L, Martorell J, et al. Description of digital fluoroscopic excretory urography in healthy New Zealand rabbits (Oryctolagus cuniculus). Vet Rec 2018;183:568.

minimal side effects in rabbits, including 1 rabbit with transient apnea and no side effects in a second study.[18] One study showed equivalent study quality using intraosseous versus intravenous administration in rabbits.[21] EU has been assessed using both intraosseous and subcutaneous administration of iodine-based contrast in Persian squirrels (*Sciurus anomalus*). Although the subcutaneous route of administration did not demonstrate the nephrogram phase adequately, it was successful in showing the pyelogram phase and filling of the ureters and bladder.[22] No adverse effects were noted.

Contrast-induced nephrotoxicosis is an uncommon side effect of contrast administration that reportedly occurs in 3% to 25% of humans and has also been reported in dogs and experimental models in rabbits.[23,24] Nevertheless, based on experimental canine models, these adverse effects seem to be of low clinical relevance.[25] Side effects of contrast administration can be exacerbated by hypovolemia and episodes of ischemia. Contrast studies should not be performed in patients that are clinically dehydrated or demonstrating oliguric renal failure.

EU can be used to determine the architecture of the corticomedullary tissue within the renal silhouette (**Fig. 7**). EU is sensitive to dilation of the collecting system that may be due to obstruction or ascending infection, although ultrasonography has widely replaced EU for this purpose. EU is the most sensitive imaging modality to detect tears or disruptions of the renal capsule and ureters, causing leakage of urine into the retroperitoneal space. EU has been used to diagnosis both ureteral ectopia[26] and ureterovesicular stenosis[27] in ferrets. EU also can be used to qualitatively estimate glomerular filtration rate (GFR).

The lower urinary tract (urinary bladder and urethra) also may be visualized with EU but with less consistency than with retrograde cystourethrography (discussed later).

CONTRAST CYSTOURETHROGRAPHY

Positive-contrast cystourethrography, also known as retrograde cystography, is accomplished by administering contrast from the distal urethra retrograde into the urinary bladder, obtaining radiographs during and after the contrast agent is administered.[28] Contrast can be easily introduced into the lower urinary tract by placing a catheter into the distal urethra and manually holding the catheter in place. Nonionic iodine-based contrast agents should be used and often diluted 1:1 or 2:1 with sterile saline. To fully distend the urethra, contrast should be actively injected into the catheter while the radiograph is taken. Small air bubbles within the contrast can be

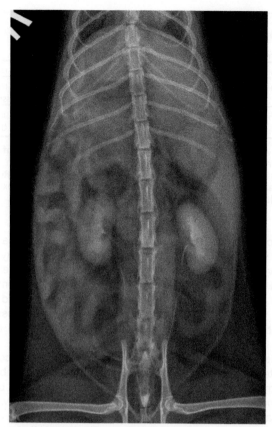

Fig. 7. Ventrodorsal radiograph of the abdomen of an adult ferret (*Mustela putorius furo*), as part of an EU study. The renal silhouettes are contrast enhanced, and contrast is visible within the normal renal pelvises and ureters. (*Courtesy of* M. Hallman, DVM, DACVR, Stillwater, OK.)

mistaken for lucent calculi, and, if identified, the image should be repeated with a second push of contrast to determine if the abnormality persists.

Positive-contrast cystourethography can be used to detect tears or disruptions within the urethra and urinary bladder or to confirm the location of the urinary bladder in the case of body wall herniation, reported in rabbits.[29,30] An adequate volume of contrast must be administered to distend the bladder, and the radiograph should be taken during active administration while the contrast is under positive pressure to identify small tears.

Radiolucent calculi, such as those composed of cysteine or urates, are identified as filling defects within the pool of contrast in the urinary bladder or urethra. Radiopaque calculi also are visible as filling defects and appear lucent compared with the surrounding opaque contrast media. Older techniques, using a combination of positive contrast and negative contrast (ie, air or gas) within the urinary bladder to increase the detection of calculi, have been widely replaced with ultrasonography.

If the bladder is fully distended with contrast, the mucosal surface can be evaluated, with irregularity and thickening of the mucosa suggesting cystitis or neoplasia. Incomplete distention of the bladder can highlight artifactual thickening that can be incorrectly interpreted as disease, and these studies should be interpreted with caution. Ultrasonography has widely replaced contrast studies for evaluation of the urinary bladder wall.

Retrograde cystourethrography may be the best method to visualize the lumen and mucosal surface of the urethra and can identify strictures, obstructions due to radiolucent calculi or seminal concretions, neoplastic mural lesions, and tears in the urethra. Again, images should be obtained while contrast is being administered with positive pressure to fully distend the lumen of the urethra. Retrograde cystourethrography has been suggested as a simple tool for diagnosis of bladder herniation in rabbits,[31] because the location of the bladder can be easily identified.

ULTRASONOGRAPHY

Ultrasonography is increasingly available in companion animal general practices and has numerous benefits over survey and contrast radiography. There are no ionizing radiation exposure to the patient or staff and no known side effects. Many patients tolerate ultrasound with minimal sedation. One important advantage of ultrasound is the ability to guide fine-needle aspirations safely and accurately. Cystocentesis for urinalysis and culture as well as fine-needle aspirates of solid masses can be performed easily with ultrasound guidance in many cases. A 1-inches, 22-gauge needle can be used in many medium-sized patients, such as rabbits and guinea pigs, with minimal sedation. Most importantly, ultrasound offers real-time images with superior visualization of soft tissue architecture and fluid-tissue interfaces. Disadvantages of ultrasound include the time required to perform the study and the dependence of study quality the operator skill and experience.

To image the urinary tract, the ventral and ventrolateral surfaces of the abdomen are clipped of hair, and a combination of alcohol and ultrasound-specific coupling gel is applied to the skin, eliminating any air between the probe's surface and surface of the skin. Fur must be clipped in order to achieve adequate skin contact but should be done prudently to minimize body heat loss by excessive clipping. A minimal amount of alcohol should be used with warmed acoustic coupling gel to maintain contact of the probe with the skin without excessively cooling the patient. High-frequency (7.5–15 MHz) curvilinear and linear transducers produce the best image quality on small patients.

Ultrasound waves cannot penetrate gas, and thus the GI tract of many herbivorous mammals can limit what will be visualized. Depending on the shape of a patient's abdomen, imaging into the last few intercostal spaces and along the lateral aspect of the sublumbar region may be needed to see around the GI tract. Fasting the patient may aid in reducing the amount of ingesta within the stomach and large intestine but often is not done in clinical cases due to potential side effects and other practical purposes. In 1 study, both fasting and administration of simethicone, to reduce GI gas accumulation, did not improve visibility of abdominal organs in rabbits.[32]

Kidneys

Normal kidneys in exotic companion mammals are smoothly marginated with well-defined corticomedullary distinction (**Fig. 8**A). In the transverse plane, the renal papilla creates a triangular or crescent shape along which lies the renal pelvis, a potential space capable of dilation during disease. Rabbits have a large amount of hyperechoic fat within the renal sinus compared with other species (**Fig. 8**B). Ferrets can have a hyperechoic band through the medulla that is considered diet related and incidental.[12]

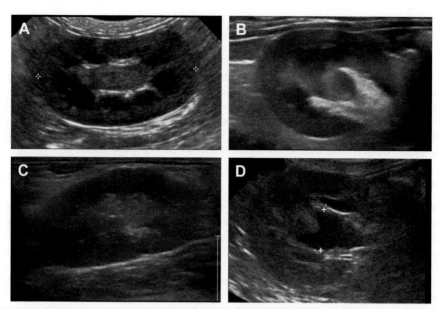

Fig. 8. (*A*) Sagittal and (*B*) transverse plane ultrasound images of the normal kidney of a rabbit (*Oryctolagus cuniculus*). Note the corticomedullary distinction and hyperechoic fat within the renal sinus surrounding the pelvis. (*C*) Sagittal plane ultrasound image of a guinea pig (*Cavia porcellus*) with chronic degenerative nephrosis. Note the irregular cortical margin, poor corticomedullary distinction, and pinpoint mineralization within the medulla. (*D*) Transverse plane ultrasound image of the kidney in a rabbit with chronic ureteral obstruction. Note the dilated anechoic renal pelvis (calipers). (*Courtesy of* M. Hallman, DVM, DACVR, Stillwater, OK.)

Acute renal injury may result in mild enlargement of the kidneys or perirenal fluid accumulation, or the kidneys may appear within normal limits. Regardless of the initial insult to the kidneys, which may include toxins, nephrotoxic antibiotics, infection (such as *Encephalitozoon cuniculi* in rabbits), chronic interstitial nephritis, or amyloidosis, chronic changes result in kidneys that are reduced in length, with irregular margination and reduced corticomedullary distinction (**Fig. 8C**).[33] Aged rats afflicted with chronic progressive nephrosis have kidneys that are enlarged compared with normal.[15]

Renal neoplasia is generally uncommon in exotic companion mammals, with renal lymphoma, sarcoma, and adenocarcinoma reported in ferrets and rabbits.[14,34] Renal neoplasms may present as single or multiple nodules or masses within renal parenchyma or with complete effacement of normal parenchyma with large, irregular kidneys and total loss of corticomedullary definition. Although ultrasound is sensitive to changes in the architecture of the kidney, these changes are often nonspecific, and ultrasonography can be used to guide tissue sampling for cytology and histopathology and definitive diagnosis.

Renal cysts are seen in many species and are a common finding in aged ferrets.[35] Renal cysts can range from a few, small incidental cysts to multiple, large cysts that destroy a significant amount of renal architecture, termed *polycystic kidney disease*.[35] Ultrasonographically, cysts are defined as having a thin round wall and anechoic content (**Fig. 9**). Cysts exhibit distal acoustic enhancement, demonstrating their fluid-filled nature. Perinephric pseudocysts, which are large accumulations of fluid beneath the

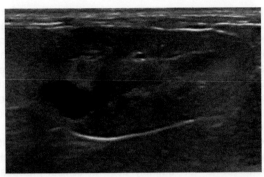

Fig. 9. Sagittal plane ultrasound image of the kidney of an adult ferret (*Mustela putorius furo*). There is a moderately sized oval anechoic cyst within the cranial pole of the kidney. (*Courtesy of* M. Hallman, DVM, DACVR, Stillwater, OK.)

renal capsule and surrounding the renal parenchyma, have been reported in a ferret with multiple parenchymal cysts.[36]

Calculi within the renal pelvis (nephrolithiasis) and within the ureters (ureterolithiasis) are a common finding in many small mammal species.[15] Calculi appear as 1 or multiple smooth or irregular hyperechoic margins with distal acoustic shadowing (**Fig. 10**). Stones that are lucent on radiographs, such as cysteine or urate origin, can be detected with ultrasound. Calculi can lead to obstruction of the urinary system or predispose to infection.

Pyelonephritis, or infection of the renal pelvis and interstitium, is often secondary to calculi within the pelvis or proximal ureter. Infection may appear as hyperechogenicity of the renal pelvis content or of the renal papilla.[33] The renal pelvis often is dilated in these cases (**Fig. 8D**). Even if the urine within the dilated pelvis is anechoic, infection secondary to obstruction cannot be ruled out sonographically, and urine culture must be pursued.

Hydronephrosis refers to dilation of the pelvis or collecting system of the kidney to such a degree that overall renal size becomes enlarged and the cortex becomes

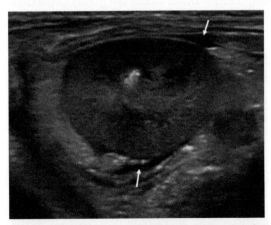

Fig. 10. Transverse plane ultrasound image of the kidney of an adult ferret (*Mustela putorius furo*). There is a small hyperechoic calculus within the renal pelvis (calipers), and a small amount of free peritoneal effusion surrounding the kidney (*arrows*). (*Courtesy of* M. Hallman, DVM, DACVR, Stillwater, OK.)

thinned. Hydronephrosis develops secondary to obstruction of a ureter or long-standing infection. Ureteral obstruction and hydronephrosis have been reported in ferrets secondary to inadvertent ureter ligation during ovariohysterectomy[14,15,37] and secondary to congenital ureterovesicular stenosis.[27] Hydronephrosis has been reported in rabbits secondary to postoperative adhesions,[38] renal pelvic neoplasia,[39] and ureterolithiasis.[40] On ultrasound examination, a hydronephrotic kidney has a large anechoic central pelvic region, and the cortex can become so thinned as to appear as a hyperechoic rim only. The pelvis of a hydronephrotic kidney can become infected or hemorrhagic, appearing hyperechoic on ultrasound.

Contrast-enhanced ultrasonography has been used in numerous studies in humans, cats, and dogs and can provide perfusion data of the kidney as well as for mass lesions.[41,42] This technique is not routinely used in clinical practice and availability may be limited. One recent study reports the use of contrast-enhanced ultrasound in the diagnosis of liver lobe torsion in a rabbit.[43]

Ureters

The normal ureters are too small to be routinely identified on ultrasound. Dilated ureters (hydroureter) are identified on ultrasound as tubular structures paralleling the aorta and caudal vena cava but without Doppler flow and are usually due to downstream obstruction from calculi (**Fig. 11**). Ureterolithiasis has been reported most commonly in guinea pigs[44,45] but can occur in any species where calculi are present.[46]

Urinary Bladder and Urethra

On ultrasound, the normal urinary bladder has a thin wall and anechoic contents and varies in size. The trigone and urethra may be located within the pelvis and not visible via a transabdominal approach. In herbivorous animals on a high-calcium diet, calcium-based crystals may be visible within the bladder, either suspended within the lumen or settling along the gravity-dependent portion of the bladder wall. Large amounts of heavy crystalline material (sludge) can be differentiated from solid structures by manual agitation of this material by gently prodding the probe against the patient's ventrum, creating a snow globe appearance of swirling bladder content (**Fig. 12**). In contrast, discrete cystic calculi are gravity dependent and create distal acoustic shadowing (**Fig. 13**).

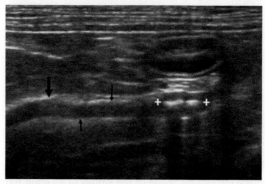

Fig. 11. Sagittal plane ultrasound image of a hydroureter. The ureter is dilated (*arrows*), with 2 small hyperechoic calculi with distal acoustic shadowing, located within the ureteral lumen distally (calipers). (*Courtesy of* M. Hallman, DVM, DACVR, Stillwater, OK.)

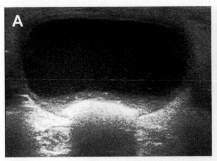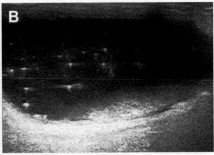

Fig. 12. Sagittal plane ultrasound images of the urinary bladder of an adult ferret (*Mustela putorius furo*). (*A*) There is gravity-dependent material within the bladder, creating a hyperechoic interface and distal acoustic shadowing. (*B*) The bladder is manually agitated by balloting the probe on the ventrum, and numerous small hyperechoic foci go into suspension, demonstrating crystalline debris instead of a single calculus. (*Courtesy of* M. Hallman, DVM, DACVR, Stillwater, OK.)

Cystitis and urethritis have been described in ferrets, guinea pigs, and African pygmy hedgehogs (*Atelerix albiventris*) and occur more commonly in females, often secondary to calculi.[14] On ultrasound, cystitis appears as a thickened irregular bladder mucosa (see **Fig. 13**; **Fig. 14**). Cystitis occurs commonly due to bacterial infection, and ultrasound can be used to guide cystocentesis for urinalysis and culture. A bladder that is mostly empty and not distended can mimic the appearance of cystitis due to normal thickening of the unstretched wall. Repeating imaging after the bladder has had time to fill can help differentiate this artifact. Ultrasonography can also be used for determining bladder location in cases of herniation (**Fig. 15**).

Neoplasia of the urinary bladder, such as transitional cell carcinoma, is rare in exotic companion mammals but has been reported in the rabbit and guinea pig.[47,48] Urinary bladder neoplasia results in asymmetric thickening of the bladder wall with an irregular mucosal margin. Severe cystitis may mimic neoplasia, and with these ultrasonographic findings, infection should be ruled out.

Only the proximal portion of the urethra is visible with transabdominal ultrasound, and disease or obstruction occurring downstream may require other modalities for diagnosis, such as survey radiographs or contrast cystourethrography. Although a distal urethral obstruction may not be visible on ultrasound, it may result in severe

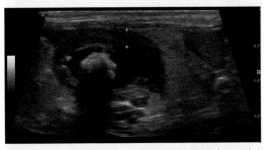

Fig. 13. Transverse ultrasound image of the urinary bladder of an adult guinea pig (*Cavia porcellus*). There is a large calculus within the lumen, with an irregular hyperechoic margin and causing distal acoustic shadowing. The urinary bladder wall is thickened, indicating concurrent cystitis (calipers). (*Image Courtesy of* S. Loeber, DVM, University of Wisconsin-Madison, Madison, WI.)

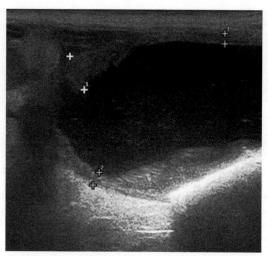

Fig. 14. Sagittal plane ultrasound images of the urinary bladder of an adult ferret (*Mustela putorius furo*). There is gravity-dependent material creating a hyperechoic interface and distal acoustic shadowing along the dorsal bladder wall. The cranioventral apical bladder wall is thickened and irregular (calipers 1) compared with the ventral and dorsal bladder wall (calipers 2 and 3), most consistent with cystitis. (*Courtesy of* M. Hallman, DVM, DACVR, Stillwater, OK.)

distention and cranial displacement of the bladder and proximal urethra, which can be identified within the abdomen sonographically. Cystic structures within the bladder and urethral wall have been reported in ferrets causing signs of dysuria.[49]

COMPUTED TOMOGRAPHY

Computed tomography (CT) is increasingly available at specialty and referral hospitals. Although the spatial resolution is slightly less than with ultrasonography or radiography, CT offers superior contrast resolution and the ability to view

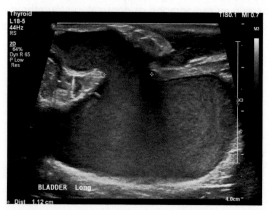

Fig. 15. Sagittal plane ultrasound image of the urinary bladder in an adult rabbit (*Oryctolagus cuniculus*). There is disruption of the ventral body wall (calipers) with herniation of a portion of the bladder into the subcutaneous tissues. Note the echogenic swirling urine content. (*Courtesy of* M. Hallman, DVM, DACVR, Stillwater, OK.)

cross-sectional slices of the patient in succession, thus removing superimposition of other tissues, namely the ingesta-filled GI tract. Machines with higher slice numbers are able to scan larger regions of tissue at 1 time, enabling studies to be performed quickly and with reduced patient motion artifact.[50] Patients may require chemical restraint, but ill or obtunded patients may be imaged with passive restraint or containment within a fiberglass container. In many exotic companion mammals, the thorax, abdomen, and skeletal structures can be imaged in 1 scan, without having to manipulate or reposition the patient, in as little as 1 minute or less.

CT can be performed before, during, and after intravenous contrast administration, in a similar fashion to radiographic EU (described previously), using the same type of contrast agents. Contrast-enhanced CT provides improved resolution of soft tissue structures and accurate assessment of the cortical, medullary, and pelvic portions of the upper urinary tract. CT with contrast also can provide structural information about the kidneys, confirm the patency of the ureters, or identify ureteral disruption (**Fig. 16**). Continuous scanning of the kidneys during and immediately after intravenous administration of an iodine-based contrast agent also can be used to generate time-attenuation curves and quantify the GFR. In cases of unilateral renal disease requiring nephrectomy, this technique may provide both detailed anatomic information for surgical planning (**Fig. 17**) as well as assessment of the amount of function the diseased kidney contributes to overall GFR.[51]

MAGNETIC RESONANCE IMAGING

Magnetic resonance imaging (MRI) provides superior soft tissue contrast and a cross-sectional assessment of anatomy without the limitation of superimposition and with no radiation exposure. Despite these advantages, MRI of the abdomen

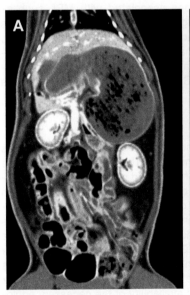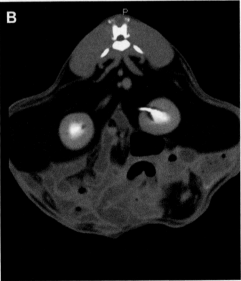

Fig. 16. CT images of the abdomen of an adult rabbit (*Oryctolagus cuniculus*) after intravenous contrast administration. (*A*) Dorsal plane image showing the cortical and inner medullary contrast enhancement of the nephrogram phase. (*B*) Transverse plane image showing the pelvic and proximal ureteral enhancement of the pyelogram phase. (*Courtesy of* M. Hallman, DVM, DACVR, Stillwater, OK.)

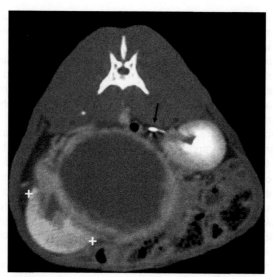

Fig. 17. Transverse plane postintravenous contrast CT image of the abdomen of an adult rabbit (*Oryctolagus cuniculus*) with a mass originating from the right kidney (calipers). The mass had characteristics of an abscess, including a non–contrast-enhancing center and a contrast-enhancing wall. *Staphylococcus aureus* was cultured. The left kidney was unaffected. Contrast is seen in the proximal left ureter (*arrow*). (*Courtesy of* M. Hallman, DVM, DACVR, Stillwater, OK.)

is infrequently performed in companion animals, often due to the relative availability of abdominal ultrasound. Additionally, limitations associated with MRI, such as cost and lack of availability, the need for a long anesthetic episode, and artifacts generated from motion of the diaphragm, all hinder the clinical use of this modality. In small patients, such as exotic companion mammals, limitations on slice thickness and image resolution also may play a part. Protocols using contrast-enhanced MRI to measure individual kidney GFR have been described in dogs and rabbits.[52,53]

NUCLEAR SCINTIGRAPHY

Nuclear scintigraphy is performed by injecting the patient with a radioisotope that is labeled for specific integration or excretion by the body. The patient is then imaged using a gamma camera, which detects regions of increased radiopharmaceutical uptake. Scintigraphic studies of the urinary system can provide dynamic information on renal function and postrenal patency.[54] The most common radioisotope used in imaging the urinary system is technetium-99m diethylenetriaminopentaacetic acid, which is filtered at the glomerulus with no tubular action and can be used to quantify GFRs. The advantage of nuclear scintigraphic evaluation of GFR over blood inulin, creatinine, or iohexol tests is that it can provide GFR information for each individual kidney as well as for the patient as a whole[55] and does not require multiple blood samples. The major disadvantages of nuclear imaging are the limited availability of the necessary equipment, the special licensing required, the increased radiation dose to the patient and handlers, and requirements for isolation. Nuclear scintigraphy is performed in rabbits in basic science research settings, but has not been commonly used in clinical practice.[56]

SUMMARY

A variety of imaging modalities are available to exotic companion mammal practitioner. Generally, techniques can be extrapolated from studies performed in cats and dogs with good success in small mammal species. The wide availability and numerous advantages of ultrasound have widely replaced the use of some modalities, such as EU in many clinical situations. CT also is becoming more readily available and provides a large amount of anatomic information very quickly. As ultrasonographic and CT studies are increasingly performed in exotic companion mammal patients, the database of information regarding the appearance of both normal and abnormal anatomy will continue to grow.

REFERENCES

1. Raidal SR, Raidal SL. Comparative renal physiology of exotic species. Vet Clin North Am Exot Anim Pract 2006;9:13–31.
2. Holz PH, Raidal SR. Comparative renal anatomy of exotic species. Vet Clin North Am Exot Anim Pract 2006;9:1–11.
3. O'Malley B. Clinical anatomy and physiology of exotic species. Edinburgh (Scotland): Elsevier Saunders; 2005.
4. Harcourt-Brown FM. Diagnosis of renal disease in rabbits. Vet Clin North Am Exot Anim Pract 2013;16:145–74.
5. Reese S, Hein J. General principles: radiography. In: Krautwald-Junghanns M, Pees M, Reese S, et al, editors. Diagnostic imaging of exotic pets. Hannover (Germany): Schlütersche; 2011. p. 144–57.
6. Balıkçı Dorotea S, Banzato T, Bellini L, et al. Kidney measures in the domestic rat: a radiographic study and a comparison to ultrasonographic reference values. J Exot Pet Med 2016;25:157–62.
7. Eshar D, Briscoe JA, Mai W. Radiographic kidney measurements in North American pet ferrets (Mustela furo). J Small Anim Pract 2013;54:15–9.
8. Dorotea SB, Banzato T, Bellini L, et al. Radiographic anatomy of dwarf rabbit abdomen with normal measurements. Bulg J Vet Med 2016;19:96–107.
9. Dimitrov R, Chaprazov T. An anatomic and contrast enhanced radiographic investigation of the rabbit kidneys, ureters, and urinary bladder. Revue de Med Vet 2012;163:469–74.
10. Banzato T, Bellini L, Contiero B, et al. Abdominal ultrasound features and reference values in 21 healthy rabbits. Vet Rec 2015;176:101.
11. Ferrari M, Carlos da Silva WA, Monteiro RV. Ultrasonographic features of the chinchilla (Chinchilla lanigera) kidney. J Exot Pet Med 2013;22:393–5.
12. Reese S. Sonoanatomy: abdomen. In: Krautwald-Junghanns M, Pees M, Reese S, et al, editors. Diagnostic imaging of exotic pets. Hannover (Germany): Schlütersche; 2011. p. 224–37.
13. Clauss M, Burger B, Liesegang A, et al. Influence of diet on calcium metabolism, tissue calcification and urinary sludge in rabbits (Oryctolagus cuniculus). J Anim Physiol Anim Nutr (Berl) 2012;96:798–807.
14. Johnson J, Brandão J, Perry S, et al. Urinary system. In: Mitchell M, Tully T, editors. Current therapy in exotic pet practice. St Louis (MO): Elsevier; 2016. p. 494–548.
15. Pollock CG. Disorders of the urinary and reproductive systems. In: Quesenberry KE, Carpenter JW, editors. Ferrets, rabbits, and rodents: clinical medicine and surgery. 3rd edition. St Louis (MO): Elsevier Saunders; 2012. p. 46–61.

16. Nwaokorie EE, Osborne CA, Lulich JP, et al. Epidemiology of struvite uroliths in ferrets: 272 cases (1981-2007). J Am Vet Med Assoc 2011;239:1319–24.

17. Vilalta L, Altuzarra R, Espada Y, et al. Description and comparison of excretory urography performed during radiography and computed tomography for evaluation of the urinary system in healthy New Zealand White rabbits (*Oryctolagus cuniculus*). Am J Vet Res 2017;78:472–81.

18. Altuzarra R, Vilalta L, Martorell J, et al. Description of digital fluoroscopic excretory urography in healthy New Zealand rabbits (Oryctolagus cuniculus). Vet Rec 2018;183:568.

19. Heuter KJ. Excretory urography. Clin Tech Small Anim Pract 2005;20:39–45.

20. Orcutt CJ. Ferret urogenital diseases. Vet Clin North Am Exot Anim Pract 2003;6: 113–38.

21. Porzio P, Pharr JW, Allen AL. Excretory urography by intraosseous injection of contrast media in a rabbit model. Vet Radiol Ultrasound 2001;42:238–43.

22. Tavana M, Peighambarzadeh S, Savojbolaghy S. Comparison between intraosseous and subcutaneous excretory urogaphy in Persian squirrels. Res Opin Anim Vet Sci 2015;5:25–9.

23. Kiss N, Hamar P. Histopathological evaluation of contrast-induced acute kidney injury rodent models. Biomed Res Int 2016;2016:15.

24. Schultz SG, Lavelle KJ, Swain R. Nephrotoxicity of radiocontrast media in ischemic renal failure in rabbits. Nephron 1982;32:113–7.

25. Kirberger RM, Cassel N, Carstens A, et al. The effects of repeated intravenous iohexol administration on renal function in healthy beagles–a preliminary report. Acta Vet Scand 2012;54:47.

26. MacNab TA, Newcomb BT, Ketz-Riley C, et al. Extramural ectopic ureter in a domestic ferret (*Mustela putorius furo*). J Exot Pet Med 2010;19:313–6.

27. Vilalta L, Dominguez E, Altuzarra R, et al. Imaging diagnosis- radiography and ultrasonography of bilateral congenital ureterovesical junction stenosis causing hydronephrosis and hydroureter in a ferret *(Mustela putorius furo)*. Vet Radiol Ultrasound 2017;58:E31–6.

28. Dimitrov R, Stamatova-Yovcheva K. Imaging anatomical radiological investigation of rabbit urinary bladder and pelvic urethra. Anim Health Prod Hyg 2015;4: 387–92.

29. Grunkemeyer VL, Sura PA, Baron ML, et al. Surgical repair of an inguinal herniation of the urinary bladder in an intact female domestic rabbit *(Oryctolagus cuniculus)*. J Exot Pet Med 2010;19:249–54.

30. Petritz OA, Guzman DS-M, Gandolfi RC, et al. Inguinal-scrotal urinary bladder hernia in an intact male domestic rabbit (*Oryctolagus cuniculus*). J Exot Pet Med 2012;21:248–54.

31. Thas I, Harcourt-Brown FM. Six cases of inguinal urinary bladder herniation in entire male domestic rabbits. J Small Anim Pract 2013;54:662–6.

32. da Silva KG, de Andrade C, Sotomaior CS. Influence of simethicone and fasting on the quality of abdominal ultrasonography in New Zealand White rabbits. Acta Vet Scand 2017;59:48.

33. Reese S, Hein J. Abdomen. In: Krautwald-Junghanns M, Pees M, Reese S, et al, editors. Diagnostic imaging of exotic pets. Hannover (Germany): Schlütersche; 2011. p. 280–97.

34. Suran JN, Wyre NR. Imaging findings in 14 domestic ferrets (*Mustela putorius furo)* with lymphoma. Vet Radiol Ultrasound 2013;54:522–31.

35. Jackson CN, Rogers AB, Maurer KJ, et al. Cystic renal disease in the domestic ferret. Comp Med 2008;58:161–7.

36. Puerto DA, Walker LM, Saunders HM. Bilateral perinephric pseudocysts and polycystic kidneys in a ferret. Vet Radiol Ultrasound 1998;39:309–12.

37. Sailler A, Risi E, Magrans J, et al. Surgical management of a pararenal pseudo-cyst in a ferret (*Mustela putorius furo*). J Exot Pet Med 2019;30:60–4.

38. Duhamelle A, Tessier E, Larrat S. Ureteral stenosis following ovariohysterectomy in a rabbit *(Oryctolagus cuniculus)*. J Exot Pet Med 2017;26:132–6.

39. Rose JB, Vergneau-Grosset C, Steffey MA, et al. Adrenalectomy and ne-phrectomy in a rabbit *(Oryctolagus cuniculus)* with adrenocortical carcinoma and renal and ureteral transitional cell carcinoma. J Exot Pet Med 2016;25: 332–41.

40. Tahas SA, Pope J, Denk D, et al. Diagnostic challenges and surgical treatment of hydroureteronephrosis in a rabbit *(Oryctolagus cuniculus)*. Vet Rec Case Rep 2017;5:e000379.

41. Liu DJX, Hesta M, Stock E, et al. Renal perfusion parameters measured by contrast-enhanced ultrasound in healthy dogs demonstrate a wide range of vari-ability in the long-term. Vet Radiol Ultrasound 2019;60:201–9.

42. Pollard R, Nyland T, Berry C, et al. Advanced ultrasound techniques. In: Mattoon J, Nyland T, editors. Small animal diagnostic ultrasound. 3rd edition. St Louis (MO): Saunders Elsevier; 2015. p. 78–93.

43. Stock E, Vanderperren K, Moeremans I, et al. Use of contrast-enhanced ultraso-nography in the diagnosis of a liver lobe torsion in a rabbit (*Oryctolagus cunicu-lus*). Vet Radiol Ultrasound 2019;1–5. https://doi.org/10.1111/vru.12709.

44. Gaschen L, Ketz C, Lang J, et al. Ultrasonographic detection of adrenal gland tumor and ureterolithiasis in a guinea pig. Vet Radiol Ultrasound 1998;39:43–6.

45. Stieger SM, Wenker C, Ziegler-Gohm D, et al. Ureterolithiasis and papilloma for-mation in the ureter of a guinea pig. Vet Radiol Ultrasound 2003;44:326–9.

46. Cojean O, Combes A, Maitre P, et al. Surgical treatment of congenital vesi-courachal diverticulum associated with ureteral and vesical calcium oxalate urolithiasis in a domestic ferret *(Mustela putorius furo)*. J Exot Pet Med 2019;29:22–6.

47. Cikanek SJ, Eshar D, Nau M, et al. Diagnosis and surgical treatment of a transi-tional cell carcinoma in the bladder apex of a pet rabbit *(Oryctolagus cuniculus)*. J Exot Pet Med 2018;27:113–7.

48. Trahan C, Mitchell W. Spontaneous transitional cell carcinoma in the urinary bladder of a strain 13 guinea pig. Lab Anim Sci 1986;36:691–3.

49. Li X, Fox JG, Erdman SE, et al. Cystic urogenital anomalies in ferrets *(Mustela pu-torius furo)*. Vet Pathol 1996;33:150–8.

50. Mackey EB, Hernandez-Divers SJ, Holland M, et al. Clinical technique: applica-tion of computed tomography in zoological medicine. J Exot Pet Med 2008;17: 198–209.

51. Zoller G, Langlois I, Alexander K. Glomerular filtration rate determination by computed tomography in two pet rabbits with renal disease. J Am Vet Med Assoc 2017;250:681–7.

52. Mehl JN, Lupke M, Brenner AC, et al. Measurement of single kidney glomerular filtration rate in dogs using dynamic contrast-enhanced magnetic resonance im-aging and the Rutland-Patlak plot technique. Acta Vet Scand 2018;60:72.

53. Annet L, Hermoye L, Peeters F, et al. Glomerular filtration rate: assessment with dynamic contrast-enhanced MRI and a cortical-compartment model in the rabbit kidney. J Magn Reson Imaging 2004;20:843–9.

54. Tyson R, Daniel GB. Renal scintigraphy in veterinary medicine. Semin Nucl Med 2014;44:35–46.
55. Kerl ME, Cook CR. Glomerular filtration rate and renal scintigraphy. Clin Tech Small Anim Pract 2005;20:31–8.
56. Jabarian V, Assadnassab G, Oskoi SD, et al. Measurement of rabbit's glomerular filtration rate (GFR) by scintigraphy. Euro J Exp Bio 2012;2:1545–9.

Amphibian Renal Disease

Christine Parker-Graham, DVM, MA[a],
Leigh A. Clayton, DVM, DAVBP (Avian), DAVBP (Reptile and Amphibian)[b],
Lisa M. Mangus, DVM, PhD, DACVP[c],*

KEYWORDS

- Amphibian • Kidney • Renal • Physiology • Pathology • Therapy
- Infectious disease • Neoplasia

KEY POINTS

- Reflective of their impressive taxonomic diversity and range of habitats, the amphibians have evolved an array of physiologic adaptations to maintain fluid homeostasis.
- Abnormal fluid accumulation in the form of hydrocoelom and/or subcutaneous edema is a common presenting sign in amphibians with renal disease.
- Bacterial and fungal infections of the amphibian renal system are usually part of a disseminated, multiorgan process, and often occur secondary to skin lesions.
- Noninfectious causes of renal disease in amphibians are mostly husbandry related. Etiologic diagnosis requires careful analysis of dietary factors and environmental conditions.
- Definitive antemortem diagnosis of renal disease in amphibians is challenging. Treatment is empirical and aimed at addressing possible underlying infection, reducing fluid accumulation, and optimizing husbandry practices.

INTRODUCTION

The amphibians are an extremely diverse, globally distributed class of vertebrates comprising more than 7000 species of anurans (frogs and toads), caudates (salamanders and newts), and caecilians with life styles ranging from fully aquatic to entirely terrestrial. In all amphibians, the urinary system functions in delicate balance with the skin to maintain fluid and electrolyte homeostasis. Given the importance of the kidneys to these vital processes, it is not surprising that renal disease frequently leads to morbidity and mortality in amphibian species. This article reviews clinically and diagnostically relevant aspects of amphibian renal anatomy and physiology, provides recommendations for diagnostic and therapeutic options, and discusses potential etiologies of renal disease in amphibian patients.

Disclosure Statement: The authors have no disclosures.
[a] US Fish and Wildlife Service, 510 Desmond Drive SE, Lacey, WA 98503, USA; [b] Animal Care, New England Aquarium, 1 Central Wharf, Boston, MA 02110, USA; [c] Department of Molecular and Comparative Pathobiology, Johns Hopkins University, 733 North Broadway, Suite 811, Baltimore, MD 21205, USA
* Corresponding author.
E-mail address: lmangus1@jhmi.edu

Table 1	
Key clinical history topics for amphibians with suspect renal disease	
Clinical History Topic	**Implications for Renal Health and Disease**
Enclosure (construction, recent changes to the system, temperature and humidity gradients, substrate types)	Nephrotoxic substances, including heavy metals and components of poly vinyl chloride glue, can leach into water from housing components and plumbing Enclosures should include microenvironments that provide variable temperature and moisture levels to promote optimal hydration Abrasive substrates can damage amphibians' skin and predispose animals to systemic bacterial and fungal infections that affect the kidneys
Water source and quality	Exposure to hypoosmotic water (eg, distilled water without additional electrolytes) can stress physiologic mechanisms that maintain fluid homeostasis and contribute to edema Water quality parameters (eg, pH, temperature, hardness) may influence toxicity of contaminants and cutaneous absorption of electrolytes
Diet (including supplements, gut-loading of prey, potentially edible plants in enclosure)	Hypovitaminosis A has been associated with squamous metaplasia of the renal tubules and lower urinary tract in toads[9] Ingestion of oxalate-rich plants has been associated with oxalate nephropathy in tadpoles and frogs High protein diet may contribute to cystic calculi formation in uricotelic species
Origin of animals in enclosure (affected and unaffected)	Viral and parasitic infections of the renal system are more likely in animals obtained from the wild New animals may introduce infectious diseases to an established system
Types of species in enclosure	Territorial species may guard water sources within a habitat, preventing other animals from accessing it

Physical Examination and Clinical Signs

Before handling the animal, the examiner should observe the patient in its enclosure, evaluating their use of vertical space, ambulation, posture, and mentation. Handling of ill amphibians should be kept to a minimum to decrease stress and the examiner should wear powder-free examination gloves rinsed with dechlorinated water. An accurate body weight is an important part of the examination, keeping in mind that body weight can vary widely based on hydration and feeding status.

Edema is a common clinical sign in amphibians with renal disease and can present as excess fluid in the coelomic cavity (hydrocoelom) and/or subcutaneous space. In anurans, fluid also accumulates in the subcutaneous lymph sacs, a condition often referred to as lymphedema (**Fig. 2**).[9] The differential diagnosis list for amphibians presenting with edema is lengthy and also includes a range of infectious and noninfectious conditions affecting the skin, cardiovascular system (including the subcutaneous lymph hearts), liver, and gastrointestinal tract, as

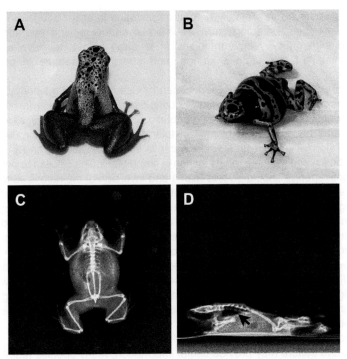

Fig. 2. Clinical edema in dendrobatid frogs. (*A*) Subcutaneous edema in the hindlimbs of a blue poison dart frog (*Dendrobates azureus*). (*B*) A yellow banded poison dart frog (*D leucomelas*) with severe hydrocoelom. (*C*) A ventrodorsal radiograph of a dyeing poison dart frog (*D tinctoris*) with severe hydrocoelom and subcutaneous edema of the limbs. (*D*) Lateral view showing compression the lung fields (*black arrow*) by coelomic fluid.

well as exposure to low-solute water. In cases of renal insufficiency, fluid accumulation results from decreased plasma oncotic pressure secondary to glomerular protein loss and/or decreased electrolyte reabsorption in the tubules. Severe edema can cause increased respiratory rate and effort, lethargy, and mobility deficits. Despite an increase in weight owing to edema, amphibians with renal disease may be in poor body condition or show signs of muscle wasting. Other clinical signs of renal disease in amphibians include lethargy, decreased appetite, and either increased or decreased urine output.

Laboratory Evaluation

Blood sampling can be difficult in many amphibians owing to their small size. In anurans of sufficient size, the ventral midline vein, femoral vein, and sublingual vein may be used for sampling; in salamanders, the ventral tail vein may be used. Cardiocentesis is a last resort option for venipuncture because this technique has been associated with cardiac arrest in amphibians.[14] Lithium heparin is the preferred anticoagulant for amphibian species because it does not result in hemolysis.[15] As in reptiles, it is estimated that up to 1% of total body weight may be collected as a blood sample in healthy amphibians. This volume is likely smaller for compromised animals.[16]

There is a paucity of published reference intervals for amphibian species. Moreover, wide variation in complete blood count and biochemistry values have been observed in clinically normal amphibians in association with seasonal changes, sex, age, breeding status, nutritional condition, and hydration. When presented with critically ill amphibians, it is often helpful to have a clinically normal animal of the same sex, age, and species to sample in parallel for comparison.

Levels of nitrogenous waste products can be used to evaluate kidney function in amphibians; however, it is important to consider species variation in nitrogenous waste production among species (ammonotelic, ureotelic, or uricotelic), as well as hydration status because amphibians can tolerate wide variation in circulating urea levels and normally retain urea when water is scarce.[10] Calcium and phosphorus may also be used to evaluate renal function in amphibians. The calcium to phosphorus ratio in most species should be less than 1 and inversion of the ratio is suggestive of hypocalcemia, renal disease, or both.[16] Total protein measurements can be helpful in identifying hypoproteinemia; however, total protein obtained by refractometry may be overestimated in amphibians because of other solids present in the blood stream, such as triglycerides and cholesterols. The biuret method used by most commercial diagnostic laboratories is a reliable method of measuring total proteins in amphibians.[10] Decreased total proteins may indicate renal disease, inappropriate diet, hepatic disease, or gastrointestinal disease. Leukocytosis, when coupled with other clinical signs of renal disease, may indicate an infectious process affecting the kidneys. Animals with leukocytosis benefit from prompt treatment with wide-spectrum antimicrobials.

For those species from which a urine sample is obtained, fluid analysis, cytology, and culture may provide useful information. Many species readily urinate when handled and the examiner should have a sterile cup or syringe available to collect urine; otherwise, amphibian patients may be encouraged to urinate by stimulating the cloaca with a moistened cotton-tipped applicator. Cellular content, presence of bacteria or fungal elements, and/or evidence of renal casts can indicate kidney disease. Because amphibians cannot concentrate urine, urine specific gravity is an indicator of plasma osmolality rather than the concentrating ability of the kidney.

Celiocentesis and lymphatic draining can be both diagnostic and therapeutic in animals with edema. Collected fluid should be submitted for fluid analysis, cytology, and bacterial and fungal culture. Fluid culture may help in ruling out bacterial infection and septicemia as a potential cause for edema. Fluid samples with low protein and low cell counts are more likely to be associated with organ failure.[9]

Diagnostic Imaging

Full-body radiographs are a helpful part of the complete workup for ill amphibians and may be useful in detecting radiodense renal or cystic calculi, mineralization of the kidneys or other soft tissue, and masses occupying the caudal coelom. Mammography and dental units are optimal for smaller amphibians, but traditional radiography units may be used, keeping in mind that fine detail will often be lost. Ultrasound examination is helpful to evaluate the kidneys, check for renal calculi, and evaluate the coelomic fluid pool.

Laparoscopy can be helpful to visualize kidneys, but is difficult in many amphibians because of their small size. A paramedian incision is preferred for laparoscopy of the kidneys. Biopsies can be collected from the kidney at that time, as well as fungal and bacterial cultures. Closure of the incision in 2 layers is advised.[17]

CLINICAL MANAGEMENT
Medications

Because of the inherent difficulty in obtaining a definitive antemortem diagnosis of renal disease in amphibians, clinical management is often empirical. Antimicrobials should be used when bacterial kidney infection is suspected. Very few pharmacokinetics studies have been conducted in amphibians, but formularies should be consulted when available. Enrofloxacin is often favored because of its broad antimicrobial spectrum and known tolerance among amphibians (**Table 2**). In a retrospective study of dendrobatid frogs housed at the National Aquarium in Baltimore, Maryland, Clancy[21] and colleagues demonstrated increased positive outcomes in edematous frogs treated with enrofloxacin versus those that did not receive enrofloxacin. At the National Aquarium, enrofloxacin is dosed at 10 to 20 mg/kg by mouth every 24 hours for at least 10 days. Micropipettes are useful for accurately dosing small amphibians. Aminoglycoside antibiotics should be avoided in amphibian patients with suspected renal disease owing to potential nephrotoxicity.

Furosemide (2–5 mg/kg by mouth every 24–48 hours) may be used to help decrease fluid accumulation in the coelom and lymph sacs in amphibians with edema.[21] In mammals, furosemide causes diuresis by decreasing ion absorption in the ascending thick loop of Henle. The mechanism of action in amphibians is unclear, but the drug may target specific ion channels in the collecting tubules.[22] Steps should be taken to ensure that amphibians treated with furosemide do not become dehydrated (ie, have appropriate soaking solutions readily available).

Allopurinol is commonly used in birds and reptiles with renal disease to decrease the production of uric acid. In ammonotelic and ureotelic amphibians, allopurinol is of little application because these species do not produce uric acid as their end nitrogenous waste product. Uricotelic species may benefit from allopurinol (10 mg/kg by mouth every 24 hours) if hyperuricemia is demonstrated or suspected.[16]

Supportive Care

During the convalescent period, careful attention should be paid to body weight and body condition of amphibian patients, because weight can fluctuate markedly with hydration and accumulation of edema fluid. Celiocentesis may be performed in amphibians with edema to decrease compression of the lungs and viscera. Fluid may also be evacuated by soaking amphibian patients in a mildly hypertonic solution, like amphibian Ringer's or 0.4% to 1.0% salt solution.[14] If these fluids are not available, one can use 1 part 0.9% saline with 2 parts 5% dextrose, 9 parts 0.9%

Table 2 Pharmacokinetic studies of enrofloxacin in amphibians			
Species	**Dose**	**Route**	**Results**
African clawed frogs (*Xenopus laevis*)	10 mg/kg	IM and SQ	Therapeutic plasma concentration maintained for $\geq$8 h
Coqui frogs (*Eleutherodactylus coqui*)	10 mg/kg	TO	Therapeutic plasma concentration maintained for $\geq$24 h
Houston toads (*Anaxyrus houstonensis*)	5 mg/L 10 mg/kg	TO and PO	Therapeutic concentrations in liver for 10 h (TO) and 24 h (PO); no adverse effects after 12 d of daily dosing

Abbreviations: IM, intramuscular; PO, oral; SQ, subcutaneous; TO, topical.
Data from Refs.[18–20]

saline to 1 part sterile water, or 4 parts lactated Ringer's solution to 1 part 5% dextrose.[14] The metabolic rate of a sick amphibian is significantly higher than that of a well conspecific; therefore, food intake and nutrition are paramount to recovery.[23] Hadfield and Whitaker[14] engage in a detailed discussion of amphibian critical nutrition.

DISEASES OF THE AMPHIBIAN RENAL SYSTEM
Viruses

Iridoviruses in the genus ranavirus cause systemic infection and significant morbidity and mortality in free-ranging populations of amphibians. Well-documented examples include tadpole edema virus, which affects premetamorphic frogs and toads; frog virus 3, which affects a wide range of anuran species; and *Ambystoma tigrinum* virus, which predominantly affects tiger salamanders. Ranavirus infections are less frequently reported in amphibians under human care, but may be underdiagnosed because secondary bacterial and fungal infections are common and, if severe, can mask underlying viral disease.[24] Similar to other visceral organs and the skin, lesions of ranavirus infection in the kidneys include hemorrhage and necrosis, particularly of the renal hematopoietic tissue.[25] Basophilic cytoplasmic inclusions bodies may also be observed, but are not a consistent finding in all species. Definitive diagnosis often requires ancillary diagnostics, such as *in situ* hybridization or polymerase chain reaction on postmortem tissue samples. Polymerase chain reaction can also be performed on premortem samples (cloacal and oral swabs) if there is a clinical suspicion of ranavirus, although this may be relatively insensitive for detecting early infections in amphibians.[25]

Lucke's renal adenocarcinoma of northern leopard frogs (*Rana pipiens*) is perhaps the most notorious virus-associated renal disease of amphibians, although it is unlikely to be encountered clinically. This neoplasm is caused by the oncogenic ranid herpesvirus 1 and exhibits a temperature-dependent cycle. Viral replication is greatest under cool, winter temperatures, whereas neoplastic proliferation occurs mainly occurs during warmer months when viral replication is greatly reduced.[26]

Bacteria

Bacterial infection of the amphibian renal system typically occurs in the context of generalized bacteremia. The majority of systemic bacterial infections in amphibians occur secondary to skin lesions and are caused by gram-negative organisms such as *Aeromonas hydrophila*, *Pseudomonas* spp., and various enterobacteria (eg, *Salmonella* and *Proteus* spp.) that are commonly found in aquatic environments.[9,16,27] Although a diagnosis of septicemia is difficult to confirm postmortem without corroborating culture results, findings such as intravascular bacterial colonies and glomerular necrosis with fibrin thrombi can be highly suggestive. Ascending bacterial infections of the urinary bladder, ureters, and renal tubules also occur in amphibians.[9]

Mycobacterial infections are common in amphibians and can result in localized or widespread inflammation affecting multiple organs, including the kidneys. Many species of nontuberculous environmental mycobacteria, including *Mycobacterium marinum*, *M chelonei*, and *M liflandii*, have been isolated from amphibians.[28] Clinical disease tends to occur in animals that are immunocompromised owing to other illness, stress, or suboptimal husbandry practices.[29] Discrete, nodular granulomas are the classic gross and histologic lesion associated with mycobacteriosis. However, depending on the chronicity of infection and numerous host and virulence factors that influence the immune response, mycobacterial infection in amphibians can also result in highly necrotizing inflammation (**Fig. 3**) or dense infiltrates of relatively small, uniform macrophages that resemble round cell neoplasia. Because of this variability, an acid-fast stain should be routine practice for any inflammatory lesion in an amphibian patient, both premortem and postmortem.

Intracellular organisms in the family *Chlamydiaceae* are increasingly recognized as emerging pathogens of amphibians. Most recent reports of chlamydiosis in amphibians have identified *Chlamydophila pneumoniae*, notable for its zoonotic potential, as the causative agent.[30,31] A novel species of *Chlamydiacea* has also been isolated from salamanders.[32] Histologically, nonsuppurative inflammation has been observed in multiple organs, including the kidneys. Granular clusters of intracellular bacteria may be seen in infiltrating macrophages and are best visualized using a Gimenez stain. Polymerase chain reaction testing is also available.

Fungi

Similar to bacterial infections, fungal infections of the amphibian renal system typically occur as part of a disseminated process and are frequently preceded by ulcerative or traumatic skin lesions. Amphibians are susceptible to infection by a wide range of filamentous, saprophytic fungi including *Fusarium* spp., *Mucor* spp., *Rhizopus* spp., and *Basidiobolus ranarum*.[33,34] There are also reports of disseminated mycoses in amphibians involving pigmented fungi (eg, *Exophiala* and *Cladosporium* spp), which can appear as round, segmented sclerotic bodies or as invasive hyphae in tissue sections (**Fig. 4**).[33] Granulomas are commonly seen grossly and microscopically in the organs of amphibians with chronic fungal disease; however, as seen in **Fig. 4**, associated inflammation can be also be mixed and necrotizing in the more acute stages of infection.

Parasites

Amphibians serve as intermediate and definitive hosts for a number of trematode species. Although encysted metacercaria are often encountered as incidental findings in the viscera of free-ranging animals, heavy parasitic burdens and those inciting robust inflammatory responses can significantly impact renal function.[34,35] Adult flukes of genera *Gorgodera*, *Gorgoderina*, and *Phyllodistomum* can be found in the urinary bladder and ureters. Infections tend to be subclinical unless burdens are heavy enough to cause urinary obstruction.

Oligochaete worms of genus *Dero* have been observed colonizing the cloaca, urinary bladder, and ureters of various anurans. These coelomate worms are members of phylum Annelida (ie, segmented worms with true coeloms). The life cycle of

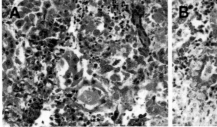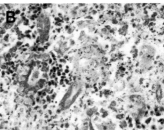

Fig. 3. Renal mycobacteriosis in an African clawed frog (*Xenopus laevis*). (*A*) Hematoxylin and eosin (400×) stain showing disruption of tubules and abundant necrotic cellular debris. (*B*) Numerous acid-fast bacilli can be seen on Ziehl-Neelsen staining (400×).

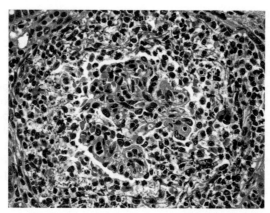

Fig. 4. Pigmented fungal infection in the kidney of a common mudpuppy (*Necturus maculosus*). Light brown fungal hyphae surround and invade a glomerulus. Fugal culture of coelomic fluid from this animal yielded *Exophiala* spp. Hematoxylin and eosin (200×) staining.

oligochaete worms involves a free-living stage within an aquatic microenvironment, such as a bromeliad plant, and there seems to be variation among subgenera as to whether they have a commensal or endoparasitic relationship with anurans, or if frogs and toads merely transfer worms from one location to the next.[36,37] Although oligocheates are typically incidental findings, large burdens of worms may lead to obstruction or rupture of the ureters.[34,36]

The myxozoa are a diverse group of microscopic metazoan parasites that have also been reported to cause illness, including renal disease, in amphibians. A myxozoan in genus *Chloromyxum* was identified in the kidneys of several wild-caught Asian horned frogs (*Megaphrys nasuta*) that died soon after import to the United States.[38] Associated lesions included renal tubular dilation, necrosis, and nonsuppurative interstitial nephritis. A novel species of myxozoan, named *Hoferellus anurae*, was identified in the urinary tracts of wild-caught frogs from multiple sites in Africa.[39] Similar to *Hoferellus* species that infect fish, *H anurae* was often associated with gross enlargement of the kidneys and multiple fluid-filled cysts. Other myxozoa, such as those in the genera *Sphaerospora,* are occasionally found in the renal tubules of free-ranging ranids and caudates with mild or no associated pathologic changes (**Fig. 5**).[40]

Neoplasia

Aside from Lucke's renal adenocarcinomas of northern leopard fogs, reports of neoplasia affecting the amphibian urinary system are uncommon. Spontaneous renal carcinomas have been described in anuran and caudate species, including African clawed frogs, an ornate horned frog (*Cyratophrys ornata*),[16] a mountain yellow-legged frog (*Rana muscosa*),[34] and a common mudpuppy (*Necturus maculosus*),[41] as well as a single caecilian (a rubber eel, *Typhlonectes natans*).[42] High rates of renal cell carcinomas have been reported in laboratory-raised Japanese and Chinese toad hybrids (*Bufo japonicus* and *B raddei*), which have been proposed as a model of renal carcinogenesis.[43] Nephroblastomas arising from embryonic mesonephric tissue have been reported in African clawed frogs,[44] fire-bellied newts (*Cynpos pyrrhogaster*),[45] and a Japanese giant salamander (*Andrias japonicus*).[46] Despite being an uncommon finding in routine practice, renal tumors should be considered as differential diagnoses for caudal coelomic masses in amphibians.

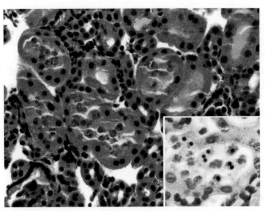

Fig. 5. Myxozoan parasites in the kidney of a green frog *(Rana clamitans)*. Several plasmodia containing developing spores are present in the renal tubules. Affected tubules are mildly dilated and epithelial cells contain eosinophilic hyaline droplets, suggestive of protein resorption. Hematoxylin and eosin (400×). Inset: On Gram stain (400×), 2 round polar capsules can be seen in mature spores, consistent with the genus *Sphaerospora*.

Nutritional and Metabolic Diseases

Renal disease associated with oxalate crystal deposition has been reported in free-ranging American bullfrog tadpoles *(Lithobates catesbeianus)*, likely secondary to ingestion of oxalate-rich plants in the environment, as well as recently metaphor-mosed wood frogs *(Lithobates sylvaticus)* that were fed boiled spinach during tadpole development.[47,48] Oxalate nephropathy has also been observed in captive waxy monkey frogs that were housed in an enclosure containing the oxalate-producing plant silver queen *(Aglaonema roebelinii)*.[49] It was suspected that crickets fed to the frogs were eating the plants before being eaten themselves. In the authors' experience, low numbers of oxalate-like crystals have occasionally been seen in the renal tubules of amphibians with otherwise normal kidneys, as well as anurans with end-stage kidney disease. The role of crystal accumulation in the latter scenario is uncertain because it could be secondary to already decreased renal function (**Fig. 6**).

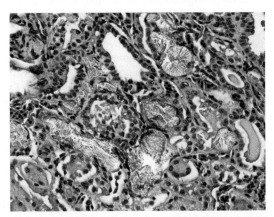

Fig. 6. Radially arranged oxalate-like crystals in the renal tubules of an American bullfrog *(Lithobates catesbeianus)* with chronic renal disease. Hematoxylin and eosin (200×) staining.

Cystic calculi have been found in some uricotelic tree frog species, including waxy monkey tree frogs (*Phyllomedusa sauvagii*).[50,51] Urolithiasis in these cases was likely due to a combination of uricotelism, a high-protein diet, dehydration, and temperature fluctuations that supported urate crystal formation. Neither renal nor systemic gout have been reported in amphibian species to date. There is a single description of localized articular gout in the digit of an American bullfrog, but the renal histology was not reported.[51]

Hypovitaminosis A has been linked to a disorder known as short tongue syndrome in captive toads.[52] In affected animals, squamous metaplasia of the epithelium and mucous glands of the tongue makes it difficult to apprehend food, leading to wasting and lethargy. Squamous metaplasia was also observed in the cloaca, urinary bladder, and renal tubules in some animals.[9,52]

Congenital and Developmental Syndromes

Multiple naturally occurring mutations in Mexican axolotls lead to a syndrome known as short toes. This phenotype is characterized by variably shortened limbs, impaired limb regeneration, and abnormal development of the urogenital tract.[53] In addition to malformed limbs, severely affected animals develop hydrocoelom and edema owing to renal insufficiency. The kidneys are grossly small and show histologic changes resembling renal dysplasia in other species.[54]

In a large zoo-managed population of Panamanian golden frogs (*Atelopus zeteki*), 8 of 9 animals affected by polycystic nephropathy died between 1 and 2 years of age and were from the same clutch, suggestive of an inherited trait or predisposition. Lesions were characterized by marked dilation of renal tubules with or without interstitial inflammation and fibrosis.[55] Polycystic nephropathy was also reported as a common cause of mortality among anurans in an *ex situ* survival assurance colony in Panama. However, in these cases the syndrome was thought to be water quality or husbandry related.[52]

Toxic Substances

Both free-ranging amphibians and those under human care are susceptible to the toxic effects of a wide range of environmental contaminants. Potentially nephrotoxic substances include heavy metals (eg, copper, cadmium, lead, zinc) that can leach into water from housing components and plumbing.[56,57] Volatile compounds in glue used for poly vinyl chloride piping can also cause toxicity and subsequent renal failure in amphibians if the glue is not fully cured or if the system is not adequately flushed before introduction of animals.[16,58] Although histologic findings such as renal tubular degeneration and/or necrosis can be suggestive of toxicity, definitive diagnosis requires a thorough historical review of husbandry conditions and potential routes of exposure, as well as measurement of toxin concentrations and water quality parameters that can influence toxicity (eg, pH, temperature, hardness). Frozen tissue samples from liver, kidney, and muscle should also be collected for analysis in cases where toxicity is suspected.

Chronic Renal Disease

Despite a multitude of potential causes of renal disease in amphibians, kidney lesions seen in amphibians submitted for necropsy are often chronic and of indeterminate etiology.[9] As in mammals, long-standing renal dysfunction in amphibians eventually culminates in widespread damage to all portions of the nephron. Such end-stage kidneys are commonly found in animals that have been clinically managed for chronic or recurrent edema. Grossly, the kidneys of amphibians with chronic renal disease are often

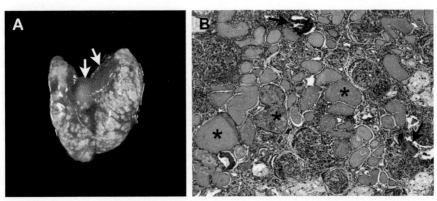

Fig. 7. Severe chronic renal disease of indeterminate etiology in a Panamanian golden frog (*Atelopus zeteki*). (*A*) Grossly, the kidneys have multifocal to coalescing areas of white discoloration. Paired, light tan structures present on the craniomedial aspects of the kidneys are the testes and adjacent Bidder's organs (*white arrows*). (*B*) Histologically, tubules are markedly dilated and contain brightly eosinophilic proteinaceous material mixed with necrotic cellular debris (*asterisks*). Glomeruli are hypercellular with synechiae formation and periglomerular fibrosis. There is also scattered mineralization (*black arrows*). Hematoxylin and eosin (100×) staining.

irregular or nodular with areas of white discoloration on the surface (**Fig. 7**A). Typical histologic changes include dilation, atrophy, and loss of renal tubules, intraluminal cellular or protein casts, glomerulosclerosis, chronic interstitial nephritis, and fibrosis (**Fig. 7**B). Cystically dilated tubules and foci of mineralization are also common.

SUMMARY

Based on the authors' experience and literature review, abnormal fluid accumulation is one of the most common presenting signs of renal insufficiency in both terrestrial and aquatic amphibians. Clinicians should keep in mind that environmental factors can contribute to renal insufficiency, or simply overload normal physiologic mechanism for maintaining fluid homeostasis, and the environment should always be reviewed and optimized as part of management. Simple medical diagnostics, such as physical examination, fluid evaluation, and cytology, can provide helpful information to guide management of individual cases. Management options, including husbandry changes and medications, can be successful in resolving abnormal fluid accumulation and it seems that amphibians, similar to other vertebrates, can have a good quality of life when suspected kidney insufficiency is present. As with other animals, clinicians should work with caregivers to understand goals of case management and quality of life factors to help guide medical choices if fluid accumulation or other clinical signs are ongoing.

REFERENCES

1. Wright KM. Anatomy for the clinician. In: Wright KM, Whitaker BR, editors. Amphibian medicine and captive husbandry. Malabar (FL): Krieger; 2001. p. 15–30.
2. Holz PH, Raidal SR. Comparative renal anatomy of exotic species. Vet Clin North Am Exot Anim Pract 2006;9:1–11.

3. Martin JA, Hillman SS. The physical movement of urine from the kidneys to the urinary bladder and bladder compliance in two anurans. Physiol Biochem Zool 2009;82:163–9.

4. Sakai T, Kawahara K. The structure of the kidney of Japanese newts, *Triturus (Cynops) pyrrhogaster*. Anat Embryol 1983;166:31–52.

5. Uchiyama M, Murakami T, Wakasugi C, et al. Structure of the kidney in the crab-eating frog, *Rana cancrivora*. J Morphol 1990;204:147–56.

6. Møbjerg N, Jespersen Å, Wilkinson M. Morphology of the kidney in the West African caecilian, *Geotrypetes seraphini* (Amphibia, Gymnophiona, Caeciliidae). J Morphol 2004;262:583–607.

7. Siegel DS, Sever DM, Aldridge RD. The pelvic kidney of male *Ambystoma maculatum* (Amphibia, urodela, ambystomatidae) with special reference to the sexual collecting ducts. J Morphol 2010;271:1422–39.

8. Morris JL. Structure and function of ciliated peritoneal funnels in the toad kidney (*Bufo marinus*). Cell Tissue Res 1981;217:599–610.

9. Pessier AP. Edematous frogs, urinary tract disease, and disorders of fluid balance in amphibians. J Exot Pet Med 2009;18:4–13.

10. Forzán MJ, Heatley J, Russell KE, et al. Clinical pathology of amphibians: a review. Vet Clin Pathol 2017;46:11–33.

11. Wright KM. Applied physiology. In: Wright KM, Whitaker BR, editors. Amphibian medicine and captive husbandry. Malabar (FL): Krieger; 2001. p. 31–4.

12. Jørgensen CB. Urea and amphibian water economy. Comp Biochem Physiol A Physiol 1997;117:161–70.

13. Shoemaker VH. Exchange of water, ions, and respiratory gases in terrestrial amphibians. In: Feder ME, Burggren WW, editors. Environmental physiology of the amphibians. Chicago: The University of Chicago Press; 1992. p. 125–50.

14. Hadfield CA, Whitaker BR. Amphibian emergency medicine and care. Sem Avian Exot Pet Med 2005;14:79–89.

15. Wright KM. Clinical techniques. In: Wright KM, Whitaker BR, editors. Amphibian medicine and captive husbandry. Malabar (FL): Krieger; 2001. p. 89–110.

16. Cecil TR. Amphibian renal disease. Vet Clin North Am Exot Anim Pract 2006;9:175–88.

17. Gentz EJ. Medicine and surgery of amphibians. ILAR J 2007;48:255–9.

18. Howard A, Papich M, Felt S, et al. The pharmacokinetics of enrofloxacin in adult African clawed frog (*Xenopus laevis*). J Am Assoc Lab Anim Sci 2010;18:800–4.

19. Valitutto M, Raphael B, Calle P, et al. Tissue concentrations of enrofloxacin and its metabolite ciprofloxacin after a single topical dose in the Coqui frog (*Eleuthrodactylus coqui*). J Herpetol Med Surg 2013;23:69–73.

20. Howard L, Crump P, Papich M. Tissue concentrations of enrofloxacin and ciprofloxacin after oral and topical treatment in Houston toads (Anaxyurus [Bufo] houstonensis). Proceedings of the Annual Conference of the American Association of Zoo Veterinarians. Salt Lake City (UT), September 28 – October 4, 2013. p. 95.

21. Clancy MM, Clayton LA, Hadfield CA. Hydrocoelom and lymphedema in dendrobatid frogs at the National Aquarium, Baltimore: 2003-2011. J Zoo Wildl Med 2015;46:18–26.

22. Møbjerg N, Larsen E, Novak I. K(+) transport in the mesonephric collecting duct system of the toad Bufo bufo: microelectrode recordings from isolated and perfused tubules. J Exp Biol 2002;205:897–904.

23. Chai N. Anurans. In: Miller R, Fowler M, editors. Fowler's zoo and wildlife medicine. St. Louis (MO): Elsevier; 2015. p. 1–12.

24. Pessier AP. Hopping over red leg: the metamorphosis of amphibian pathology. Vet Pathol 2017;54:355–7.

25. Forzán MJ, Jones KM, Ariel E, et al. Pathogenesis of frog virus 3 (Ranavirus, Iridoviridae) infection in wood frogs (Rana sylvatica). Vet Pathol 2017;54:531–48.

26. McKinnell RG, Carlson DL. Luckeé renal adenocarcinoma, an anuran neoplasm: studies at the interface of pathology, virology, and differentiation competence. J Cell Physiol 1997;173:115–8.

27. Densmore CL, Green DE. Diseases of amphibians. ILAR J 2007;48:235–54.

28. Martinho F. Amphibian mycobacteriosis. Vet Clin North Am Exot Anim Pract 2012; 15:113–9.

29. Klaphake E. Bacterial and parasitic diseases of amphibians. Vet Clin North Am Exot Anim Pract 2009;12:597–608.

30. Berger L, Volp K, Mathews S, et al. Chlamydia pneumoniae in a free-ranging giant barred frog (Mixophyes iteratus) from Australia. J Clin Microbiol 1999;37: 2378–80.

31. Reed KD, Ruth GR, Meyer JA, et al. Chlamydia pneumoniae infection in a breeding colony of African clawed frogs (Xenopus tropicalis). Emerg Infect Dis 2000;6:196–9.

32. Martel A, Adriaensen C, Bogaerts S, et al. Novel chlamydiaceae disease in captive salamanders. Emerg Infect Dis 2012;18:1020–2.

33. Parè JA. Fungal diseases of amphibians: an overview. Vet Clin North Am Exot Anim Pract 2003;6:315–26.

34. Pessier AP. Amphibia. In: Terio KA, McAloose D, St. Leger J, editors. Pathology of wildlife and zoo animals. London: Academic Press; 2018. p. 915–44.

35. Holland MP, Skelly DK, Kashgarian M, et al. Echinostome infection in green frogs (Rana clamitans) is stage and age dependent. J Zool 2007;271:455–62.

36. Andrews JM, Childress JN, Iakovidis TJ, et al. Elucidating the life history and ecological aspects of Allodero hylae (Annelida: Clitellata: Naididae), a parasitic oligochaete of invasive Cuban tree frogs in Florida. J Parasitol 2015;101:275–81.

37. Lopez LCS, Rodrigues PJTFP, Rios RI. Frogs and snakes as phoretic dispersal agents of bromeliad ostracods (Limnocytheridae: Elpidium) and annelids (Naididae: Dero). Biotropica 1999;31:705–8.

38. Duncan AE, Garner MM, Bartholomew JL, et al. Renal myxosporidiasis in Asian horned frogs (Megophrys nasuta). J Zoo Wildl Med 2004;35:381–6.

39. Mutschmann F. Pathological changes in African hyperoliid frogs due to a myxosporidian infection with a new species of Hoferellus (Myxozoa). Dis Aquat Organ 2004;60:215–22.

40. Eiras JC. An overview on the myxosporean parasites in amphibians and reptiles. Acta Parasitol 2005;50:267–75.

41. Green DE, Harshbarger JC. Spontaneous neoplasia in amphibia. In: Wright KM, Whitaker BR, editors. Amphibian medicine and captive husbandry. Malabar (FL): Krieger; 2001. p. 335–400.

42. Mylniczenko ND. A medical health survey of diseases in captive caecilian amphibians. J Herpetol Med Surg 2018;16:120–8.

43. Masahito P, Nishioka M, Kondo Y, et al. Polycystic kidney and renal cell carcinoma in Japanese and Chinese toad hybrids. Int J Cancer 2003;103:1–4.

44. Meyer-Rochow VB, Asashima M, Moro SD. Nephroblastoma in the clawed frog Xenopus laevis. J Exp Anim Sci 1991;34:225–8.

45. Zwart P. A nephroblastoma in a fire-bellied newt, Cynops pyrrhogaster. Cancer Res 1970;30:2691–4.

46. Kawasumi T, Kudo T, Une Y. Spontaneous nephroblastoma in a Japanese giant salamander (*Andrias japonicus*). J Vet Med Sci 2012;74:673–5.

47. Tokiwa T, Kadekaru S, Ito M, et al. Oxalate nephropathy in free-living American bullfrog tadpoles. Dis Aquat Organ 2015;116:199–203.

48. Forzán MJ, Ferguson LV, Smith TG. Calcium oxalate nephrolithiasis and tubular necrosis in recent metamorphs of *Rana sylvatica* (*Lithobates sylvaticus*) fed spinach during the premetamorphic (tadpole) stage. Vet Pathol 2015;52:384–7.

49. Wright KM. Nutritional disorders. In: Wright KM, Whitaker BR, editors. Amphibian medicine and captive husbandry. Malabar (FL): Krieger; 2001. p. 73–88.

50. Archibald KE, Minter LJ, Dombrowski DS, et al. Cystic urolithiasis in captive waxy monkey frogs (*Phyllomedusa sauvagii*). J Zoo Wildl Med 2015;46:105–12.

51. Wright KM. Idiopathic syndromes. In: Wright KM, Whitaker BR, editors. Amphibian medicine and captive husbandry. Malabar (FL): Krieger; 2001. p. 239–42.

52. Pessier AP, Baitchman EJ, Crump P, et al. Causes of mortality in anuran amphibians from an *ex situ* survival assurance colony in Panama. Zoo Biol 2014;33: 516–26.

53. Sato K, Chernoff EAG. The short toes mutation of the axolotl. Dev Growth Differ 2007;49:469–78.

54. Washabaugh CH, Del Rio-Tsonis K, Tsonis PA. Variable manifestations in the short toes (s) mutation of the axolotl. J Morphol 1993;218:107–14.

55. Eustace R, Wack A, Mangus L, et al. Causes of mortality in captive Panamanian golden frogs (Atelopus zeteki) at the Maryland Zoo in Baltimore, 2001-2013. J Zoo Wildl Med 2018;49:324–34.

56. Blaustein AR, Romansic JM, Kiesecker JM, et al. Ultraviolet radiation, toxic chemicals and amphibian population declines. Divers Distrib 2003;9:123–40.

57. Browne RK, Odum RA, Herman T, et al. Facility design and associated services for the study of amphibians. ILAR J 2007;48:188–202.

58. Diana SG, Beasely VB, Wright KM. Clinical toxicology. In: Wright KM, Whitaker BR, editors. Amphibian medicine and captive husbandry. Malabar (FL): Krieger; 2001. p. 223–32.

Renal Disease in Teleost Patients

E. Scott Weber III, VMD, MSc, DACVPM, Cert Aquatic Vet WAVMA*

KEYWORDS

- Teleost • Corpuscles of stannius • Mesonephric • Proliferative kidney disease
- Polycystic kidney disease • Aminoglycoside toxicity

KEY POINTS

- The kidney in teleost fish is divided into an anterior head kidney responsible for immunologic and hematologic functions; the posterior trunk kidney analogous in function to other vertebrates for glomerular filtration.
- On necropsy, this functional duality of the fish kidney makes it a vital tissue for obtaining microbiologic cultures for infectious agents, especially during disease outbreaks.
- Because the gills are responsible for removing most nitrogenous waste, sodium, and chloride, serum renal panels are not as helpful for diagnosing or estimating the severity of renal disease.
- Renal repair and nephrogenesis can occur throughout the life of the animal, allowing fish to fully recover from renal pathology.
- Fish are an important laboratory model for mammalian renal diseases, including polycystic kidney disease.

INTRODUCTION

Aquatic animals are used for research, raised in aquaculture and mariculture for profitable production, maintained in public aquaria and zoos for display, stocked for commercial and sports fisheries, and kept as pets in home aquaria and garden ponds. Fish are the largest class of vertebrates and most recent estimates place the number of species at 60,147, with the number of valid genera at 5184 and the number of valid species at 35,064. Since 2000, more than 7700 new species have been added with 419 recently included in 2018.[1] The number of fish kept as pets in the United States is estimated at 139.2 million freshwater fish and another 18.8 million marine or saltwater animals, maintained in more than 12% of US households.[2]

As veterinarians, we can apply our expertise to optimize aquatic animal health and provide diagnostic, clinical, and surgical support for these aquatic patients. A growing

Disclosure Statement: No conflicts of interest.
Veterinary Information Network
* 85 Spring Run Road, White Marsh Hollow, Conestoga, PA 17516.
E-mail address: sharkdoc01@gmail.com

number of veterinarians are studying to improve their knowledge of the anatomy, physiology, and husbandry for this class of vertebrates so they can successfully impart clients with greater awareness, knowledge, and understanding of their responsibility to provide compassionate and responsible veterinary care and welfare considerations for aquatic animals. The following information provides some insight into renal function of fish by briefly examining anatomy and physiology and describing associated renal tissues, such as the corpuscles of Stannius, inter-renal gland, chromaffin cells, and anterior kidney. Renal function in fish is compared and contrasted with other vertebrates and unique attributes of the piscine kidney as relevant laboratory models for renal diseases in other animals, including humans, are described. Finally, we briefly summarize several infectious and noninfectious renal diseases seen in fish, focusing on pets and ornamental pond animals.

BASIC ANATOMY AND PHYSIOLOGY OF THE FISH KIDNEY

The 3 main classes of fishes are the bony fish Osteichthyes infraclass teleosts (96% of all extant species), the cartilaginous fishes such as sharks and rays referred to as Chondrichthyes, and the hagfishes (Agnatha). Because most pet fish are teleosts, these animals are the primary example unless otherwise noted.

Anatomy

The fish kidney runs cranial to caudal just ventral to the vertebrate in the retroperitoneal space. The teleost kidney is a complex organ that may be composed of the pronephric anterior or cephalic kidney, inter-renal tissue, chromaffin cells, corpuscles of Stannius, the opistonephric/mesonephric posterior or trunk kidney, renal juxtaglomerular cells, urinary ducts, urinary bladders in some species, and a urogenital aperture.[3] Both the cephalic and trunk kidney have endothelium-lined sinusoidal spaces that are important for fish immunology.

The anterior or head kidney contains inter-renal tissue and chromaffin cells and in some species is contiguous with the caudal or trunk kidney, depending on embryologic and developmental differences per species.[4] Primitive species tend to have less grossly morphologic separation of the head and trunk kidney, yet both sections are readily differentiated with histopathologic evaluation.

Unique to fish, the anterior kidney serves primarily an immunologic and hematologic function with a large population of macrophages and erythrocyte production centers. Researchers have demonstrated that the area occupied by macrophage aggregates in the anterior kidney positively correlates with the health status in salmonids and may negatively suggest immune compromise caused by such factors as stress and acute bacterial infection.[5] Inter-renal tissue in fish has been described as comparable in structure with the zona intermedia of the rat adrenal cortex,[6] whereas chromaffin cells are homologous with the adrenal medulla.[7] Both of these adrenal-like tissues are dispersed close to blood vessels in the cephalic kidney.[8] Thyroid follicles are also found in the cephalic kidney and are postulated as a normal occurrence required for immune signaling.[9]

The corpuscles of Stannius are located in the middle of the kidney marking the transition between cephalic and caudal regions. Originally thought to be analogous to the adrenal gland in mammals, embryologic development suggests this tissue arises from the pronephric duct.[10] Subsequently, the corpuscles of Stannius have been shown to be an important endocrine gland regulating calcium blood levels in both marine and freshwater fish,[11] although the corpuscles of Stannius seem to be more active in some marine species.[12] These and other findings suggest the corpuscles of Stannius are likely to be a precursor to the mammalian parathyroid gland.[13]

The caudal kidney is most analogous histologically and functionally to the mammalian kidney, but the piscine kidney serves primarily an osmoregulatory function, because the gills are responsible for most sodium, chloride, and nitrogenous waste excretion.[14] In comparison with mammalian kidneys, teleost kidneys can have hematopoietic centers in both the head and trunk kidney. Additionally, fish renal tissue does not have a cortical medullary structure and there is a dual blood supply consisting of renal arteries and a renal portal system flowing from the lymph and blood.

The functional components of the teleost nephron consist of a Bowman's capsule, glomerulus, renal tubule demarcated as the proximal tubule I and II, distal tubule, connecting tubule, and collecting duct.[15] Some marine fish lack glomeruli,[16] although elasmobranchs have been shown to have a more developed nephron used for urea reabsorption that contains an intermediate tubule lacking in teleosts.[17] The fish glomeruli are supplied by venous blood from the renal portal system and lack a loop of Henle used in mammals, birds, and reptiles for water and ion, mostly Na^+, Cl^-, K^+, Ca^{2+} and HCO_3^- resorption.[18] This blood circulation raises concerns about administering injectable pharmacologic agents and antibiotics into the tail of fish that are processed through the kidney, which may render the agents inactive before complete systemic circulation.

The renin–angiotensin system appeared first in primitive forms during the early evolution of bony fishes. Zebrafish (Danio rerio) are perhaps the most studied fish model and are shown to have 2 distinct morphologic populations of mesonephric renin cells that function similarly to mammals.[19] Later research confirmed marine elasmobranchs also possess a renin–angiotensin system,[20] and studies using river ray (Potamotrygon humerosa) renal corpuscles suggests mesonephric renin cells respond to renin–angiotensin system-mediated challenges in a similar manner to mammals demonstrating conservation of the physiologic actions of the renin–angiotensin system across vertebrates.[21]

Physiology

On the most basic level, freshwater fish are hypertonic and are constantly trying to excrete water. Marine species are hypotonic and need to prevent dehydration and to retain water and excrete ions. Therefore, kidney function of freshwater teleosts for water regulation in osmotic balance differs dramatically from marine teleosts requiring water retention and excretion of divalent cations (magnesium and SO_4), inorganic phosphate, and hydronium.[22,23] There is a more in-depth review for veterinarians in Osmoregulation in Fish: Mechanisms and Clinical implications by Greenwell and colleagues[24] Glomerular filtration rates vary greatly among species, but based on function most freshwater species of teleost have a higher glomerular filtration rate than marine species.[25] Because of the different environmental demands of freshwater versus marine environments, the tubule and collecting ducts are impermeable in freshwater species needing to retain divalent cations while these same structures are permeable in marine species to allow these excess cations to be excreted (**Table 1**). Some fish are euryhaline and are capable of adjusting to a wide range of salinity. These species have different mechanisms for dealing with fast and sudden environmental changes in salinity.

Most elasmobranchs commonly kept in public aquaria or as pets have a different osmoregulatory mechanism. Cartilaginous fish retain circulating organic salts, urea, and trimethylamine oxide, making them hyperosmotic to seawater.[17] Being hyperosmotic allows their kidneys to regulate water similar to freshwater teleosts, and

Table 1
Renal physiology and osmoregulation in freshwater versus marine fish

	Freshwater Species	Marine Species
Osmoregulation	Hypertonic to the environment: Constantly trying to excrete water	Hypotonic to the environment: Need to prevent dehydration and retain water while excreting ions
GFR	Higher	Lower
Nephron structure	Tubules and collecting ducts are impermeable, reflecting the need to retain divalent cations	Tubules and collecting ducts are permeable to allow excess cations to be excreted.

Abbreviation: GFR, glomerular filtration rate.

inorganic salts from seawater are excreted via a specialized organ called the rectal gland.[17]

These physiologic differences make standard veterinary renal serum panels unreliable for diagnosing renal disease in fish. As an example, the gill is primarily responsible for removal of nitrogenous waste and is vital for sodium and chloride regulation obviating the value of many of these parameters such as Na, Cl, and blood urea nitrogen for renal pathology.[14]

Renal Regeneration

Research has shown that fish kidneys can repair renal injury in several species, such as goldfish (*Carassius auratus*), zebrafish, catfish, trout, tilapia, and the aglomerular toadfish.[26,27] Although mammalian kidneys can repair the tubular epithelium of the nephron, nephrogenesis cannot occur in adult mammals, whereas fish are capable of growing nephrons de novo throughout their life. More recently, the migration of nephron progenitor cells has been studied showing development of functional nephrons after transplantation.[28] From embryogenesis to adulthood, zebrafish share several similarities with the anatomy and physiology of the mammalian kidney, making this species an important research model for understanding nephrogenesis pathways.[27] Through the use of genetically targeted knockouts and knockdowns regularly used in research, zebrafish are a model for understanding the molecular pathogenesis of several human renal disease and syndromes, and this species may be valuable for testing and developing new therapies.[3,29]

INFECTIOUS DISEASES OF FISH

Because the head and trunk kidney have endothelium-lined sinusoidal spaces lined with phagocytic mononuclear cells, the fish kidney is the most common organ used for microbiological culture and molecular diagnostics for infectious agents in fish disease outbreaks. A majority of systemic infectious agents often cause anterior or posterior kidney pathology. Descriptions of taking a sterile kidney cultures and samples from fish are readily available in several fish pathology references (**Fig. 1**).[30,31]

In freshwater fish, the most common clinical sign associated with renal disease is coelomic ascites marked by coelomic distension. Ascites can be associated with possibly swimming and buoyancy deficits owing to renal and fluid mass effects. Clients and fish hobbyists refer to coelomic distension as dropsy, often misattributing this nonspecific term as a disease (**Fig. 2**). Another common term used by clients and fish hobbyists is pine coning, which refers to rapid acute coelomic ascites causing

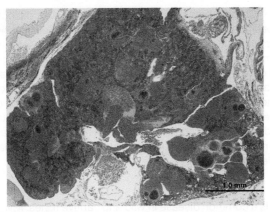

Fig. 1. A histopathology slide showing sepsis of unknown etiology in the anterior kidney.

the scales to lift up making the skin of the fish resemble a pinecone. Care must be taken not to conflate these colloquial terms as disease, because many fish aquarists and hobbyists ask for specific treatments using these descriptors without any diagnosis. When performing a fish necropsy, performing a kidney culture, completing renal histopathology, and saving fresh or frozen kidney tissue can greatly improve the odds of obtaining an accurate diagnosis.

Bacterial Infection

Bacteria from many common bacterial diseases are also routinely isolated from the fish kidney including common pathogens such as *Aeromonas sp.* from koi, goldfish, and salmonids and *Edwardsiella* spp. from freshwater catfish.

Bacterial kidney disease

Bacterial kidney disease is a chronic infection caused by the gram-positive bacterium, *Renibacterium salmoninarum*. Bacterial kidney disease occurs in a variety of salmonids and the entire Salmonidae family is considered susceptible.[32] As fish pathogens, gram-positive infections are generally slower growing and marked with intracellular

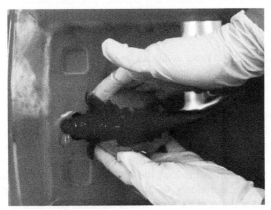

Fig. 2. A goldfish/koi hybrid showing severe coelomic distention caused by ascites dropsy from polycystic kidney disease.

bacterial invasion. Chronic granulomas form in many tissues associated with heavy macrophage populations, but external lesions are seldom a clinical sign of infection.[32] Some of the nonspecific clinical signs that may occur during bacterial kidney disease include anemia, melanosis, and exophthalmos. On gross necropsy, gray-white lesions can be identified on several visceral organs, most notably both the anterior and posterior kidney. Intracellular gram-positive rods can be found within macrophages. Diagnosis can be made via a kidney culture or with several molecular diagnostic tests, including enzyme-linked immunosorbent assay (ELISA), immunofluorescence antibody testing, and polymerase chain reaction (PCR). Although not approved for use in food fish, erythromycin has been successfully used to treat bacterial kidney disease in adult or juvenile salmonids.

Mycobacteriosis

Mycobacteriosis is a common disease in wild and captive fishes. *Mycobacterium* spp. are ubiquitous in aquatic environments and many species of marine and freshwater fish are susceptible. Mycobacteria cause problems in ornamental marine and freshwater fish trade worldwide and are an insidious problem. Bataillon and coworkers[33] first reported mycobacteriosis in 1897 in a common carp. Several species of atypical mycobacteria have been isolated from marine and freshwater fish. The 3 most common etiologic agents found in pet fish to date include *Mycobacterium marinum*, *M fortuitum,* and *M chelonae.*

Transmission of the causative agent is primarily through consumption of contaminated feed, contaminated water, or aquatic detritus, and cannibalism of infected fish. Environmental conditions favorable to this pathogen include low levels of dissolved oxygen, low pH, high organic loads, and warm water. Many species of freshwater and marine fish can be infected in water temperatures ranging from temperate, including the common goldfish.[34]

Affected fish are listless, lethargic, and isolate themselves from other fish.[34] Some animals may have exophthalmia, coelomic ascites, and inflammation of the skin. Deep skin ulcers may develop over granulomas within skeletal muscle. Sometimes pigment alterations occur, such as a lightning or darkening of the chromatophores. Scoliosis or other bone deformities can also occur, although this effect is less common in fish.

Gross necropsy lesions caused by mycobacteriosis can be gray-white to tan miliary granulomas, that are found in virtually any parenchymatous tissue. The spleen, kidney, and liver are the most common organs affected. Enlarged organs, coelomitis, and generalized edema may be present. Red, slightly elevated scales or ulcers may be seen in the skin.

There are no antemortem tests available for diagnosing atypical mycobacteriosis in fish. Histopathology with Fite's acid-fast stain is the current method of choice when paired with clinical findings (**Fig. 3**). Culture of affected tissues coupled with molecular testing is the gold standard, but can take several months and sometimes will only provide the genus. PCR of infected tissues is both a sensitive and accurate confirmatory test for mycobacteriosis, offering rapid turnaround, although it is also expensive.

There is currently no effective treatment, although several experimental regimens have been described; however, they lack histopathology and clinical follow-up. Another caveat with treatment is that the antimicrobials required, and the duration of treatment for mycobacteriosis in an aquarium or pond, lends to accidental discharge of treated water and pathogen, and potential overdosing of the antibiotics, which may lead to antibiotic resistance. Management and avoidance are the only control for mycobacterial outbreaks in aquaria or aquaculture.

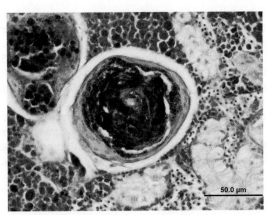

Fig. 3. Fite's acid-fast staining of the posterior kidney showing numerous acid-fast organisms presumed to be of *Mycobacteria* sp. from an Australian rainbow fish (*Melanotaenia fluviatilis*).

Atypical mycobacteriosis is zoonotic and can cause infections in humans and other mammals. Tuberculoid infections in humans using public swimming pools was first reported in 1939 in Sweden.[35] US cases of *M marinum*, also associated with public swimming pools, emerged in 1951,[36] and the causative organism *M balnei* was identified in 1954.[37] Recently, *M fortuitum* has been implicated in pneumonia in a cat.[38]

Today, mycobacteriosis is commonly referred to as fish tank granuloma and a misnomer is fish handler's disease, which historically referred to rashes caused by the bacteria *Erysipelothrix rhusiopathiae*, although the term is now loosely used to describe rashes caused by any pathogen after handling fish. All fish should be managed as if they may contain mycobacteriosis, especially abantids and rainbow fishes. Gloves are recommended when handling potentially infected fish or cleaning suspect aquaria. People who have cuts on their hands or those who are immunosuppressed are at greatest risk.

Mycobacteriosis also has One Health implications, posing an environmental threat to the wild fisheries and posing a potential zoonotic risk for commercial and sport fishing personnel. In 1997, the first cases of mycobacteriosis began surfacing in wild striped bass (*Morone saxatalis*) in the Chesapeake and after bay-wide health surveillance in 1998, it was estimated that 60% of striped bass in the Chesapeake Bay had this disease.[39,40]

Viral Infection

Many systemic viral and fungal pathogens cause pathology of either or both the anterior and posterior kidney.

Cyprinid herpesvirus

Koi herpesvirus (KHV) and goldfish herpesvirus (GHV) and their respective etiologic agents of cyprinid herpesvirus 3 and cyprinid herpesvirus-2 are 2 diseases that poise an economic threat to both industry and hobbyists. Before virus isolation, researchers named the disease carp interstitial nephritis and gill necrosis virus because of the renal pathology associated with these infections.[41] KHV is a reportable disease to the World Organisation for Animal Health and the US Department of Agriculture. These diseases may occur during the cooler months of spring and fall when water temperatures most commonly range between 70°F and 78°F (21.1–25.6°C).[42] Water temperature is a key factor in disease control, but exposing infected koi, carp, or goldfish to temperatures greater than 80°F (26.7°C) during an outbreak can cause fish to become lifelong latent carriers of their respective viruses.[42]

Both KHV and GHV are believed to have appeared between 1995 and 1996. KHV caused mass mortalities of wild and domestic koi and common carp (*Cyprinus carpio*), and the first published report of virus isolation from infected koi in the United States and Israel was in 1998.[43]

Diseases caused by both pathogens are similar with gross lesions of necrotic gill tissue, patchy skin sometimes with hemorrhages, and sunken eyes. On necropsy, infected fish have swelling of the kidney and spleen sometimes accompanied by diffuse coelomic hemorrhage. GHV is also marked by anemia with necrosis of the cranial kidney.[44]

Diagnosis for both KHV and GHV is made using histopathology combined with PCR testing of fresh or frozen gill and kidney biopsies.[45,46] Virus isolation is the gold standard from freshly euthanized or dead fish, but can take several weeks for confirmation and is not readily available at many diagnostic laboratories.

Because of latency and a carrier state that can last for 9 years, control of KHV and GHV is complicated.[47] There is currently no treatment and the best prevention. Proper quarantine and testing and certification programs at the producer, breeder, and distributor level are vital to managing these pathogens. Conventional PCR, ELISA, and real-time TaqMan PCR to test for viral DNA of GHV and KHV and host antibody response are available at some aquatic animal diagnostic laboratories, but interpretation of test results require experience.[45,46]

KHV ELISA is extremely sensitive and may be used as a screening tool, especially for populations of koi. This test may have false positives that can be eliminated via serial sampling.[48] Some available commercial ELISAs have been described in peer-reviewed scientific literature and testing methodologies have been validated.[48] ELISA should be used for nonclinical fish because during outbreaks, approximately 2 to 3 weeks is required to develop appropriate antibodies for detection by ELISA.[49]

PCR looks specifically for viral nucleic acid. TaqMan PCR is the test of choice during clinical outbreaks of disease. This test can be coupled with virus isolation to help determine the geographic strain of KHV present. To control KHV, there must be standardization both internationally and nationally by the World Organisation for Animal Health or US Department of Agriculture Animal and Plant Health Inspection Service.

The future may hold promise for development of vaccine programs successful in other countries such as Israel for KHV.[50] Before any such programs are accepted in the United States, the vaccine's efficacy and impact on testing or surveillance must be fully vetted and thorough risk analysis, cost effectiveness, and the practical supply, distribution, and application of the vaccine will have to be worked out.

Parasitic Disease

Renal nematode and trematode infections have been identified in fish. Several external protozoan infections have caused systemic illness such as *Tetrahymena* sp. isolated from the kidneys of freshwater fish and *Uronema* sp. from marine fish have been found in severe infections.

Proliferative kidney disease

Although the acronym PKD is commonly used in human and small animal medicine to refer to polycystic kidney disease, in fish medicine and among fish biologist PKD is associated with proliferative kidney disease of salmonids. Proliferative kidney disease is a disease caused by the myxozoan parasite *Tetracapsuloides bryosalmonae*[51] and has been identified in California hatcheries and wild stocks from the Merced River in California.[52,53] Similar to other myxozoan disease in fish, the parasite life cycle requires an oligochaete intermediary. The rainbow trout (*Onchorynchus gairdneri*) serves as a dead end host. Clinical signs include a swollen coelom, anemia, and exophthalmos with high mortalities occurring in warm weather or heavily fed fish in aquaculture or hatchery settings. Although many organs can be infected, the most profound lesions are associated with the kidney. The kidney first becomes red and enlarged and then turns a gray color. There is a loss of excretory tissue and arteritis of the small vessels feeding the kidney. If fish survive to colder months, the kidney can regenerate. Early reports suggested treatment with malachite green could impart immunity on stocks of fish, but as with other myxozoans management and prevention takes precedent.

Polycystic kidney disease

Polycystic kidney disease can occur in pond-raised common and fancy goldfish varieties and is caused by infection with one of several species of myxozoans, the most common being *Hoferellus carassii* (**Fig. 4**).[54] There is a similar disease in common carp, rarely seen in koi, caused by *Sphaerospora renicola*.[55] Fish present with coelomic distension and may have impaired buoyancy. Based on clinical cases, usually only a few fish present with clinical signs. This finding is supported by the first studies conducted in a wild population of goldfish in which 5 out of 80 animals exhibited clinical signs.[56] In a pond case reported from New Zealand, nearly 30% of fish were affected.[57] This disease occurs in earthen ponds because the causative myxozoan parasite requires an aquatic oligochaete worm to complete its life cycle.[58] Diagnosis is generally made on necropsy and histopathology by observing the parasites. There is no known treatment. Management for this pathogen involves decreasing the area for oligochaete worms that reside in the pond. Ultraviolet sterilization may be beneficial in killing the infective stage before attaching to the fish, as demonstrated with other myxozoan parasites.[59] Pond renovations may include using concrete or inert rubber or plastic liners to decrease sediment accumulation and facilitate cleaning. Actively removing detritus and sediment in the ponds a couple times per year may also be helpful.

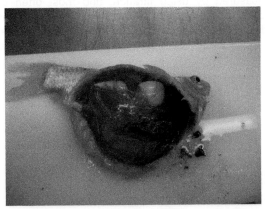

Fig. 4. Necropsy of a goldfish (*Carassius auratus*) with polycystic kidney disease caused by the myxozoan *Hoferellus carassii*.

NONINFECTIOUS DISEASES OF FISH
Polycystic Kidney Disease

Polycystic kidney disease is commonly seen in a variety of fish. There is a well-described model of polycystic kidney disease in zebrafish created using a genetic knockdown model[60] and in a pc mutant of medaka (*Oryzias latipes*),[61] but in most species the cause remains unknown. Clinically, this disease is regularly seen in comet and fancy goldfish. The appropriate diagnostic workup for a fish presenting with coelomic ascites consists of a detailed history, water quality analysis, physical examination, radiographs, ultrasound examination, and hematology. Because the teleost kidney is the only organ that lies directly below the spine on radiographs, any ventral displacement of the swim bladder is indicative of renal enlargement (**Fig. 5**). Fluid-filled cysts can be readily imaged using ultrasound examination, and the cysts can be aspirated for fluid analysis using ultrasound guidance. Laparoscopic renal biopsy can also be performed in an anesthetized animal.[62] If no etiologic cause is found, a presumptive diagnosis of idiopathic polycystic kidney disease can be made. Fluid-filled cysts that are causing buoyancy or swimming problems can be drained, using ultrasound-guided fluid centesis. Fluid removal will only give temporary relief and the fluid will return anywhere from several days to several months depending on the severity of renal pathology. The condition is progressive and leads to the eventual death of the animal. There are currently no known medical treatments nor are any peer-reviewed reports of surgical correction.

Water Quality

Every veterinary case in aquatic animal medicine begins with a thorough history and water quality analysis. Alkalinity and hardness are 2 water quality parameters often confused. Hardness is the sum of the multivalent cations in solution, whereas alkalinity is a measure of the solution's ability to neutralize acids (bicarbonate or HCO_3^- ions and carbonate CO_3^{2-} ions). In natural water systems, calcium carbonate is usually present and acts as a buffering agent. The 2 main cations are Ca^{2+} and Mg, with the former usually present at 10 times the amount of the latter. Other cations that can be found include barium, strontium, iron, copper, zinc, cobalt, nickel, aluminum, and others depending on water source, pollution, and geology. These cations occur as hydroxides, carbonates, and bicarbonates, but also to a lesser degree as sulfates, chlorides, silicates, phosphates, and borates.

Hardness is measured by using titration, and most often accomplished by adding drops to solicit a color change after a primary chelation $CaCO_3$ in the water with egtazic acid followed by drop-wise addition of EDTA to chelate the calcium and magnesium. Both are measured in degrees of carbonate hardness where 1

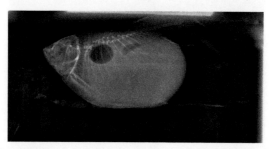

Fig. 5. A right lateral radiograph showing ventral and cranial displacement of the swim bladder from an undiagnosed renal mass in a fancy goldfish (*Carassius auratus*).

degree of carbonate hardness equals 17.86 mg calcium carbonate per liter of water. Alkalinity and hardness can also be measured as $CaCO_3$ mg/kL or parts per million (ppm) for convenience of reporting a single number to represent multiple chemicals and for ease in calculating a solution's carbonate and noncarbonate hardness.

There are negative and positive effects associated with increased hardness in freshwater environments. In general, an increase of hardness can help osmotic balance, because increased Ca^{2+} results in a decrease in cell permeability leading to less cellular ion loss. In contrast, animals from soft water environments expend more energy to prevent ion loss across cell membranes that are more permeable. The net effect of calcium serum levels results in increased calcitonin regulation for homeostasis by the corpuscles of Stannius.[63] Commonly kept freshwater fish have a wide range of hardness requirements with many South American Amazon species preferring soft water at 0 to 30 ppm, while Rift Lake cichlids from Africa prefer hardness values from 170 to 220 ppm. For the average mixed freshwater community tanks or outdoor koi or goldfish pond levels from 75 to 125 ppm are considered optimal.

As hardness exceeds 300 ppm bicarbonates cannot be excreted, causing serum metabolic alkalosis. High hardness values can also lead to the pathologic accumulation of Ca^{2+} concretions in the kidneys called nephrocalcinosis (**Fig. 6**), which can cause both acute and chronic effects on aquatic animal health. The calcification observed in renal calcinosis of rainbow trout was identified as calcium salts deposited within necrotic tissue, differentiating this as a dystrophic rather than metastatic process.[64]

Toxic Exposure

Fish are susceptible to aminoglycoside toxicity. A typical case presentation is a koi that has been treated empirically for external ulcers, with or without veterinary consultation using an injectable aminoglycoside. The fish can present with healing or nonhealing ulcers, most often coupled with coelomic ascites. These cases can result in anything from full recovery to death, depending on the dose and duration of aminoglycoside administration and underlying systemic bacterial infection. Clients often obtain theses antibiotics from a veterinarian who typically does not treat fish and defers to the experience of the pond owner. The author only uses aminoglycosides based on

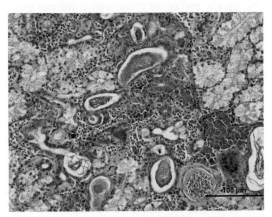

Fig. 6. A histopathology slide showing nephrocalcinosis in a brown trout (*Salmo trutta*) caused by prolonged exposure to increased water hardness.

antibiotic resistance and sensitivity that clinically indicates these antibiotics are the appropriate treatment choice, and the dose needs to be based on actual fish weight. Many hobbyists attempt to dose systemic antibiotics based on a guesstimate of weight based on the length of the fish based on online data for healthy koi without consideration of body condition.

In zebrafish, researchers have demonstrated that gentamicin can cause a decrease in the glomerular filtration rate, and some chemotherapeutic agents such as cisplatin result in histologic changes and a decrease in renal function in larval zebrafish.[65] Further research supporting the author's observations of koi recovering after showing clinical signs of renal damage was documented in the freshwater goldfish, C auratus.[66,67] Gentamicin-induced necrosis of proximal tubular epithelial cells was induced using a single intracoelomic injection of 50 mg/kg gentamicin in goldfish. Animals humanely killed at several day intervals over a 21-day period showed repair of injured nephrons with regeneration along the basement membrane several days after injection and new nephrons 2 to 3 weeks after injection.[66,67]

Other chemicals and toxins have been implicated in causing renal pathology in fish, sometimes necessitating an advanced water quality analysis to identify the toxin. It is strongly suggested to freeze an additional 500 mL water sample when responding to an outbreak so water chemical analysis can be included in the diagnostic evaluation.

Goldish exposed to a single dose of the solvent hexachlorobutadiene developed polycystic kidneys within 70 days.[68] Reimschuessel and colleagues[69] also demonstrated that fish fed a combination of melamine and cyanuric acid developed melamine-cyanurate complex renal crystals, similar to those associated with feline renal pathology after ingestion. Renal pathology was also observed in the rosy barb fish (*Puntius conchonius*) exposed chronically to methoxyethyl mercuric chloride, a common industrial and agricultural pollutant found in waterways,[70] and other mercury compounds caused renal epithelia necrosis in stinging catfish (*Heteropneustes fossilis*).[71] Malathion toxicity observed in spotted snakehead (*Channa punctatus*) caused renal necrosis and tubule edema.[72] The number of toxins causing renal pathology is too great to include in its entirety in this article, but clinicians should be aware that many chemical insults can lead to signs of renal disease in fish.

Neoplasia

Different types of renal cancer can occur in fish with or without exposure to a carcinogenic compound. A renal cystic adenocarcinoma in a flowerhorn cichlid[73] and renal adenocarcinoma in an oscar (*Astronotus ocellatus*, Agassiz) has been reported.[74] A nephroblastoma was observed in bester sturgeon, a cultured hybrid of *Huso huso* × *Acipenser ruthenus*.[75] The most comprehensive list of renal neoplasms can be found in a review by Lombardini and colleagues,[76] which includes rare cases of spontaneous renal tubular cell tumors as well as bladder and collecting duct neoplasms. There currently are no peer-reviewed references for treatment of urinary tract neoplasms in any fish species, but if these cancers can be more quickly and readily diagnosed, veterinary oncology principles from other animal models could be applied.

Nutritional Deficiencies

The sheer number of fish in the pet trade (approximately 470 freshwater species and between 1700 and 2300 marine fish species)[77–79] make it near impossible for any one individual to have a complete understanding of the environmental and nutritional requirements for the vast majority of animals available for retail. As we gain experience keeping and rearing a variety of species, we can better understand and optimize their environmental and nutritional requirements.

There are some examples of nutritional deficiencies causing renal disease in fish. Deficiencies of biotin and pantothenic acid in lake trout (*Salvelinus namaycush*) revealed a far greater glycogen deposition in renal tubules of biotin deficient animals, whereas fish fed neither biotin nor pantothenic acid exhibited greater renal tubular necrosis.[80]

Renal tubular calcium oxalate crystals have been associated with a reversible condition caused by deficiencies of the fat-soluble vitamins A and E and lipid peroxidation in cultured marine clownfish (*Amphiprion ocellaris*).[81] Bladder stones composed of calcium, inorganic phosphate, and magnesium salts have been found at necropsy or have been surgically removed from some marine species of pufferfish and burrfish by the author. These bladder stones may be dietary or environmental in origin, although no peer-reviewed references are currently found.

SUMMARY

Teleost fish are susceptible to several infectious and noninfectious causes of renal disease. Even when presented with a freshly deceased animal, the clinician can gather important diagnostics via a sterile kidney microbiological culture and water quality analysis for the benefit of the population of an aquarium, outdoor pond, or hatchery. An approach for diagnosing and treating renal disease in fish requires an understanding of the comparative differences in renal anatomy and physiology of these patients to provide a practical, and successful clinical outcome. Although identifying and treating renal diseases in aquatic animals is challenging, the knowledge we can gain from fish, especially with their potential for nephrogenesis following renal injury, may prove instrumental in managing renal disease in humans and other companion animals.[82]

REFERENCES

1. Fricke R, Eschmeyer WN, van der Laan R, editors. Eschmeyer 's catalog of fishes: genera, species, references. 2019. Available at: http://researcharchive.calacademy. org/research/ichthyology/catalog/fishcatmain.asp. Accessed February 1, 2019.
2. American Pet Products Association. APPA National Pet Owners Survey. In: APPA website. 2017-2018. Available at: https://americanpetproducts.org/Uploads/ MemServices/GPE2017_NPOS_Seminar.pdf. Accessed February 1, 2019.
3. Drummond IA. Kidney development and disease in the zebrafish. J Am Soc Nephrol 2005;16:299–304.
4. Abdel-Aziz EH, Ali TE, Abdu SB, et al. Chromaffin cells and interrenal tissue in the head kidney of the grouper, *Epinephilus tauvina* (Teleostei, Serranidae): a morphological (optical and ultrastructural) study. J Appl Ichthyol 2010;26:522–7.
5. Gregori M, Miragliotta V, Leotta R, et al. Morphometric evaluation of interrenal gland and kidney macrophages aggregates in normal healthy rainbow trout (*Oncorhynchus mykiss*) and after bacterial challenge with Yersinia ruckeri. Vet Med Int 2014;2014:210625.
6. Ogawa M. Fine structure of the corpuscles of Stannius and the interrenal tissue in goldfish, Carassius auratus. Z Zellforsch Mikrosk Anat 1967;81:174–89.
7. Sampour M. The study of adrenal chromaffin of fish, *Carassius auratus* (Toleostei). Pak J Biol Sci 2008;11:1032–6.
8. Withes PC. Endocrinology (adrenal glands). Comparative animal physiology. Fort Worth: Saunders College; 1992. p. 548–52.

9. Geven E, Klaren P. The teleost head kidney: integrating thyroid and immune signalling. Dev Comp Immunol 2017;66:73–83.

10. Huot E. Preliminaire sur l'origine des capsules surrénales des poissons lophobranches. C. R. Hebd. Seances Acad. Sci. Ser. D Paris 1898;126:49–50.

11. Frederic DG. The development and phylogeny of the corpuscle of Stannius in Ganoid and Teleostean fishes. J Morphol 2005;70:41–67.

12. Bedjargi PC, Kulkarni RS. Studies on differences in number, location and size of the corpuscles of stannius in freshwater and seawater fishes. International Journal of Pure and Applied Zoology 2014;2(2):171–4.

13. Greenwood MP, Flik G, Wagner GF, et al. The corpuscles of Stannius, calcium-sensing receptor, and stanniocalcin: responses to calcimimetics and physiological challenges. Endocrinology 2009;150:3002–10.

14. Ip YK, Shit FC. Ammonia production, excretion, toxicity, and defense in fish: a review. Front Physiol 2010;1:134.

15. Sakai T. The structure of the kidney from the freshwater teleost Carassius auratus. Anat Embryol 1985;171:31–9.

16. Beyenbach KW. Kidneys sans glomeruli. Am J Physiol Renal Physiol 2004;286:F811–27.

17. Hyodo S, Kakumura K, Takagi W, et al. Morphological and functional characteristics of the kidney of cartilaginous fishes: with special reference to urea reabsorption. Am J Physiol Regul Integr Comp Physiol 2014;307:R1381–95.

18. Morya R, Kumar K, Kumar P. Anatomical and physiological similarities of kidney in different experimental animals used for basic studies. J Clin Exp Nephrol 2018;3:9.

19. Rider SA, Christian HC, Mullins LJ, et al. Zebrafish mesonephric renin cells are functionally conserved and comprise two distinct morphological populations. Am J Physiol Renal Physiol 2017;312:F778–90.

20. Lacy ER, Reale E. The presence of a juxtaglomerular apparatus in elasmobranch fish. Anat Embryol 1990;182:249–62.

21. Lacy ER, Reale E. A unique juxtaglomerular apparatus in the river ray, Potamotrygon humerosa, a freshwater stingray. Zoomorphology 2017;137:155–64.

22. Evans DH. Teleost fish osmoregulation: what have we learned since August Krogh, Homer Smith, and Ancel keys. Am J Physiol Regul Integr Comp Physiol 2008;295:R704–13.

23. Grafflin AL. Renal function in marine teleosts: IV. The excretion of inorganic phosphate in the sculpin. Biol Bull 1936;71:360–74.

24. Greenwell MG, Sherrill J, Clayton LA. Osmoregulation in fish. Mechanisms and clinical implications. Vet Clin North Am Exot Anim Pract 2003;6:169–89.

25. Nishimura H, Imai M. Control of renal function in freshwater and marine teleosts. Fed Proc 1982;41:2355–60.

26. Reimschuessel R. A fish model of renal regeneration and development. ILAR J 2001;42:285–91.

27. Gerlach GF, Wingert RA. Kidney organogenesis in the zebrafish: insights into vertebrate nephrogenesis and regeneration. Wiley Interdiscip Rev Dev Biol 2013;2:559–85.

28. Davidson AJW. Kidney regeneration in fish. Nephron Exp Nephrol 2014;126:45.

29. Santoriello C, Zon LI. Hooked! Modeling human disease in zebrafish. J Clin Invest 2012;122:2337–43.

30. Reimschuessel R, May EB, Bennett RO, et al. Tropical fish medicine. Necropsy examination of fish. Vet Clin North Am Small Anim Pract 1988;18:427–33.

31. Weber ESP, Govett P. Parasitology and necropsy of fish. Compendium 2009; 31:E12.

32. Fryer JL, Sanders JE. Bacterial kidney disease of salmonid fish. Annu Rev Microbiol 1981;35:273–98.

33. Bataillon E, Dubard R, Terre U. Un nouveau type de tuberculose. C R Seances Soc Biol Fil 1897;49:446–9.

34. Talaat AM, Trucksis M, Kane AS, et al. Pathogenicity of *Mycobacterium fortuitum* and *Mycobacterium smegmatis* to goldfish, *Carassius auratus*. Vet Microbiol 1999;66:151–64.

35. Groenheit R, Ghebremichael S, Pennhag A, et al. Mycobacterium tuberculosis strains potentially involved in the TB epidemic in Sweden a century ago. PLoS One 2012;7:e46848.

36. Norden A, Linnell F. A new type of pathogenic mycobacterium. Nature 1951; 168:826.

37. Linell F, Norden A. *Mycobacterium balnei* new acid-fast bacillus occurring in swimming pools and capable of producing skin lesions in humans. Acta Tuberc Scand Suppl 1954;33:1–84.

38. Couto SS, Artacho CA. *Mycobacterium fortuitum* pneumonia in a cat and the role of lipid in the pathogenesis of atypical mycobacterial infections. Vet Pathol 2007; 44:543–6.

39. Gauthier DT, Rhodes MW. Mycobacteriosis in fishes: a review. Vet J 2009;180: 33–47.

40. Spotte S. Candiru: life and legend of the bloodsucking catfishes. Berkeley (CA): Creative Arts Book Co.; 2002.

41. Pikarsky E, Ronen A, Abramowitz J, et al. Pathogenesis of acute viral disease induced in fish by carp interstitial nephritis and gill necrosis virus. J Virol 2004; 78:9544–51.

42. Gilad O, Yun S, Adkison MA, et al. Molecular comparison of isolates of an emerging fish pathogen, koi herpesvirus, and the effect of water temperature on mortality of experimentally infected koi. J Gen Virol 2003;84:2661–7.

43. Hedrick RP, Gilad O, Yun S, et al. A herpesvirus associated with mass mortality of juvenile and adult koi, a strain of common carp. J Aquat Anim Health 2000;12: 44–57.

44. Goodwin AE, Sadler J, Merry GE, et al. Herpesviral haematopoietic necrosis virus (CyHV-2) infection: case studies from commercial goldfish farms. J Fish Dis 2009; 32:271–8.

45. Goodwin AE, Khoo L, LaPatra SE. Goldfish hematopoietic necrosis herpesvirus (cyprinid herpesvirus 2) in the USA: molecular confirmation of isolates from diseased fish. J Aquat Anim Health 2006;18:11–8.

46. Gilad O, Yun SC, Zagmutt-Vergara FJ, et al. Concentrations of a koi herpesvirus (KHV) in tissues of experimentally infected *Cyprinus carpio* koi as assessed by real-time TaqMan PCR. Dis Aquat Organ 2004;60:179–87.

47. Goodwin AE, Merry GE, Sadler J. Detection of the herpesviral hematopoietic necrosis disease agent (Cyprinid herpesvirus 2) in moribund and healthy goldfish: validation of a quantitative PCR diagnostic method. J Aquat Anim Health 2006;69: 137–43.

48. Adkison MA, Gilad O, Hedrick RP. An enzyme linked immunosorbent assay (ELISA) for detection of antibodies to the koi herpesvirus (KHV) in the serum of koi, *Cyprinus carpio*. Fish Pathol 2005;40:53–62.

49. O'Connor MR, Farver TB, Weber ES III, et al. Protective immunity of a modified-live cyprinid herpesvirus 3 vaccine in koi (*Cyprinus carpio* koi) 13 months after vaccination. Am J Vet Res 2014;75:905–11.

50. Weber ES III, Malm KV, Yun SC, et al. Efficacy and safety of a modified-live cyprinid herpesvirus 3 vaccine in koi (*Cyprinus carpio* koi) for prevention of koi herpesvirus disease. Am J Vet Res 2014;75:899–904.

51. Morris DJ, Adams A. Transmission of *Tetracapsuloides bryosalmonae* (Myxozoa: Malacosporea), the causative organism of salmonid proliferative kidney disease, to the freshwater bryozoan *Fredericella sultana*. Parasitology 2006;133:701–9.

52. Hedrick RP, MacConnell E, De Kinkelin P. Proliferative kidney disease of salmonid fish. Annu Rev Fish Dis 1993;3:277–90.

53. Foott JS, Stone R, Nichols K. Proliferative kidney disease (*Tetracapsuloides bryosalmonae*) in Merced River hatchery juvenile Chinook salmon: mortality and performance impairment in 2005 smolts. Calif Fish Game 2007;93:57.

54. El-Matbouli M, Fischer-Scherl T, Hoffmann RW. Transmission of *Hoferellus carassii* Achmerov, 1960 to goldfish *Carassius auratus* via an aquatic oligochaete. Bull Eur Assn Fish 1992;12:54–6.

55. Eszterbauer E, Szekely C. Molecular phylogeny of the kidney-parasitic Sphaerospora renicola from common carp (*Cyprinus carpio*) and *Sphaerospora sp.* from goldfish (*Carassius carassius auratus*). Acta Vet Hung 2004;52:469–78.

56. Munkittrick KR, Moccia RD, Leatherland JF. Polycystic kidney disease in goldfish (*Carassius auratus*) from Hamilton Harbour, Lake Ontario, Canada. Vet Pathol 1985;22:232–7.

57. Gill JM. Polycystic kidney disease in goldfish (*Carassius auratus*). N Z Vet J 1994; 42:77.

58. Trouillier A, El-Matbouli M, Hoffmann RW. A new look at the life-cycle of *Hoferellus carassii* in the goldfish (*Carassius auratus auratus*) and its relation to kidney enlargement disease (KED). Folia Parasitol 1996;43:173–87.

59. Hoffman GL. Disinfection of contaminated water by ultraviolet irradiation, with emphasis on whirling disease (*Myxosoma cerebralis*) and its effect on fish. Trans Am Fish Soc 1974;103:541–50.

60. Huang L, Xiao A, Wecker A, et al. A possible zebrafish model of polycystic kidney disease: knockdown of wnt5a causes cysts in zebrafish kidneys. J Vis Exp 2014; 2. https://doi.org/10.3791/52156.

61. Mochizuki E, Fukuta K, Tada T, et al. Fish mesonephric model of polycystic kidney disease in medaka (*Oryzias latipes*) pc mutant. Kidney Int 2005;68:23–34.

62. Stetter MD. Laparoscopic surgery in teleost fish. Proceedings of the 33rd Annual IAAAM Conference. Hosted by ZooMarine, Albufeira, Portugal, May 4–8, 2002.

63. McDonald M. The interaction of environmental calcium and low pH on the physiology of the rainbow trout, *Salmo Gairdneri*: I. Branchial and renal net ion and H+ fluxes. J Exp Biol 1983;102:123–40.

64. Harrison JG, Richards RH. The pathology and histopathology of nephrocalcinosis in rainbow trout *Salmo gairdneri* Richardson in fresh water. J Fish Dis 1979; 2:1–12.

65. Hentschel DM, Park KM, Cilenti L, et al. Acute renal failure in zebrafish: a novel system to study a complex disease. Am J Physiol Renal Physiol 2005;288: F923–9.

66. Reimschuessel R, Williams D. Development of new nephrons in adult kidneys following gentamicin-induced nephrotoxicity. Ren Fail 1995;17:101–6.

67. Salice CJ, Rokous JS, Kane AS, et al. New nephron development in goldfish (*Carassius auratus*) kidneys following repeated gentamicin-induced nephrotoxicosis. Comp Med 2001;51:56–9.
68. Reimschuessel R, Kane AS. A possible teleost model for polycystic kidney disease. Proceedings of the 24th Annual IAAAM Conference. Hosted by John G Shedd Aquarium, Chicago, Illinois, May 16–20, 1993.
69. Reimschuessel R, Gieseker CM, Miller RA, et al. Evaluation of the renal effects of experimental feeding of melamine and cyanuric acid to fish and pigs. Am J Vet Res 2008;69:1217–28.
70. Gill TS, Pant JC, Tewari H. Branchial and renal pathology in the fish exposed chronically to methoxy ethyl mercuric chloride. Bull Environ Contam Toxicol 1988;41:241–6.
71. Bano Y, Hasan M. Histopathological lesions in the body organs of cat-fish (*Heteropneustes fossilis*) following mercury intoxication. J Environ Sci Health B 1990;25: 67–85.
72. Magar RS, Shaikh A. Effect of malathion toxicity on detoxifying organ of fresh water fish *Channa Punctatus*. Int J Pharmaceut Chem Biol Sci 2013;3:723–8.
73. Rahmati-Holasoo H, Shokrpoor S, Masoudifard M, et al. Renal cystic adenocarcinoma in a flowerhorn cichlid with metastatic involvement of the spleen. J Aquat Anim Health 2017;29:158–64.
74. Rahmati-Holasoo H, Shokrpoor S, Masoudifard M, et al. Telangiectatic osteosarcoma and renal adenocarcinoma in an Oscar (*Astronotus ocellatus*, Agassiz): diagnostic imaging and immunohistochemical study. J Fish Dis 2018;41:1165–72.
75. Rahmati-Holasoo H, Soltani M, Masoudifard M, et al. Nephroblastoma in bester sturgeon, a cultured hybrid of *Huso huso* × *Acipenser ruthenus*: diagnostic imaging, clinical and histopathological study. J Fish Dis 2018;41:1093–101.
76. Lombardini ED, Hard GC, Harshbarger JC. Neoplasms of the urinary tract in fish. Vet Pathol 2014;51:1000–12.
77. Rhyne AL, Tlusty MF, Szczebak JT, et al. Expanding our understanding of the trade in marine aquarium animals. Peer J 2017;5:e2949.
78. Hensen RR, Ploeg A, Fossa SA. Standard names for freshwater fishes in the ornamental aquatic industry, vol. 5. The Netherlands: OFI Educational Publication; 2010. p. 145.
79. Yi Y. Tracking a moving target: ornamental fish in the pet trade. 2015. https://doi.org/10.13140/RG.2.1.1938.0646.
80. Poston HA, Page JW. Gross and histological signs of dietary deficiencies of biotin and pantothenic acid in lake trout, *Salvelinus namaycush*. Cornell Vet 1982;72: 242–61.
81. Blazer VS, Wolke RE. Ceroid deposition, retinal degeneration and renal calcium oxalate crystals in cultured clownfish, *Amphiprion ocellaris*. J Fish Dis 1983;6: 365–76.
82. Elmonem MAA, Berlingerio SP, van den Heuvel LPWJ, et al. Genetic renal diseases: the emerging role of zebrafish models. Cells 2018;7:130.